Major League
Careers Cut Short

Major League Careers Cut Short

Leading Players Gone by 30

CHARLES F. FABER

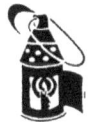

McFarland & Company, Inc., Publishers
Jefferson, North Carolina, and London

Also of interest are the following works from McFarland: *Baseball Ratings: The All-Time Best Players at Each Position, 1876 to the Present*, 3d ed. (2008) by Charles F. Faber; *Spitballers: The Last Legal Hurlers of the Wet One* (2006) by Charles F. Faber and Richard B. Faber; *The American Presidents Ranked by Performance* (2000, softcover 2006) by Charles F. Faber and Richard B. Faber; *Baseball Pioneers: Ratings of Nineteenth Century Players* (1997) by Charles F. Faber

LIBRARY OF CONGRESS CATALOGUING-IN-PUBLICATION DATA

Faber, Charles F.
 Major league careers cut short : leading players gone by 30 / Charles F. Faber.
     p.   cm.
 Includes bibliographical references and index.

 ISBN 978-0-7864-4743-5
 softcover : 50# alkaline paper ∞

 1. Baseball players — United States — Death. 2. Baseball players — United States — Biography. 3. Baseball — United States — History. 4. Death — Causes. I. Title.
 GV865.A1.F286   2011
 796.357092'2 — dc22 [B]   2010040888

British Library cataloguing data are available

© 2011 Charles F. Faber. All rights reserved

No part of this book may be reproduced or transmitted in any form or by any means, electronic or mechanical, including photocopying or recording, or by any information storage and retrieval system, without permission in writing from the publisher.

Front cover: Ross Youngs of the New York Giants, 1923 (Library of Congress)

Manufactured in the United States of America

McFarland & Company, Inc., Publishers
  Box 611, Jefferson, North Carolina 28640
  www.mcfarlandpub.com

For Jay

Acknowledgments

Frequently it said that writing is lonely work. I have not found that to be the case. From the conception of this undertaking, I have been in almost constant communication with friends and family. As always, my son, Daniel Faber, provided encouragement and helpful suggestions. As I completed a first draft of each of the biographical sketches in the book, I sent a copy to my son-in-law, Jay Webb, who responded with thoughtful and constructive criticism. The quality of the finished work owes much to his insightful questions and comments. My daughter, Deborah Webb, and grandson, Zachariah Webb, read the entire manuscript and suggested further improvements. Both were very helpful in dealing with various computer glitches.

Patricia D. Kelly, the photo archivist at the National Baseball Hall of Fame and Museum, provided many of the photographs used in the book and granted permission for their use. The research staff at that institution graciously furnished player files containing valuable information.

I appreciate the contributions of my colleagues in the Society for American Baseball Research (SABR). The SABR online research program is indispensable for a work of this nature. Other online resources, credited in the text, were equally useful.

Finally, I acknowledge the contributions of other friends and members of my family. Without their love, help and encouragement, no book of mine would ever have been published.

Table of Contents

Acknowledgments — vi
Preface — 1
Abbreviations — 2

Part One: Leading Position Players — 3
   Chicken Wolf — 4
   Bill Lange — 9
   Ross Youngs — 15
   Benny Kauff — 20
   Freddie Lindstrom — 25
   Bob Horner — 31
   Ray Chapman — 34
   Carlos May — 38
   Happy Felsch — 42

Part Two: Leading Pitchers — 49
   Amos Rusie — 50
   Sandy Koufax — 55
   Sadie McMahon — 61
   Addie Joss — 65
   Bob Caruthers — 70
   Win Mercer — 76

Part Three: All Position Players — 81
   First Basemen — 82

Second Basemen	94
Shortstops	112
Third Basemen	123
Catchers	136
Right Fielders	142
Center Fielders	158
Left Fielders	172
Part Four: All Pitchers	**182**
Appendix	273
Notes	275
Bibliography	281
Index	285

Preface

Millions of boys have dreamed of playing major league baseball. To participate, perhaps to star, in the national pastime was their fondest aspiration. In their view, what could be more heroic than to hit a game-winning home run or strike out an opposing slugger with the bases loaded? Since 1876, approximately 16,000 young men have had at least a taste of glory by appearing in big league games, many of them only a few times. By the end of the 2009 season, out of the millions who have aspired, fewer than three thousand individuals have had the good fortune to be a major league regular for five or more seasons.[1] Most of these reached the big leagues in their late teens or early twenties, peaked in their late twenties, and played into their mid or late thirties. The median age at which they hung up their spikes was 35. However, there have been 197 young men who played in their last big league contest at the age of 30 or younger. One of them actually pitched seven years in the big leagues and played in his final major league game at the age of 22.

This is a book about the lives of those 197 men — the ones who participated *as a player* in their final game in "The Show" before their 31st birthday. Some of them continued in the majors in some other capacity, such as a manager, coach or umpire. Many played baseball well beyond the age of 30 in the minor leagues, in Japan, or elsewhere. These men are included among the 197 so long as they played in no major league games after their 31st birthday. Why did their careers end too soon? The reasons are as varied as the men themselves: Killed when hit by a pitch; suicide; fatal illness; injury; banishment from the sport; inability to adjust to a change in the pitching distance; objections by a future father-in-law to his daughter marrying a ballplayer; and declining ability are some of the reasons for early departure from the field of dreams. Some hopes were dashed by the demons of drug abuse, alcoholism or mental illness. Other players left voluntarily because they had visions of greener pastures in another field. Included are five players who have been enshrined in the Hall of Fame in Cooperstown. Several others were well on their way toward immortality when their careers came to a premature end.

This book is divided into four parts. Part One contains biographical sketches of nine of the best eligible position players. Part Two profiles six of the better pitchers. Parts Three and Four are alphabetical listings of all other eligible position players and pitchers, respectively, along with shorter profiles of each. These entries contain all essential information, condensed into a few paragraphs. Ratings and rankings are included where appropriate. The entire book is intended to give the reader a better perspective on those players whose careers ended too soon.

Abbreviations

AA	American Association	**NLCS**	National League Championship Series
ABL	Australian Baseball League	**NWL**	Northwestern League
AL	American League	**OBP**	On-Base percentage
BA	Batting Average	**PCL**	Pacific Coast League
ERA	Earned Run Cverage	**Pct.**	Percentage
FL	Federal League	**PL**	Players League
G	Games played	**R**	Runs scored
GM	General Manager	**RBI**	Runs Batted In
IP	Innings Pitched	**SA**	Southern Association
L	Games lost	**SABR**	Society for American Baseball Research
MVP	Most Valuable Player	**SB**	Stolen Base
NA	National Association	**SO**	Strike Outs
NAACP	National Association for the Advancement of Colored People	**UA**	Union Association
		W	Games won
NAIA	National Association of Intercollegiate Athletics	**WA**	Western Association
		WHIP	Walks plus Hits per Innings Pitched
NCAA	National Collegiate Athletic Association	**WL**	Western League
NL	National League		

PART ONE

Leading Position Players

Anyone who logged a significant amount of time in the major leagues was a very good baseball player. After all, many millions have striven, but only a few thousand have reached the top rung of their chosen profession. However, among the 107 position players who played their last major league game at the age of thirty or younger, some stand out as being more talented than others. In Part One, biographical sketches are presented of the highest-ranked position players, according to Faber System ratings.[1] Primary sources for statistical data are *The Baseball Encyclopedia*[2] and *Baseball-Reference*,[3] supplemented as necessary by other works. Sources do not always agree on some data, such as the date of birth or the number of stolen bases in a particular year. After making an effort to determine which source is more likely to be accurate, the present writer has used his own judgment in determining which data to use.

When different spellings of a name are found, the one most frequently used by contemporaries is normally used. One exception to this rule is the spelling of Pittsburgh. The modern spelling is used consistently, although the final "h" was regularly omitted until well into the twentieth century.

A major source of accounts of games is *Newspaper Archives*.[4] Often the same article appears in several different newspapers, probably as a result of papers using the same press service. In such cases, only one of multiple sources is cited. All players with five or more eligible seasons are rated by the Faber System. *Total Baseball*[5] rates nearly every player in the history of major league baseball. Bill James[6] ranks the top 125 of all time at each position. From these ratings it is possible to infer rankings for the players listed in this book, although none of the analysts did so explicitly.

The nine most productive players profiled in Part One are also included in the alphabetical list of players in Part Three. In that section, concise summaries of essential information about the 107 eligible players are presented, along with an occasional interesting anecdote.

CHICKEN WOLF

It was a remarkable quartet of friends who grew up together on the west side of Louisville in the years following the Civil War — Pete, Willie, and the twins John and Phil. By 1880 the teenagers formed the nucleus of an outstanding semi-pro baseball team called the Eclipse. Pete was nearly a year older and much bigger and stronger than his buddies. Willie could not hit the ball as far as Pete, but he excelled in many facets of the game. The twins rounded out a fearsome foursome of future major leaguers from a small city on the banks of the Ohio River. Before one crucial game their manager instructed the players to eat lightly, but Willie's appetite got the better of him and he consumed a huge quantity of stewed chicken. During the game Willie committed several errors in the field. Pete blamed the miscues on the feast of chicken and nicknamed the miscreant "Chicken." The name stuck, and for many years Willie was known as Chicken Wolf.

William Van Winkle Wolf was born in Louisville on May 12, 1862, the son of German immigrants Barbara and Andrew Wolf. Willie learned to play baseball with his neighborhood friends, including Pete Browning and the Reccius brothers, John and Phil. The semi-pro club had been founded by Billy Reccius, older brother of the twins, in the mid–1870s. The club took up a collection at each game and split the proceeds among the players. By 1881 the club began paying salaries to the players. About this time they were joined by a young man from Cincinnati named Joe Crotty. (According to the 1880 census, Crotty was living in Cincinnati with his widowed mother, an immigrant from Ireland. His occupation was listed as "Base Ballist.") In 1882 the American Association (AA) was formed as a second major league, in competition with thte National League. The Eclipse were granted a franchise in the new circuit, and soon changed their name to the Louisville Colonels.

According to eminent baseball historian David Nemec, "The most vibrant and freewheeling time in baseball history came during the years between 1882 and 1891 when the upstart American Association fought the National League tooth and nail for the right to coexist as a major league."[7] The two leagues competed on nearly an equal basis for a decade, fighting off a challenge by the Union Association in 1884 and the Players League in 1890.

Opposite: **William Van Winkle "Chicken" Wolf was one of the greatest stars of the nineteenth century. Of all the players whose major league careers ended at the age of 30 or younger, Wolf ranks number one in Faber System points (National Baseball Hall of Fame Library, Cooperstown, New York).**

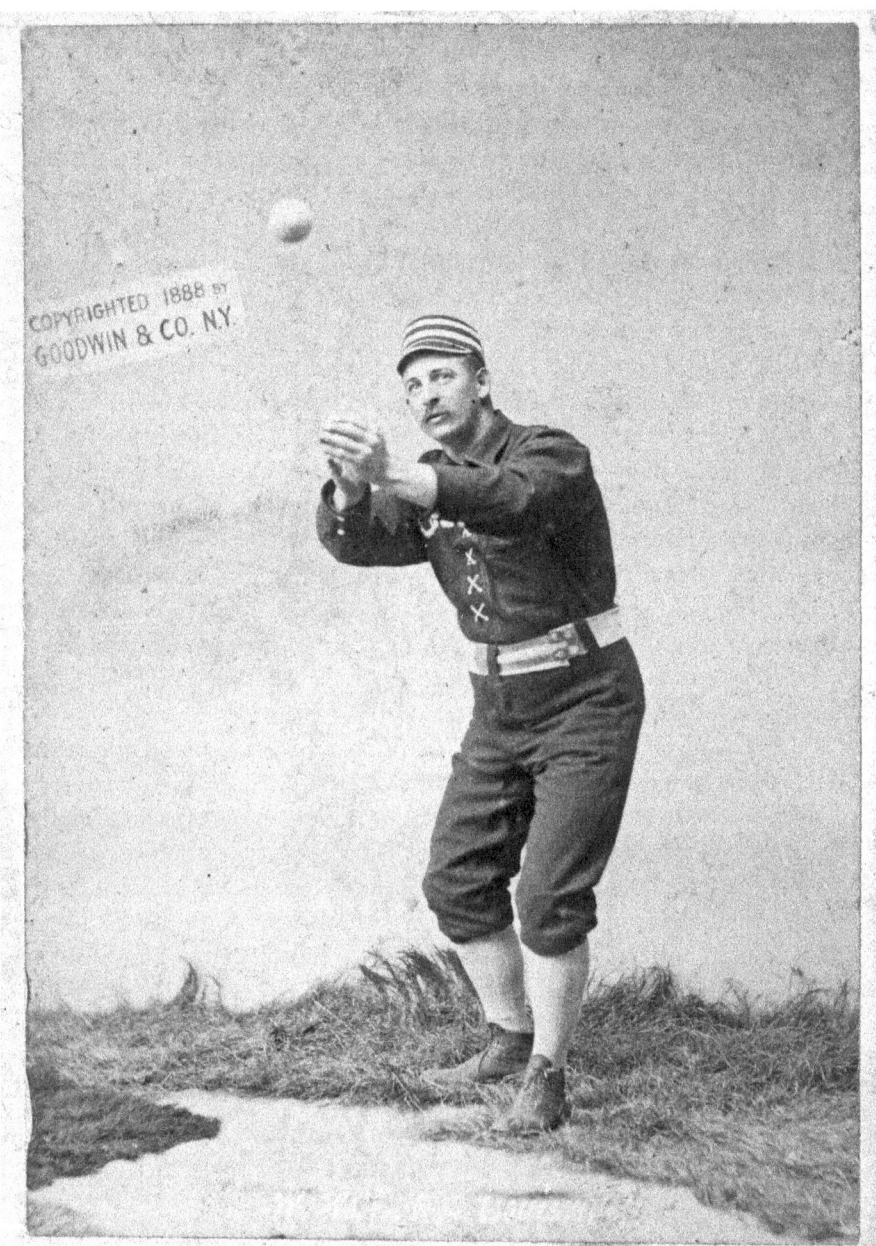

However, the loss of key players to the latter doomed the AA. It survived only one more year until it gave up the ghost and its surviving clubs joined the National League in 1892. The major league career of Chicken Wolf spanned these ten "vibrant" years. Of all the players in the storied history of the American Association, no other man played as many games in the loop as did Wolf.

Among the reasons the AA gained instant credibility were the exploits of Pete Browning. Known as the "Louisville Slugger" and "the Gladiator," he became the new league's greatest hitter. Legend has it that the first modern barrel-shaped bat was made for him.[8] Hillerich and Bradsby named their Louisville Slugger bats in his honor. Pete was joined on the Louisville entry in the AA by Chicken Wolf, John Reccius and, for a short time, Joe Crotty. Later in the first season Phil Reccius came aboard. The young men made their major league debuts at a tender age. At the beginning of the 1882 season Crotty was 21, Browning was 20, while Wolf and the twins were all teenagers at 19.[9] According to *Sporting Life,* Wolf was the lowest-paid professional baseball player in the history of the sport. Louisville paid him only $9 per week.[10] That was a great bargain! Although Crotty and the twins had less than stellar major league careers, Wolf remained in the American Association as long as that league existed.

Although he logged games at every position on the field (including pitcher), Wolf was mainly a right fielder. Evidently his fielding improved since the day he acquired the nickname Chicken. Playing in the outfield alongside the inept Browning (whose nickname of Gladiator was partly due to his battles with fly balls hit in his direction), Wolf had to cover a lot of ground. He led the AA in outfield range in each of his first two seasons in the majors. He led the league in outfield assists in 1882 and in double plays by an outfielder in 1883. According to the Faber System he was the league's best fielding outfielder four times — in 1882, 1886, 1887, and 1891.[11] In other words, he was tops in American Association's first year, its last year, and twice in between. In three of those seasons his combined batting and fielding achievements earned him the most points of any AA right fielder. For a career, the Faber System ranks him as the seventh-best major league right fielder of all time in fielding points per season.[12]

As a hitter Wolf was better than the average major leaguer, but he had one season that was truly outstanding. In 1890 he led the American Association with a .365 batting average, 197 hits, and 260 total bases. That season he also hit 29 doubles, banged out four home runs, and stole 46 bases. Palmer and Gillette named him their ex post facto Most Valuable Player in the American Association for 1890. His heroics helped Louisville win its first and only major league pennant. As the Colonels had finished in last place the previous season, the team became the first team in the majors to go from last place to first in a span of one year. Admittedly, Louisville was helped by the defection of some players on rival teams to the new Players League, but it was still quite an accomplishment. Perhaps getting out from under the shadow of Browning, who was one of the defectors, helped Wolf. (After the Gladiator left, Wolf's teammates started calling him Jimmy. The reason for this is not known, but some modern-day reference books still use the name Jimmy Wolf, although the majority prefer the appellation Chicken.) After that one season of glory the club from the Falls City never fared that well again. The Association folded after the 1891 season, and the Colonels transferred to the National League, where they languished in the second division until merging with the Pittsburgh Pirates after the 1899 season.

After the end of the 1890 season the AA champion Colonels faced the National League champion Brooklyn Dodgers in what was sometimes called a World's Series. The two teams battled each other as well as inclement weather over a period of several days, with three wins each and one tie, before a forecast of snow caused the cancellation of what should have been the deciding contest. Wolf played well in the series, leading the regulars with a .360 average, garnering fourteen total bases and driving in eight runs.[13] Nevertheless, it had to be a disappointing conclusion to his most productive season.

During Louisville's ten years in the American Association, Wolf played in more than 97 percent of the club's games. He holds the AA record for most games played (1195); most hits (1438); most doubles (214); most triples (109); and most total bases (1921).

Despite his nickname, Chicken Wolf was not a colorful character. He simply showed up day after day, did his job, and did it well. However, he was involved in one incident that gained considerable publicity. On an August day in 1886, Louisville and Cincinnati were tied, 3–3, in the 11th inning. Wolf hit a long drive to center field. Ab Powell, the Redlegs center fielder, raced to pick up the ball. Just as he reached for the pellet, a stray dog grabbed Powell by the leg and would not let go. With the dog hanging on to him, Powell was unable to make a throw and Wolf circled the bases for an inside-the-park, game-winning home run.

Wolf's other brush with notoriety came during the disastrous 1889 season. During those times many clubs did not employ a manager in the sense that term is used today. Most teams had a captain, to whom certain managerial duties were assigned. The season opened with Dude Easterbrook as captain. The captain started fining players who did not follow his instructions. Among those fined was second baseman Dan Shannon, who protested the ten-dollar assessment. Wolf came verbally to the second sacker's defense, whereupon

Easterbrook fined Wolf ten dollars. When Wolf refused to back down, the captain upped the fine to forty dollars, a substantial amount in view of 1889 ballplayer salaries. Wolf appealed to the team owner, Mordecai Davidson. Within a week Easterbrook was fired, and the team selected Wolf as its new captain. Under Wolf's management, things did not improve. Davidson started fining players for errors in the field. This led to what has been called the first players strike in major league history, as six players sat out.[14] The crisis ended when Davidson sold the club and Wolf resigned as captain.

Following the demise of the American Association Wolf wanted to stay in baseball. He started the 1892 season with the Syracuse-Utica Stars of the Eastern League. Later that summer he played three games with the St. Louis National League club. His final major league appearance came with St. Louis on August 21, 1892. After playing for Buffalo in the Eastern League in 1893, Wolf returned to Louisville. In June 1894 he got a job with the city fire department. The 1900 census showed William V. Wolf, an engine driver for the fire department, living with his wife, Carrie, and their sons, William and Milton, ages ten and two, respectively, on Twentieth Street near the West Walnut Street neighborhood where he had lived as a child.

In 1901 his horse-drawn vehicle was involved in a serious accident. Rushing to the scene of a fire, his engine collided with a pushcart at the corner of Walnut and Eighteenth streets. Thrown out of the engine, he hit his head on the cobblestone street and then was dragged by the horses for some distance. The head injury caused him to become mentally unbalanced and he was institutionalized for most of the rest of his life. For a time in 1901 he was confined in the Lakeland Insane Asylum near Louisville. Ironically, two of his ex-teammates also were committed to the same place a few years later. Pete Browning's many years of heavy drinking and improperly treated mastoiditis led to diminished mental capacity. He was mistakenly diagnosed as insane and spent two weeks at Lakeland in 1905. It has been reported that John Reccius later spent time in the same institution.[15] It seems incredible that three boyhood friends would grow up together, play baseball on the same major league team, and later spent time in the same mental institution. "Truth is stranger than fiction" may be a cliché, but it certainly applies in the case of these three Kentuckians.

To make Wolf's final years even more unhappy, one of his sons died in 1901, shortly after the fire engine accident. Suffering from the head injury, Wolf continued to experience declining health. William Van Winkle Wolf died May 16, 1903, just four days after his 41st birthday. He was buried in the Cave Hill Cemetery in Louisville. Although his name is not well known to modern baseball fans, Chicken Wolf deserves to be remembered as one of the greatest stars of the nineteenth century.

His major league record: **Bold** indicates league leader.

Year	Age	Club	G	AB	R	H	HR	RBI	BA	OBP
1882	19	Louisville AA	78	318	46	95	0	n.a.	.299	.318
1883	20	Louisville AA	**98**	389	59	102	1	n.a.	.262	.272
1884	21	Louisville AA	110	**486**	79	146	3	73	.300	.310
1885	22	Louisville AA	**112**	483	79	141	1	52	.292	.309
1886	23	Louisville AA	130	545	93	148	3	61	.272	.310
1887	24	Louisville AA	137	569	103	160	2	102	.282	.331
1888	25	Louisville AA	128	538	80	154	0	67	.286	.320
1889	26	Louisville AA	130	546	72	159	3	57	.291	.333
1890	27	Louisville AA	134	543	100	**197**	4	98	**.363**	.421
1891	28	Louisville AA	138	528	67	136	1	81	.256	.320
1892	29	St. Louis NL	3	14	1	2	0	1	.143	.143
TOTAL			1198	4959	779	1440	18	592	.290	.327

Wolf's postseason record:

Year	Age	Club	G	AB	R	H	HR	RBI	BA	OBP
1890	28	Louisville AA	7	25	4	9	0	8	.360	.429

His minor league record:

Year	Age	Club	League	G	AB	H	BA
1892	29	Syracuse	Eastern League	27	16	24	.209
1893	30	Buffalo	Eastern League	114	94	161	.343

Of all the players whose major league careers ended at the age of thirty or younger, Chicken Wolf ranks number one in Faber System points. *Total Baseball* ranks him sixth in this group.

BILL LANGE

In 1936 King Edward VIII gave up his throne to wed the woman he loved. Thirty-seven years earlier a young man who held Chicago in the palm of his hand gave up his career for the same reason. The handsome young baseball star, one of the most popular players ever to grace the Windy City, faced an ultimatum from his future father-in-law. He had to either give up the game of baseball or abandon his plans to marry. Bill Lange chose marriage, and baseball lost one of its most talented athletes.

William Alexander Lange was born in San Francisco on June 6, 1861, the sixth of the seven children of German immigrants Mary and Charles Lange. For many years the elder Lange was a soldier stationed at the Presidio, and it was in this San Francisco neighborhood that his son learned the game of base-

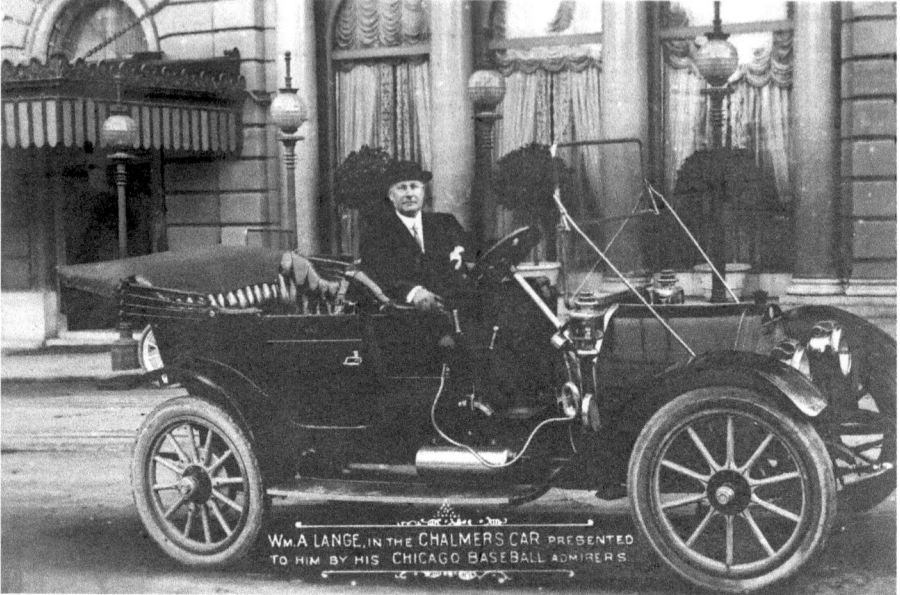

Bill Lange is shown seated in a Chalmers automobile presented to him by Chicago fans. Lange gave up his baseball career because his future father-in-law objected to his daughter marrying a ballplayer (National Baseball Hall of Fame Library, Cooperstown, New York).

ball. As a teenager Bill began his professional baseball career as a catcher and second baseman at Port Townsend, Washington, where he hit higher than .300 in 1889 and 1890. In 1891 he moved up to Seattle of the Pacific Northwestern League, where he again hit over .300 and had a record of four wins and seven losses as a pitcher. He started the next season with the same club but the league disbanded in August, and Bill finished the year with Oakland in the California League. That was the end of his minor league career, for he joined the Chicago Colts in the National League in 1893, never to return to the bushes.

Lange's minor league record:

Year	Age	Club	League	G	R	H	BA
1891	19	Seattle	Pacific Northwest	36	17	39	.305
1892	20	Seattle	Pacific Northwest	57	54	67	.303
		Oakland	California	53	42	57	.277

At the start of the 1893 season, Lange was 21 years old with four years of minor league experience. During that first season in the majors he played mainly second base and outfield, and hit .281, the only time in his major league career that he hit less than .319. In 1894 Bill became the Colts' regular center fielder and remained as such for the rest of his days in Chicago, albeit with an occasional start at another spot. At one time or another he played all of the infield and outfield positions as well as catcher. He never pitched in the majors, although he had tried his hand in the pitcher's box as a teenager back in Seattle.

The term "five-tool player" was not used in Lange's day, but he had all the tools. He hit for average and with power, had great speed on the bases, possessed a strong arm, and was one of the league's best fielders. He had a lifetime .330 average in the majors. Chicago has had a team in the National League since the inception of the circuit in 1876, but no Chicago player (whether as a White Stocking, Colt, Orphan, Cub or any other appellation) has ever topped Bill's .389 batting average of 1895, his 84 stolen bases in 1896, or his lifetime total of 399 or 400 sacks swiped. For many years he was credited with 100 stolen bases in 1896, but modern researchers have corrected that figure to 84.[16]

Standing nearly 6' 2" and weighing close to 200 pounds, Lange was considered a big man in a time when the average ballplayer was smaller in stature than today's counterpart. For this reason, he was nicknamed "Big Bill." More frequently, he was called "Little Eva." The source of that moniker is not known, but it was frequently used in the 1890s.

Other than leading the National League in stolen bases with 73 in 1897, Little Eva was not a league leader — never a batting champion or a home run king. However, he was frequently near the leaders. In 1895, for example, he ranked in the top five in batting average, on-base percentage, slugging percentage, home runs, and stolen bases — all in the same season. In addition to leading the league in stolen bases once, he was second twice, and fifth once. According to the Faber System, he was the National League's best fielding center fielder in 1898.[17]

Beyond the numbers, however, Lange's stature is attested to by the praise of men who saw him play. Hall of Fame pitcher, manager, and executive Clark Griffith named him to his all-time all-star team. Another Hall of Famer, baseball pioneer Al Spalding, also placed Little Eva on his all-time team, ranking him ahead of Tris Speaker, saying, "Both men could go back or to either side equally well. Both were lightning fast in handling ground balls. But no man I ever saw could go forward and get a low line drive like Lange."[18] Tim Murnane, arguably the most respected sportswriter of the era, also placed Lange on his all-time team. Al Spink, founding editor of *The Sporting News*, wrote that Lange was "Ty Cobb enlarged, fully as great in speed, batting skill and baserunning."[19] Although William Akin never saw Lange play, he identified him as the greatest defensive center fielder of the 1890s: "In the absence of logically compelling statistical evidence, the impression of contemporary observers must be given greater weight. The evidence points to Bill Lange of Chicago."[20]

Baseball researcher and writer Bill James is effusive in his praise of Lange. He writes, "Bill Lange was probably the greatest all-around athlete to play major league baseball in the nineteenth century."[21] James also suggests that in many ways Lange could be considered as a nineteenth-century Mickey Mantle.[22]

In what ways did Lange resemble Mickey Mantle? At least three possibilities exist: his phenomenal baseball talent; his incredible popularity; and his flamboyant lifestyle. Although it is difficult to compare players from different eras, it seems clear that Lange matched or even exceeded Mantle in hitting for average, fielding, and base running. However, Mantle's prodigious home run clouting gave him a dominance that Little Eva never achieved. As for popularity, Lange may have indeed been Mantle's equal. Akin quotes the *Chicago Tribune* as stating that Lange was "the most popular man who ever wore a Chicago uniform." Akin wrote that Little Eva's personality mirrored the spirit of the Gay Nineties: "Fun-loving and carefree, he had a fondness for practical jokes, women, and nightlife." Does that sound like Mantle?

With such a large public presence, Lange inevitably became the subject of colorful anecdotes. One story that persisted for years tells of Big Bill crashing through a wooden fence to make a game-saving catch. Although the tale is apocryphal, it still appears in print from time to time. Another anecdote has not been debunked. According to this story, Lange wanted to delay reporting for spring training in 1897 long enough to attend the world's heavyweight boxing championship match between James Corbett and Bob Fitzsimmons in Carson City, Nevada, on March 17. To stall for time Lange demanded an extra $500. To his surprise, the team met his demand with two conditions — he was to keep the bonus a secret and report immediately. Wealthier but stymied, Big Bill had to come up with another delaying tactic. He invented a twisted ankle and attended the fight, where Fitzsimmons won the championship. Apparently the bad ankle healed in time for Lange to lead the league in stolen bases that season.

After that Lange played two more seasons before he had to make the choice between marriage and baseball. He chose marriage, and his playing days were over at the age of 28. (The table below gives his age at the beginning of each season. He turned 28 in June of his final year in the majors.)

Lange's major league record: **Bold** indicates league leader.

Year	Age	Club	League	G	AB	R	H	HR	RBI	SB	BA	OBP
1893	21	Chicago	NL	117	469	92	132	8	88	47	.281	.358
1894	22	Chicago	NL	113	449	86	146	6	91	66	.325	.402
1895	23	Chicago	NL	123	478	120	186	10	98	67	.389	.456
1896	24	Chicago	NL	122	469	114	153	4	92	84	.326	.414
1897	25	Chicago	NL	118	479	119	163	5	83	73	.340	.406
1898	26	Chicago	NL	113	442	79	141	5	69	22	.319	.377
1899	27	Chicago	NL	107	416	81	135	1	58	41	.325	.416
TOTAL				813	3202	691	1056	39	579	400	.330	.400

Lange returned to San Francisco, married Grace Giselman, and entered the real estate business, at which he apparently was successful. Both the 1900 and 1910 censuses showed the couple residing with a live-in Chinese servant next door to Grace's parents, Anna and William Giselman, on Golden Gate Avenue. Unfortunately for the romantic tale of the man who gave up his career for the woman he loved, the marriage ended in divorce in 1913. Grace charged her husband with extreme mental cruelty. According to her testimony, the marriage had been a happy one for thirteen years. Then Lange started staying out late at night and frequenting fashionable clubs and dansants without her. She testified that he moved to the Olympic Club, deserting his home entirely. Bill did not appear in court to contest the suit. The 1920 census showed the divorced Grace living with her widowed mother.

After his retirement Lange stayed in California, turning down repeated offers to return to the big leagues as a player. He retained an interest in baseball, however. Since 1902 the National Association of Professional Baseball Leagues had governed the minor leagues. In 1907 the NAPBL declared the California State League an "outlaw" league for harboring former major league players who had been blacklisted for violating the reserve clause. A national commission was created to try to dissolve the outlaw league. Lange was recruited to use his influence among local sportswriters to speed up the process. The effort was successful as the California State League ceased operations in 1909.

John McGraw, manager of the New York Giants, employed Lange as his chief European scout, hoping to discover future Giants across the ocean. In 1919 Ban Johnson called upon Lange to establish an International Baseball League in Europe that could compete against the American League pennant winner in a different kind of World Series. This effort was unsuccessful, but it possibly explains why Lange was not included in the United States census of 1920. He may have been in Europe at the time. Lange located no potential Giants for McGraw in Europe, but he found at least two close to home in California's Bay Area — one of whom exited baseball in shame and one who entered the Hall of Fame. The most heralded of these prospects was Jim

O'Connell, who was known as "the Babe Ruth of the Pacific Coast League" when he played for the San Francisco Seals. The *New York Times* reported:

> Bill Lange, the former big league star ... gave Manager McGraw earnest advice about young O'Connell last spring. Lange ... wanted McGraw to bring home this rare slice of Western bacon, and the Giants' manager has been squinting toward San Francisco ever since. The story is that McGraw signed a blank check when the season was still young and sent it to Lange, who presented it to Charles Graham, manager of the Seals, with permission to select such figures as appealed to him and write them on the face of the check.[23]

Graham did not take advantage of that generous offer, but at the end of the season sold O'Connell to the Giants for $75,000, the highest price ever paid to that date for a minor league player.

In common with many other young phenoms, O'Connell failed to live up to the hype when he reached the majors. In a two-year big league career he appeared in a total of 139 games for the Giants. On September 27, 1924, with the Giants needing only one more victory to clinch the National League pennant, O'Connell approached Heinie Sand, shortstop for the opposition Philadelphia Phillies, and offered him five hundred dollars if he would not bear down too hard. Sand reported the incident to his manager, who informed baseball authorities. O'Connell admitted offering the bribe and claimed he got the idea from his coach, Cozy Dolan, and named several teammates whom he claimed were going to contribute to the pot. Commissioner Kenesaw Mountain Landis investigated and banned O'Connell and Dolan from baseball for life. He exonerated the other Giant players.

Another young man whom Lange recommended to the Giants fared much better. His nephew, George "Highpockets" Kelly, son of Bill's sister Mary, had a stellar career in "the Show" and was elected to the National Baseball Hall of Fame in Cooperstown.

If the nephew deserves a plaque in Cooperstown, what about the uncle who had a shorter but more spectacular career? The evidence is mixed. In order to admit Lange, the Hall would have to waive the rule requiring ten years of service to be eligible. It has already done this for Addie Joss and others. Is Little Eva worthy? Nine Hall of Fame inductees had careers that spanned the years 1893–1899, when Lange was in the majors.[24] His performance at the plate was better than some but not as good as most of the nine. During those seven years the anointed immortals compiled a collective batting average of .353, an on-base percentage of .427, scored an average of 811 runs, knocked in 607, and hit 35 home runs. All of those numbers except home runs are higher than Lange's. Of course, his stolen base total far exceeded their average of 245 steals. In the field Lange's stats compared favorably with those of the six other patrollers of the outer garden; he was better than most, ranking second behind only Big Ed Delahanty.[25]

William Alexander Lange died in San Francisco on July 23, 1950, at the age of 79. His obituary in the *New York Times*, relying on information available at the time, incorrectly credits him with a record 100 base thefts.[26]

According to the Faber System, Bill Lange is ranked second among all major league players whose careers ended at the age of thirty or younger. *Total Baseball* places him in a tie for ninth. Bill James ranks him first among center fielders. Little Eva may never be enshrined in Cooperstown, but he will be long remembered by those who appreciate his exploits on the field.

ROSS YOUNGS

Some consider him one of the best 100 ballplayers of all time. Legendary John McGraw, the winningest National League manager ever, called him "the best outfielder I ever saw." And McGraw had seen the best during his more than 40 years as player or manager in the major leagues. When the object of McGraw's praise was named to the Baseball Hall of Fame, most fans approved of the selection: others shook their heads in disbelief. "Who is this Ross Youngs? I never heard of him." When they learned the new inductee was the man they knew as Pep Young, many changed their tune. "Ah, yes. Pep Young, maybe he does belong in Cooperstown." During his playing career Ross was referred to as "Young" by his contemporaries. Recent writers have restored the final letter to his surname and call him "Youngs," which was his original name.

Royce Middlebrook Youngs was born April 10, 1897, in Shiner, a small town in Lavaca County, Texas, the second of the three sons of Henrietta Middlebrook and Stonewall Jackson Youngs, a sometime-railroad man, rancher, and cotton buyer. The family moved to San Antonio when Ross, as he was known from early childhood, was still a lad. He attended high school at West Texas Military Institute, where he excelled in sports, leading his baseball team to the 1913 state championship and starring as a quarterback on the football team. According to the *New York Times*, he was also a basketball and track star in high school.[27] A Texas reporter wrote that Ross received football scholarship offers from major colleges around the nation but wanted to pursue a professional baseball career.[28] He played ten games for Austin of the Texas League in 1914. In 1915 he played for two ill-fated clubs—Brenham in the Middle Texas League, which folded on June 30, and Waxahachie in the Central Texas Trolley League, which disbanded on July 24. He returned to San Antonio and played semi-pro ball for the rest of the season.

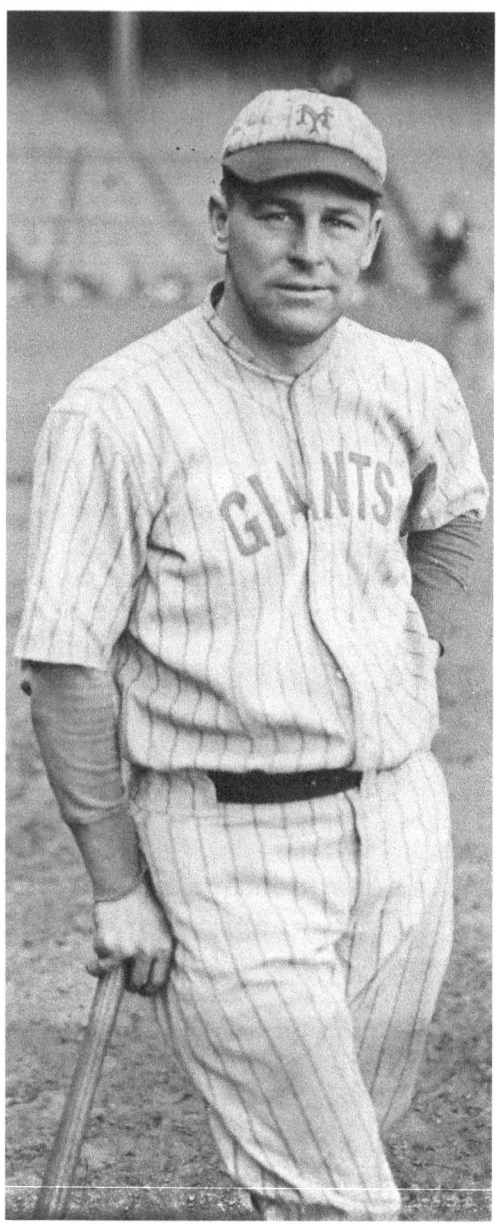

In 1916 he was signed by a viable professional club and made the most of the opportunity. Playing for the Sherman (Texas) team in the Western Association, he won the league's batting championship with a .362 average, and led the league with 195 hits and 103 runs scored for a team that played only 137 games. Dick Kinsella, the famous scout, saw Youngs play in Sherman and recommended him to the Giants. On August 14, 1916, he was sold to the New York Giants for $2000—quite a bargain, as this is the same club that paid $75,000 for the ill-fated Jimmy O'Connell a few years later.

The first time McGraw saw Youngs in a spring training game in Martin, Texas, he hung the nickname "Pep" on him. Pep is short for pepper, which signified the young man's hustle. The Giants had a working arrangement with the Rochester Hustlers of the International League. McGraw sent Ross to Rochester, and told manager Mickey Doolan, "I am giving you one of the greatest players I've ever seen. Play him in the outfield. If anything happens to him, I'm holding you responsible. Do not mess

Ross Youngs, sometimes known as "Pep" Young, was a Hall of Fame outfielder for the New York Giants. He compiled a .322 lifetime batting average and was considered by John McGraw as the best outfielder he had ever seen. His career ended prematurely when he died of a kidney disease at the age of 30 (Library of Congress).

this kid up."²⁹ Mess him up Doolan certainly did not. At Rochester Youngs hit .356, second only to the great Nap Lajoie, who was winding up his playing days in the minors after a brilliant career of 21 years as one of the brightest stars in the major leagues. Youngs had 180 hits, scored 85 runs, and stole 34 bases for the Hustlers. He was called up by the Giants on September 25, 1917, making his major league debut at the age of 20. For the next nine years he was the Giants' regular right fielder, earning a reputation as an outstanding defensive player and finishing in the top five in at least one offensive category every year until slowed by illness in 1925.

From 1918 through 1925 Youngs was in the top five in batting average three times; in on-base percentage five times; in slugging once; in runs scored five times; in hits three times; in total bases once; in doubles three times; in runs batted in once; in bases on balls five times; and in stolen bases once. In 1919 he led the National League in doubles, and paced the circuit in runs scored in 1923. In 1920 and again in 1922 he led the loop in assists and in errors by a right fielder. Alan Asnen attributed Youngs's errors to his "over-enthusiastic defensive style."³⁰ According to the Faber System, Youngs was the best rightfielder in the NL in both 1923 and 1924.³¹

The New York Giants won the National League pennant four straight times, from 1921 through 1924, the only club in the circuit to accomplish that feat. Youngs was an integral part of each of those teams. His exploits in the World Series enhanced his reputation. In the third game of the 1921 Series, he became the first player in the history of the Fall Classic to connect for two hits in one inning. While that feat has since been duplicated, the nature of those hits has not been matched. A double and a triple in the same inning have never been hit by any other World Series participant. Pep's triple came with the bases loaded in the seventh inning of a game in which the Giants overcame a 4–0 Yankee lead to win, 13–5. In the final game of the Series, Youngs was instrumental in the Giants winning the world's championship and sending the Yankees down to defeat in the first World Series in which they participated. In the first inning Dave Bancroft walked. Youngs followed with another base on balls, despite the Yankees vigorously protesting the call on ball four. Youngs's walk pushed Bancroft into scoring position at second base. Bancroft scored the only run of the game when Roger Peckinpaugh booted George Kelly's grounder and the ball rolled all the way to the outfield. In trying to identify the hero of the Series, a *Washington Post* writer suggested several names, including Youngs, of whom he wrote: "Ross Youngs was always dangerous at the plate and on the paths. He was robbed of at least three decisive hits by sensational Yankee fielding plays."³²

Youngs hit .280 in the 1921 World Series, but he added nearly a hundred points to that average in 1922, hitting .375 as the Giants won their second consecutive world's championship over the Yankees, four games to none. He hit .348 as the Yanks turned the tables on their cross-town rivals to win their first world's title in 1923. In 1924 a different opponent faced the Giants in the Fall Classic, as Walter Johnson finally got a chance to pitch in a World Series. Youngs hit only .185 as the Giants fell to the Washington Senators, four games to three.

Just before the Giants clinched the 1924 pennant, Jimmy O'Connell approached Heinie Sand, a player for the Pittsburgh Pirates, offering him $500 if he did not try too hard against the Giants. Sand reported the attempted bribe. During the subsequent investigation, O'Connell tried to implicate some of his teammates, including Youngs. Baseball Commissioner Landis exonerated Youngs but banished O'Connell from Organized Baseball for life.

In 1925 Youngs' skills started to decline. For the first and only time in his major league career he hit lower than .300. He began to suffer from virus infections, stomach ailments, and headaches, but he persevered. In 1926 his health became so bad that McGraw hired a male nurse to travel with the team. Nevertheless, Ross hit .306 in 95 games for the Giants before he finally called it quits. His final game was on August 10, 1926, at the age of 29. He had only a little over fourteen months to live.

His major league record: **Bold** indicates league leader

Year	Age	Club	League	G	AB	R	H	HR	RBI	SB	BA	OBP
1917	20	New York	NL	7	26	5	9	0	1	1	.346	.370
1918	21	New York	NL	121	474	70	143	1	25	10	.302	.368
1919	22	New York	NL	130	489	73	152	2	43	24	.311	.384
1920	23	New York	NL	153	581	92	204	6	78	18	.351	.427
1921	24	New York	NL	141	504	90	165	3	102	21	.327	.411
1922	25	New York	NL	149	559	105	185	7	86	17	.331	.398
1923	26	New York	NL	152	596	**121**	200	3	87	13	.336	.412
1924	27	New York	NL	133	526	112	187	10	74	11	.356	.441
1925	28	New York	NL	130	500	82	132	6	53	17	.264	.354
1926	29	New York	NL	95	372	62	114	4	43	21	.306	.372
TOTAL				1211	4627	812	1491	42	592	153	.322	.399

During his last two seasons, Youngs not only had health concerns but also personal problems. In October 1924 he married Dorothy Pienecke, a young woman from Brooklyn whom he had met at a resort hotel in the Berkshires. The Giants made a post-season trip to England to play before royalty. The newlyweds honeymooned in Europe. When they returned to San Antonio for the offseason, conflict developed between the bride and her mother-in-law. By the time their daughter, Caroline, was born in December 1925, the couple had separated. Ross never saw his daughter. He filed for divorce but never followed through on the suit.

In an interview from his hospital room in December 1926, Youngs assured a San Antonio newspaper reporter that he would be fully recovered and back in right field for the Giants in 1927. "I'll probably be out [of the hospital] next week. A little exercise and a lot of careful going, and these kinks I suddenly developed will be ironed out. Don't let anybody kid you about that right field job next season. I'll be in it as usual."[33] Whether this was bravado or what Ross really believed is not known. The reporter expressed no skepticism. Youngs blamed his problems on his tonsils and a wisdom tooth, both of which he had removed. He also mentioned "a cold that settled in his kidneys."

Youngs did get of the hospital for a time in the summer of 1927, but he never made it back to the ball field. On October 22, 1927, he died in a San Antonio hospital from Bright's disease. Now referred to as chronic nephritis, it is a kidney ailment for which there is no known cure. Ross Youngs is buried in Mission Burial Park South in San Antonio.

In 1928 a plaque was placed on the right field wall of the Polo Grounds to honor Youngs. It read: "A brave untrammeled spirit of the diamond, who brought glory to himself and his team by his strong, aggressive, courageous play. He won the admiration of the nation's fans, the love and esteem of his friends and teammates and the respect of his opponents. He played the game." The present whereabouts of the plaque is unknown. His nephew thought the tablet was supposed to be moved to San Francisco when the Giants franchise transferred there in 1958, but it disappeared during the move.[34]

After Bill Terry replaced John McGraw as manager of the Giants in 1932, the ex-skipper returned to his former office to retrieve two framed photographs from the wall. One was of the great pitcher Christy Mathewson. The other was of Mac's favorite outfielder, Pep Young.

In 1972 Youngs was elected to the National Baseball Hall of Fame in Cooperstown by the Veterans Committee. The drive to get him selected was spearheaded by Ford Frick, former sportswriter, National League president, and commissioner of baseball. Frick said, "Everyone has Cobb, Ruth and Speaker on his all-time outfield. But, somehow, I've got to find a place for Pep Young. Don't ask me to take one out; I've just got to get Pep in there somewhere."[35]

Is Youngs worthy of enshrinement in Cooperstown? His name appears on a list of the dozen Hall of Famers with the fewest Faber System points. This does not mean that Youngs does not belong in the Hall, only that there are some who are more deserving but have yet to be honored.[36] Youngs had an advantage in that he played in New York, the media capital of the baseball world, he appeared on baseball's biggest stage with four consecutive World

Series engagements, and he was a protégé of the famous John McGraw, who promoted him at every opportunity. On the other hand, these advantages are offset by the briefness of Pep's career; no player in the twentieth century accumulated as many Faber System points as Youngs without playing in more games than the Giants star.

Perhaps the last word should go to Ritter and Honig, who included him in their book *The 100 Greatest Baseball Players of All Time*. They wrote that a player of truly exceptional talent but with a career curtailed by injury or illness should still, despite lacking career statistics that would quantitatively rank him with the all-time greats, be included in their list of the greatest players.[37] Ross Youngs is ranked third by the Faber System among position players whose major league career ended before their 31st birthday. *Total Baseball* places him in a tie for first with Benny Kauff. James ranks him first among right fielders.

BENNY KAUFF

Hailed as the most heralded young player of his generation, he burst upon the baseball scene like a comet. The second coming of Ty Cobb, some said. In his first full season in the major leagues, he won the league batting championship. To prove it was not a fluke, he won it again the next year. The term five-tool player might well have been invented to describe him. Hit for average: he won two batting championships and posted a lifetime average of .311. Hit for power: he led the league in total bases his first year and in slugging average his second. Speed and base running skills: he led the league in stolen bases his first two seasons. Fielding: he led the league's outfielders in total chances in his sophomore season. Throwing: during that same year he threw out more base runners than any other outfielder on the circuit. He played the majority of his career on baseball's biggest stage—in New York—and for Gotham's most celebrated team of the era—the Giants. He was a World Series star. Yet he will never be inducted to the Baseball Hall of Fame. The story of Benny Kauff is a tale of incredible promise and a crushing downfall.

Benjamin Michael Kauff was born on January 5, 1890, in Pomeroy, a small town on the Ohio River in Meigs County in the southeastern part of Ohio. He was the oldest child of Hannah and William Kauff, a coal miner. Young Benny quit school at the age of 11 to join his father in the mines. Coal mining is hard work, and for seven years the lad toiled in the dust and grime, until he discovered that baseball offered a means of escape. After playing weekends for area amateur teams, he joined the Parkersville club of the Virginia

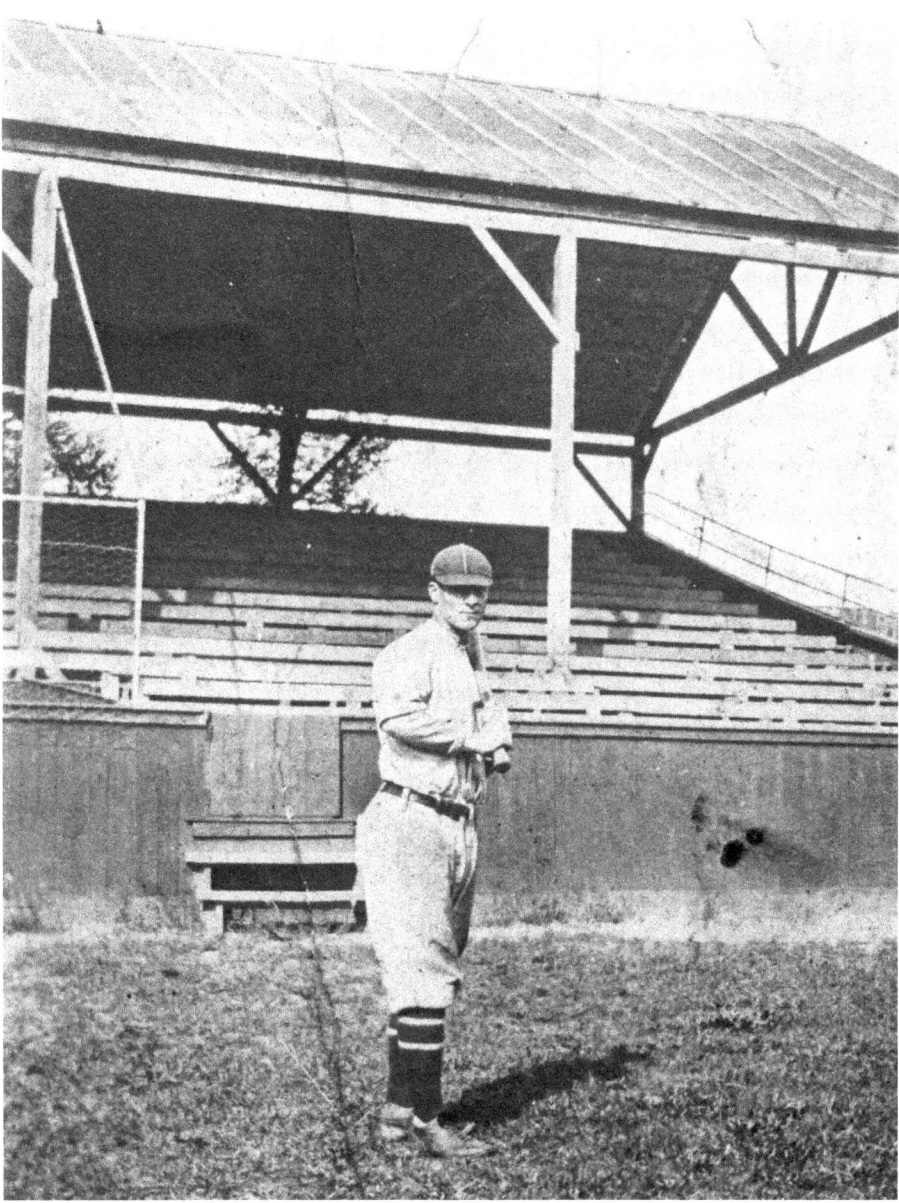

Benny Kauff was the most heralded young player of his generation. In 1914, at the age of 24, he led the Federal League in batting average, on-base percentage, runs scored, hits, and stolen bases. The next year he again won the batting, on-base, and stolen base crowns. In 1920 he was indicted on auto theft charges. Although the jury found him not guilty, Commissioner Landis banned him from baseball for life (Library of Congress).

Valley League in 1910 against the wishes of his father, who thought there was a better future in the mines than on the baseball field. Benny led the league with a .336 batting average and 36 stolen bases.

The New York Highlanders invited the 21-year-old Kauff to spring training in 1911 and sent him down to Bridgeport of the Connecticut State League, where he gained a reputation as one of the league's promising young players. In 1912 the Highlanders gave him his first taste of regular-season major league ball. After appearing in five games he was farmed out to Hartford for two seasons. In 1913 he led the Eastern Association with 176 hits and a .345 batting average. The St. Louis Cardinals grabbed him and placed him with the Indianapolis club of the American Association, where they planned to keep him until they were ready to call him up to the majors.

Before the 1914 season opened, the Federal League declared itself a major league and started signing players from the rosters of the more-established loops. The Indianapolis Hoosiers of the new circuit offered Kauff an amount that doubled his previous salary. Benny accepted and quickly became a sensation. In his first season he led the league in batting, runs scored, hits, on-base percentage, and stolen bases. According to the Faber System he was the loop's best right fielder, both in fielding and in combined fielding and hitting prowess.[38] He was the Federal League Hitter of the Year and Player of the Year.[39] He led the nation in hyperbole. An article in *The Sporting News* raved, "Kauff is the premier slugger, premier fielder, premier base stealer and best all around player in the league. He is being called a second Ty Cobb, yet there are many who will say that within next season Kauff will play rings around the Georgia Peach."[40]

Urged on by a press agent who thought the publicity would be good for the new league, Kauff readily agreed with those who called him a second Ty Cobb. He dressed himself in a fancy wardrobe, adorned with diamond rings and diamond tiepins, and said he was at least the equal of Cobb, if not his superior. His teammates were impressed by his ability to chew tobacco, smoke a cigar, and drink a beer at the same time, without interruption to any of the three pursuits.[41]

Benny's braggadocio did not go over well with everyone. Although he was immensely popular and the press loved his act, some of the other ballplayers and fans developed a strong dislike of the young star.

After the 1914 season the Indianapolis franchise was shifted to Newark and Kauff was transferred to Brooklyn in payment of some debts owed by the former Hoosier owner. Benny thought he should be a free agent and signed with the New York Giants of the National League. When the Giants took the field against the Boston Braves the afternoon of the signing, the Braves refused to play, claiming Kauff was ineligible because he had signed with the outlaw Federal League. The NL president, John Tener, agreed and voided the contract. As a result, Kauff played for the Brooklyn Tip Tops in the FL in 1915 and reinforced his image as the league's best player by leading the circuit in batting average, on-base percentage, slugging average, and stolen bases, as well as excelling in the outfield. Playing mostly center field, he led the league in Faber System points at that position. Of course, he was also tops in hitting and fielding combined.[42] For the second straight year he was the Faber System Hitter of the Year and Player of the Year in the Federal League.[43]

When the Federal League folded after the 1915 season, Kauff applied for and received reinstatement in Organized Baseball. Again he signed with the Giants, this time to a valid contract. Sportswriter Frank Graham described Benny's first appearance at the Giants' spring training camp: "He wore a loudly-striped silk shirt, an expensive blue suit, patent leather shoes, a fur-collared overcoat, and a derby hat. He was adorned with a huge diamond stickpin, an equally huge diamond ring and a gold watch encrusted with diamonds, and he had roughly $7500 in his pockets."[44]

Still not overcome by false modesty, Kauff proclaimed, "I'll hit so many balls into the grandstand that the management will have to put up screens in front to protect the fans and save the money that lost balls would cost."[45]

One sportswriter came to Benny's defense, writing that he was misquoted and misrepresented when he broke into the National League. Jack Veiock, sports editor for *International News*, wrote:

> He is not the most brilliant player in the league. He isn't a second Ty Cobb and he isn't a second Tris Speaker, but he's Benny Kauff, and before he outlives his usefulness in the big leagues his name is going to be written in the baseball hall of fame many times over. Kauff is a wonderful player, combining all-around ability with a happy disposition and an unusual love of baseball for the game itself. He would rather win than eat, and, oh, how he loves to hammer the ball.[46]

Benny's first season with the Giants was a disappointment, but he recovered and hit higher than .300 again in 1917. He helped McGraw's men get to the World Series against the Chicago White Sox in 1917, where he was first a goat and then a hero. In the third inning of the first game, Kauff tried to make a shoestring catch of a pop fly by Fred McMullin, but the ball bounded away for an RBI double, giving Chicago a 1–0 lead en route to an eventual 2–1 win. To top it off Kauff went hitless, not only in that game, but also in Games Two and Three. In the fourth inning of the fourth game Kauff came to the plate 0-for-13, taking a terrific riding from the Chicago bench. He faced Red Faber, who was to win a record-tying three games in that Fall

Classic and was working on a perfect game at that point. Kauff touched the redhead for an inside-the-park homer. In the eighth inning Benny hit one out of the park off reliever Dave Danforth. He accounted for three of the New York runs in a 5–0 victory.

In 1918 Kauff was again hitting higher than .300 when the draft board called him up. He went on active duty on June 21, and logged only 67 games for the Giants that season. He received his army discharge in February 1919, early enough to be assured of a full campaign the year of the big Black Sox scandal. He had a good year, finishing second in the NL in home runs and fourth in runs batted in, but he was no longer seen as another Ty Cobb, rather only as a very good ballplayer. The Black Sox disgrace contributed to Kauff's downfall. Two of the fixers claimed Kauff had taken part in the scheme, but no evidence was presented to back up the allegations.

Gamblers were rife not only in Chicago but in New York as well as other places. Two players on the Giants, Hal Chase and Heinie Zimmerman, attempted to fix some games. They tried to bribe several teammates, including Kauff, to help them. Benny immediately reported the attempt to his manager, John McGraw. Although Kauff acted with integrity in this matter, rumors of his alleged dishonesty began to circulate. Two different incidents, both of which he was innocent, besmirched his reputation.

Then came the crowning blow. Kauff, his brother-in-law, and a teammate had gone into a Manhattan automobile accessory business in the offseason. In February 1920 Kauff was indicted on auto theft charges. The complaint alleged that Benny and his associates had stolen a Cadillac from a West End parking lot, then fitted it with a new paint job, new tires, and a new license plate before selling it for $1800. Kauff denied the charges, claiming he was unaware the car was stolen when he re-sold it. Baseball commissioner Kenesaw Mountain Landis suspended Kauff pending resolution of the charges. The investigation dragged on for months and did not go to trial until May 1921. The trial lasted five days, but it took the jury less than an hour to return a not-guilty verdict.

Upon his acquittal Kauff expected to be reinstated. However, Landis, disregarding the jury's verdict, banned Kauff permanently from Organized Baseball. Benny was innocent in the eyes of the law, but Landis had his own views. Benny appealed to the New York State Supreme Court for a permanent injunction against the ban. The court concluded it had no grounds to act on the request, although Justice E. G. Whitaker agreed that "an apparent injustice has been done the plaintiff."[47] Benny Kauff's baseball career was over at the age of thirty.

His major league record: **Bold** indicates league leader.

Year	Age	Club	League	G	AB	R	H	HR	RBI	SB	BA	OBP
1912	22	New York	AL	5	11	4	3	0	2	1	.273	.429
1914	24	Indianapolis	FL	154	571	120	211	8	95	75	**.370**	**.447**
1915	25	Brooklyn	FL	136	485	92	165	12	83	55	**.343**	**.446**
1916	26	New York	NL	154	552	71	146	9	74	40	.264	.348
1917	27	New York	NL	153	559	89	172	5	68	30	.308	.379
1918	28	New York	NL	67	270	41	85	2	39	9	.315	.355
1919	29	New York	NL	135	491	73	136	10	67	21	.277	.334
1920	30	New York	NL	55	157	31	43	3	26	3	.274	.380
TOTAL				859	3094	521	961	49	454	234	.311	.389

On March 19, 1919, when he was 29 and his bride was 19, Benny married Hazel Cassley in Lancaster, Ohio. They had one child, Robert. After he was expelled from the major leagues, Kauff played for a while for semi-pro teams in Ohio, including the Coshocton Regulars. When his playing career concluded, Kauff settled his family in Columbus, Ohio. The 1930 census showed them living in that city. Benny's occupation was listed as used car salesman. After suffering a cerebral hemorrhage, Benjamin Kauff died in Columbus on November 17, 1961, at the age of 71. His obituary stated he was a salesman for John Lyman Company at the time of his death and that he had been a scout for the New York Giants for 22 years. He is buried in Union Cemetery in Columbus.

Among position players who played their last major league game at the age of thirty or younger, Kauff is ranked fourth by the Faber System. *Total Baseball* has him tied for first with Ross Youngs. James lowered his ranking for subjective factors and places him third among center fielders.

FREDDIE LINDSTROM

Someone once wrote that his rise to fame was meteoric, and like a meteor his flame burned out quickly. Certainly his rise was rapid. At 16 he was playing in the highest classification of minor league baseball. Two years later he became the youngest player ever to appear in the World Series, a distinction he still holds. He was known as the "boy wonder" of the major leagues. For several years his star shined brightly in the National League. When his stardom faded, the afterglow was strong enough to secure the election of Freddie Lindstrom to the National Baseball Hall of Fame in Cooperstown, despite the objections of his detractors.

Frederick Anthony Lindstrom was born on the southwest side of Chicago on November 21, 1905, the son of Mary Sweeney and Fred C. Lindstrom, a plumber. His maternal grandparents were Irish immigrants, while his paternal

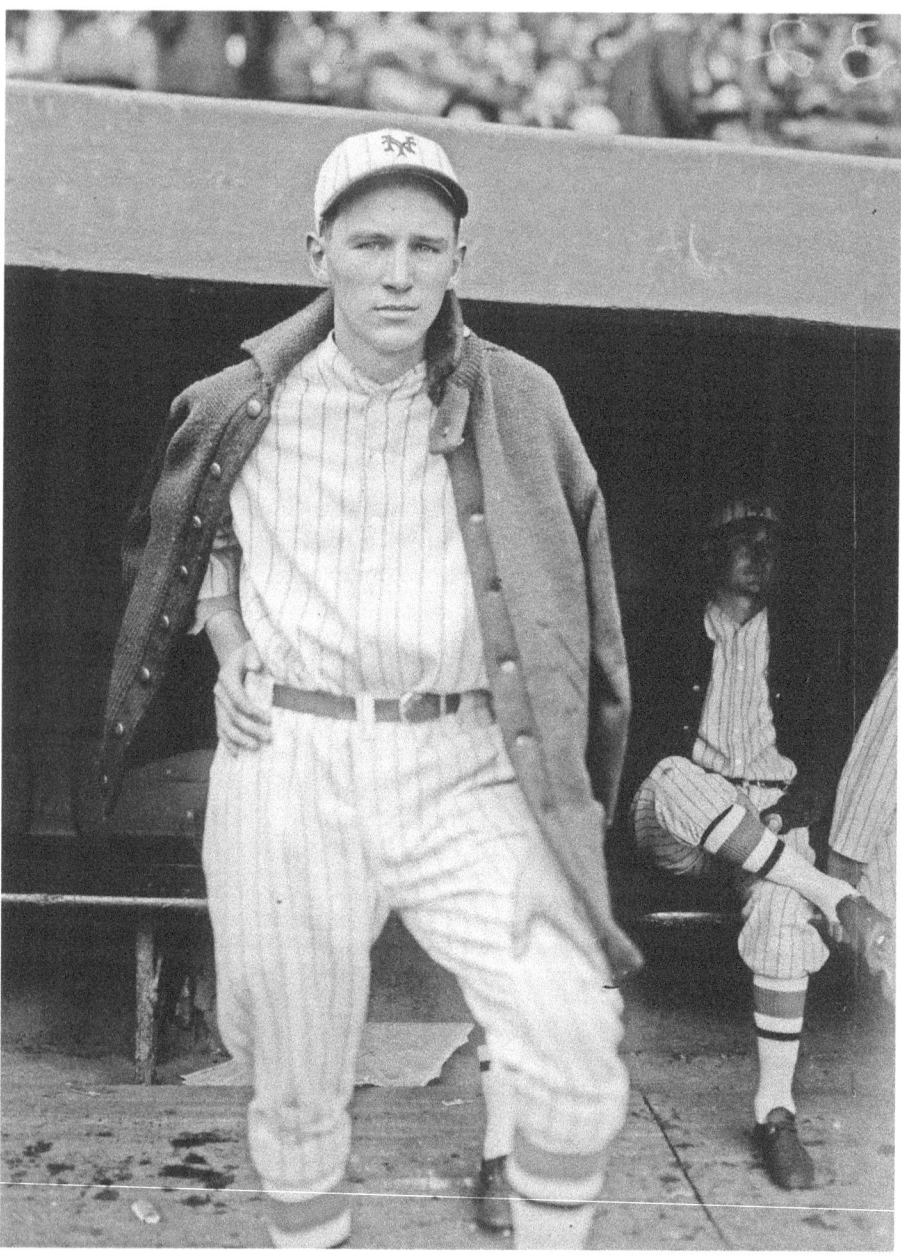

The youngest player ever to appear in a World Series, Freddie Lindstrom was the unfortunate victim of two bad bounces and became the goat of the 1924 Series. He overcame that humiliating start and posted a .311 batting average in a career that led to Cooperstown (Library of Congress).

grandparents came from Sweden. At some point the lad changed his middle name from Anthony to Charles. Freddie grew up a White Sox fan and reportedly was devastated when his hero, Shoeless Joe Jackson, was implicated in the Black Sox scandal of 1919.

After starting high school at Tilden, Freddie transferred to Loyola Academy, where he became a schoolboy star. A scout from the New York Giants watched Freddie bang out four extra-base hits against Lake View High School and signed him to a contract for $300 per month. He was assigned to the Toledo Mud Hens of the American Association, where the 16 year old hit higher than .300 in 18 games in the fall of 1922. He was back at Toledo the following year until the Giants purchased his contract on September 18, 1923.

His minor league record:

Year	Age	Club	G	AB	R	H	HR	RBI	BA
1922	16	Toledo AA	15	23	3	7	1	0	.304
1923	17	Toledo AA	147	581	77	157	1	39	.270

In his first season in the major leagues, Lindstrom was involved in some of the more memorable events of his career. Heinie Groh was the Giants' regular third baseman that year but late in the season he tore up his knee and Lindy replaced him at the hot corner. Freddie became the youngest player ever to appear in a World Series game at the age of 18 years, 10 months, and 13 days, a record that has never been broken. In Game 2 of the Series against the Washington Senators, he made seven assists, a single-game World Series record that stood for 26 years. The "boy wonder" recorded four hits off Walter Johnson, arguably the game's greatest pitcher.

It was in Game 7 that Lindy gained his infamy. With the best-of-seven series tied three games apiece, this game would decide the world championship. In the eighth inning the Giants were leading 3–1, but the Senators loaded the bases with two outs. Washington's player-manager Bucky Harris slammed a sharp grounder toward third base. Just as Freddie was about to field it, the ball took a wicked hop over his head and two runs scored to tie the game.

The game remained tied into extra innings. In the twelfth inning with runners on first and second and one out, Earl McNeeley slashed a grounder toward Lindstrom at third. Amazingly, the ball hit a pebble or a clod of dirt, perhaps the same one that had deflected the hit by Harris four innings earlier. The ball bounded into left field for a base hit and Muddy Ruel raced home with the winning run. The Washington Senators won their first World Series, and Freddie Lindstrom was the goat of the Series.

Some observers thought Providence had a hand in the miscues. Clark

Griffith, owner of the Senators, said, "God was on our side in that one. Else how did those pebbles get in front of Lindstrom, not once, but twice?"[48]

Heinie Groh was not sure whether to blame the Lord or fate. He told Lawrence Ritter, "I guess the good Lord just didn't want us to win that game, that's all there is to it." Later in the same interview he said, "It wasn't Freddie's fault. It could have happened to anybody. He never had a chance to get the ball. It was Fate, that's all. Fate and a pebble."[49]

Lindstrom recovered quickly from the World Series disaster. In 1925 he had what Bill James called the second-best season ever by a 19-year-old third baseman.[50] He improved over the next several years. From 1926 through 1931 Freddie hit .300 or better every single year. In 1928 he led the league with 231 hits and matched that total two years later to become only the second player in National League history to have two seasons with more than 230 hits. He came in second to "Sunny" Jim Bottomley in the voting for the NL Most Valuable Player award in 1928. In 1930 Lindstrom became the first third baseman in the twentieth century to hit twenty home runs in a season. In that year he had a personal high with a .379 batting average. This is somewhat less impressive than it may seem, for 1930 is considered to be the year when the liveliest ball ever was used in the major leagues. The batting average for the league as a whole, including pitchers, was .303. Lindstrom's average was fifth best in the circuit, as Bill Terry became the last National Leaguer to hit .400 in a season.

Although not generally regarded as an outstanding defensive third baseman, Lindstrom was more than adequate at that position. In 1928 he won Faber System accolades as the top fielding third sacker in the National League, and he topped the circuit in combined hitting and fielding points in that season and again in 1930.[51]

During the 1931 season Lindy broke his ankle sliding into third base and also suffered back problems, limiting his activity to only 78 games, mostly in the outfield. For the rest of his career he mainly patrolled the outer garden, logging time at all three outfield positions. Bill James thought Freddie's play in the outfield was worthy of a Gold Glove in 1933.[52]

When John McGraw retired as manager of the Giants in 1932, Lindstrom had played his entire major league career in the shadow of Coogan's Bluff. He thought he was Mac's favorite player and that he should succeed the old man as skipper. When the position went to Bill Terry, Freddie was bitter. Worse, he was outspoken in his reaction. "It was the worst mistake I ever made," Lindstrom told a reporter a quarter of a century later. "I know that now. The only trouble is you don't get wise until you get old.... If I could have just accepted that setback it'd have worked out in time. I'm sure I'd have managed some club. It was just a matter of waiting. But I fouled the whole thing up — forever."[53]

After his tirade against the Giants for not getting the managerial post, Lindstrom was traded to the Pittsburgh Pirates. He had a good year in 1933, hitting higher than .300 for the seventh and last time in his major league career. After the 1934 season he was traded again, this time to the Chicago Cubs, where he hoped to play out his career. But it was not to be. After an injury to his knee and an ineffective season at Wrigley Field, he was released by the Cubs in January 1936. A week later he was signed as a free agent by the Brooklyn Dodgers. After playing only a few games for the Dodgers, Lindstrom asked for and received his release. He played his last major league game on May 1, 1936, at the age of 30.

His major league record: **Bold** indicates league leader.

Year	Age	Club	G	AB	R	H	HR	RBI	BA	OBP
1924	18	New York NL	52	79	19	20	0	4	.253	.314
1925	19	New York NL	104	356	43	102	4	33	.287	.332
1926	20	New York NL	140	543	90	164	9	76	.302	,351
1927	21	New York NL	138	562	107	172	7	58	.306	.354
1928	22	New York NL	153	646	99	**231**	14	107	.358	.383
1929	23	New York NL	130	549	99	175	15	91	.319	.354
1930	24	New York NL	148	609	127	231	22	106	.379	.425
1931	25	New York NL	78	303	38	91	5	36	.300	.356
1932	26	New York NL	144	595	83	161	15	92	.271	.303
1933	27	Pittsburgh NL	138	538	70	167	5	55	.310	.350
1934	28	Pittsburgh NL	97	383	59	111	4	49	.290	.333
1935	29	Chicago NL	90	342	49	94	3	62	.275	.297
1936	30	Brooklyn NL	26	106	12	28	0	10	.297	.302
TOTAL			1438	5611	895	1747	103	779	.311	.351

After his retirement as a player, Lindstrom tried to catch on as a manager. He was an unsuccessful contender to follow Casey Stengel as the Brooklyn manager in 1936. When that job went to the old spitballer, Burleigh Grimes, Freddie applied for Burleigh's former role with the Louisville Colonels of the American Association. Failing to nab that position, Lindy set his sights a little lower and became manager of the Knoxville Smokies of the Southern Association. After two last-place finishes in Knoxville in 1940 and 1941, he spent one season as skipper of the Fort Smith Giants of the Western Association. Although the Giants finished the regular season in third place, they won the 1942 league championship by defeating the Topeka Owls, four games to three. The Association suspended play in 1943 because of World War II.

Sportswriter Henry McLemore penned a tale that was widely circulated in the 1930s and purported to show that Lindstrom's mind was always on baseball, even when he was at the race track. McLemore accompanied Freddie to Hialeah one January day in 1936. Before the seventh race Freddie purchased a $2 ticket on a horse named Lawmaker. According to the story, Lawmaker challenged for the lead as the steeds headed down the stretch. Freddie jumped on a chair and screamed, "Come on baby! Lawdy, lawdy, lawdy! Run for me, you dog you. Run for me." As the horses neared the finish line, it appeared that Lawmaker might be caught at the wire. The old ballplayer shouted, "Slide for it, Lawmaker, slide." Lawmaker made it without sliding, but when the jubilant Lindstrom went to cash his ticket, he discovered he had mistakenly torn it up. McLemore wrote that Lindy's bad luck had followed him all the way from Brooklyn to Florida.[54]

In 1947 Lindstrom became baseball coach at Northwestern University of the Big Ten Conference. He coached the Wildcats for 14 years until he resigned on May 12, 1961, to accept an appointment as postmaster at Evanston, Illinois.

In 1976 Freddie Lindstrom was elected to the National Baseball Hall of Fame by the Veterans Committee. An intensive lobbying campaign by his son, Andy, and the fact that former teammate Frankie Frisch headed the Veterans Committee at the time may have contributed to his selection, which proved to be very controversial. Bill James, for example, wrote, "His selection to the Hall of Fame, while it ignores players like Ken Boyer, Ron Santo, Ed Yost and Stan Hack, was a bad joke."[55]

Only two players enshrined in Cooperstown have fewer Faber System points than Lindstorm.[56] They are Rick Ferrell and Tony Lazzeri. However, only four third basemen in the history of the game have amassed more points in fewer games than Lindstrom.[57] Given his relatively short playing career, perhaps his induction in the Hall of Fame is not as unreasonable as it at first appears. As unpopular as Lindy's selection may have been with the writers, it was welcomed by his friends and relatives. About sixty-two of them made the trek from the Chicago area to Cooperstown for the ceremony.

In addition to Andy, Lindstrom had another son, Charles William Lindstrom, who went by "Chuck," a catcher who had exactly one major league appearance — with the Chicago White Sox on September 28, 1958. Freddie's first marriage ended in a divorce at Miami in 1935. In 1937 he honeymooned in Las Vegas with his new bride, 21-year-old Frances Udaloff of Los Angeles.

After living for ten years in New Port Richey, Florida, Lindstrom returned to Chicago. He died at Mercy Hospital following a long illness on October 4, 1981, at the age of 75. Among all non-pitchers whose major league careers ended at the age of thirty or younger, Lindstrom ranks fifth in Faber System points and is tied for ninth in *Total Baseball*'s ratings. James ranks him first among third basemen.

BOB HORNER

Without playing a single inning in the minor leagues, he went straight from the campus of Arizona State University to the Show. His big league career got off to a blazing start. In his first major league game he hit a home run off Bert Blyleven. At the end of the season he was named the National League Rookie of the Year for 1978, an honor to match the Golden Spikes Award he had won in the spring as the best amateur baseball player in the country. He remains the only athlete to win these prestigious awards in the same calendar year. Three times he hit 30 or more home runs in a season, despite battling injuries year after year. Finally a shoulder injury that refused to heal caused him to give up the game he loved. Rather than risk further injury, Bob Horner retired without reaching his full potential.

James Robert Horner was born on August 6, 1957, in Junction City, Kansas, but grew up in Glendale, Arizona, where he starred at Apollo High School. Based on his high school record and freshman year in college at Arizona State, the Oakland Athletics drafted him in the fifteenth round of the 1975 amateur draft. Preferring to continue his college career, he did not sign with the A's. At Arizona State Horner was named to *The Sporting News* College All-American team in both 1977 and 1978. Playing second base Bob led the Sun Devils to the College World Series title in 1977. The next year he switched to third base and was named MVP of the College World Series as Arizona State finished as national runners-up. He set a College World Series record with twenty runs batted in during the 1976–78 classics.[58]

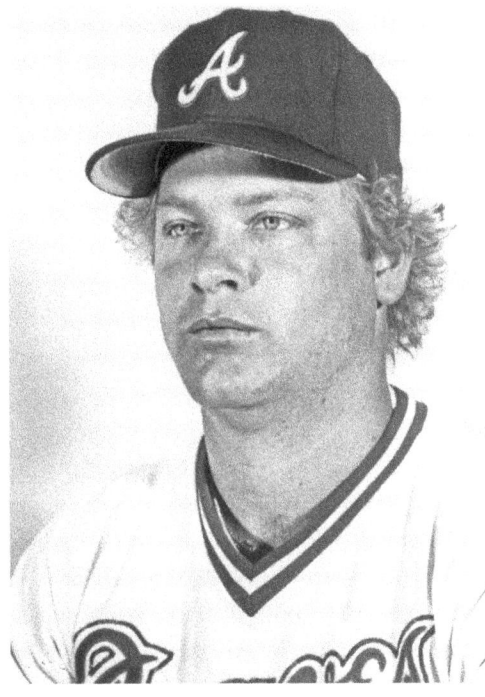

Bob Horner was the first overall pick in the 1978 amateur draft and became National League Rookie of the Year that season. Hampered by injuries, he never reached his full potential and retired at the age of 30 (National Baseball Hall of Fame Library, Cooperstown, New York).

During his college career he set an NCAA record with 58 home runs for the Sun Devils.

He was the first overall pick in the amateur draft in the spring of 1978. The Braves had first shot at him because they had had the worst record in the National League the previous season. Despite missing much of the season with a shoulder injury, Horner hit 25 home runs in 89 games and beat out Ozzie Smith for NL Rookie of the Year honors, one of the few times the rookie award went to a member of a last-place team. In his next two seasons Bob again battled recurring shoulder and leg injuries. Despite missing 79 games during the two seasons, he hit more than 30 home runs in each campaign. After the strike-shortened season of 1981, he again hit more than 30 homers in 1982. Bob was named to the NL All-Star team in 1982, but was hitless in his one at-bat.

Injuries continued to hamper Horner. In his entire big league career he never had a single year when he didn't miss games because of injuries. In August 1983 he fractured his right wrist while sliding into a base and missed the rest of the season. In May 1984 he broke the same wrist while diving for a ball at third base and was sidelined for almost the entire season, appearing in only 32 games. Never regarded highly for his fielding prowess at the hot corner, Horner was hampered by injuries to the point that he played mainly at first base for the remainder of his career. Despite missing so many games because of injuries, by the end of his tenure with the Braves he had hit more home runs in Atlanta than any other player except Hank Aaron and Dale Murphy. One of the highlights of his career came on July 6, 1986, when he hit four home runs in a game against the Montreal Expos, becoming the eleventh man in major league history to accomplish that feat.

When the Braves were unwilling to meet the slugger's salary demands for the 1987 season, Bob opted for free agency. No other major league club offered Bob what he thought he was worth, so he headed overseas to Japan. The Yakult Swallows gave him a one-year $2.4 million contract. Horner got off to a great start with the Swallows, hitting six home runs in his first four games.[59] Naturally, he became immensely popular among the baseball-loving Japanese fans. When school was out in Irving, Texas, where his family was living at the time, Bob's wife, Chris, and their two sons, Tyler and Trent, then six and four, respectively, flew to Tokyo to join him.[60] Even with his family with him and receiving the adoration of the fans, Bob found the cultural shock disconcerting and was eager to return to the United States. His unhappiness with Japan increased when the press turned on him, bringing up stories of weight problems, excessive beer drinking, and too many injuries, and hitting him hard when he claimed a sore shoulder prevented him from taking infield practice.⁶¹ At the end of the season he signed as a free agent with the St. Louis Cardinals for a reported base salary of $950,000, less than half of what he received in Japan.

To some observers Horner appeared seriously overweight when he returned from Japan. The Cardinals put a weight clause in his contract, although he claimed his weight was not a problem. He said he had the same clause in his last contract with the Atlanta Braves.⁶² Bob played 60 relatively unproductive games for the Cardinals before making his last major league appearance on June 18, 1988, at the age of 30.

His major league record:

Year	Age	Club	G	AB	R	H	HR	RBI	BA	OBP
1978	20	Atlanta NL	89	323	50	86	23	63	.266	.313
1979	21	Atlanta NL	121	487	66	153	33	98	.314	.346
1980	22	Atlanta NL	124	463	81	124	35	89	.268	.307
1981	23	Atlanta NL	79	300	42	83	15	42	.277	.345
1982	24	Atlanta NL	140	499	85	130	32	97	.261	.350
1983	25	Atlanta NL	104	386	75	117	20	68	.303	.383
1984	26	Atlanta NL	32	113	15	31	3	19	.274	.349
1985	27	Atlanta NL	130	483	61	129	27	89	.267	.333
1986	28	Atlanta NL	141	517	70	141	27	87	.273	.336
1988	30	St. Louis NL	60	206	15	53	3	33	.257	.348
TOTAL			1020	3777	560	1047	218	685	.277	.340

The Cardinals released Horner on December 21, 1988. During spring training in 1989 the Baltimore Orioles gave him a tryout at their camp in Florida. After trying for a few days to make the club as a non-roster free agent, the injury-riddled slugger called it quits because his shoulder had not healed sufficiently from an operation the previous summer. "I couldn't focus on making the club because I was always worried about the shoulder so much," he said. "One thing I didn't want to do was go out and do something major to it and have a broken down arm the rest of my life. I've got children I want to raise and teach sports to. The last thing they need is a crippled father."⁶³

When asked if he thought he might ever play again, Horner said, "Right now I have no plans except to go back to Dallas and be with my family and let my shoulder heal."⁶⁴ On July 4, 2006, Bob Horner was inducted into the College Baseball Hall of Fame as a member of its inaugural class. He is ranked by the Faber System as the sixth-best position player to leave the major leagues at the age of thirty or younger. *Total Baseball* ranks him eighteenth. James places him third among third basemen.

RAY CHAPMAN

It was a dark and rainy day in New York that 16th day of August 1920. For the young man who led off the fifth inning of a game between the Yankees and the Cleveland Indians at the Polo Grounds that afternoon, however, life was bright and sunny. The future appeared even brighter, for his club was in the thick of a pennant fight and the fulfillment of his dream of playing in a World Series seemed possible, even probable. Life had already been good to young Ray Chapman. Recently married to the daughter of a millionaire and exceedingly popular with fans and teammates alike, he was acknowledged as one of the best shortstops in all of baseball, perhaps the best ever to play for Cleveland. With the count one ball and one strike, a fastball delivered by Carl Mays sailed high and inside. Chapman's dreams, career, and life were over.

Raymond Johnson Chapman was born on January 15, 1891, on a farm near Beaver Dam in Ohio County, Kentucky. In 1905 he moved with his parents, Barbara and Everette Chapman, to Herrin, in the southern Illinois coal mining country. At the age of 18 Ray played his first organized baseball for a semi-pro club in nearby Mount Vernon. The next year he went to Springfield, the state capital, where he played every position except pitcher and catcher. Don Jensen quoted one of his Springfield teammates as saying: "He was a very flashy player, and he could run. He was a beautiful runner, the way he could pick up his knees. He was very fast, had a good arm, and was a good fielder, although at times a little erratic. And he was very jolly, a jolly guy. Always, laughing, talking, singing."[65]

In 1911 Chapman went to Davenport of the Class B Three-I League, where he hit .293, scored 75 runs, and stole 50 bases. Near the end of the season Cleveland purchased his contract and assigned him to Toledo. The Mud Hens were members of the American Association, the highest classification in the minor leagues at the time. In 1912, he batted .310 for the Mud Hens, scored 101 runs, and stole 49 bases in 140 games, enough to earn a promotion to the big leagues.

"Chappie," as he was known, made his major league debut on August 30, 1912. In competition with Ivy Olson and Roger Peckinpaugh for the shortstop position, Ray emerged victorious. In 1913 he teamed with legendary second baseman Nap Lajoie in the middle of the infield. Although hampered by injuries in 1914 and 1916, he remained the club's regular shortstop until the time of his death. Between the two injury-plagued seasons, he led the American League in games played with 154 in 1915. He led again in 1917 with 156.

In 1918 he paced the American League in both runs and walks with 84 of each. Thrice he led the junior circuit in sacrifice hits. An excellent baserunner, he topped the Indians in stolen bases five times, including a club-record 52 thefts in 1917. In an exhibition game against the Braves in Boston on Tim Murnane Day, September 27, 1917, he won a trophy for the fastest time circling the bases at 14 seconds.[66]

In the field he excelled, leading the American League in putouts three times and in assists once. In total chances per game he was the league's best on four occasions. The Faber System showed he was the circuit's best fielding shortstop and the best overall (hitting and fielding combined) in 1915, 1917, 1918, and again in 1920.[67] After the end of the war-shortened 1918 season Chapman enrolled in the Naval Auxiliary Reserve as a seaman, second class. He spent three months on a steamer on the Great Lakes and captained naval reserve baseball and football teams. He was a sprinter on the track squad and ran the 100-yard dash in 10 seconds flat. After the armistice on November 11, 1918, Chappie was released from the navy and rejoined the Indians for the 1919 season. After the season Ray married Kathleen Daly, daughter of the president of the East Ohio Gas Company. He thought briefly about retiring, but his friend Tris Speaker had been named manager of the Indians and Chappie did not want to let him down. Furthermore, there was a chance the Tribe could grab that long desired, but elusive, American League pennant in 1920.

In mid–August 1920 the Indians and the Yankees, led by Babe Ruth, were fighting for their first American League pennant, along with the defending champion Chicago White Sox. The Indians had a slight lead. Chapman was having one of his best years, hitting .304 with 97 runs scored on the day of the fateful game. Cleveland was leading, 3–0, when Ray led off the fifth inning. With the count one ball and one strike, he crouched over the plate, waiting for the next pitch. A fellow Kentuckian, Carl Mays, threw a sidearm or underhand pitch, high and tight, aiming for the inside corner of the plate. Chapman did not move.

The ball struck him in the head with a "sickening thud" and rolled out toward the pitcher's mound. Mays fielded the ball and threw to first base, apparently thinking the ball had hit the bat. First baseman Wally Pipp started to throw the ball around the infield, then he glanced home. He saw Chapman on his knees, his face contorted, blood streaming from his left ear. Yankee catcher Muddy Ruel tried to catch Chapman as his knees buckled. Umpire Tommy Connolly ran toward the stands yelling for a doctor. Two doctors came to the aid of the stricken man, applied ice, and revived him. Ray started walking toward the clubhouse, but his knees gave way and two teammates carried him the rest of the way. He was taken to St. Lawrence Hospital, where

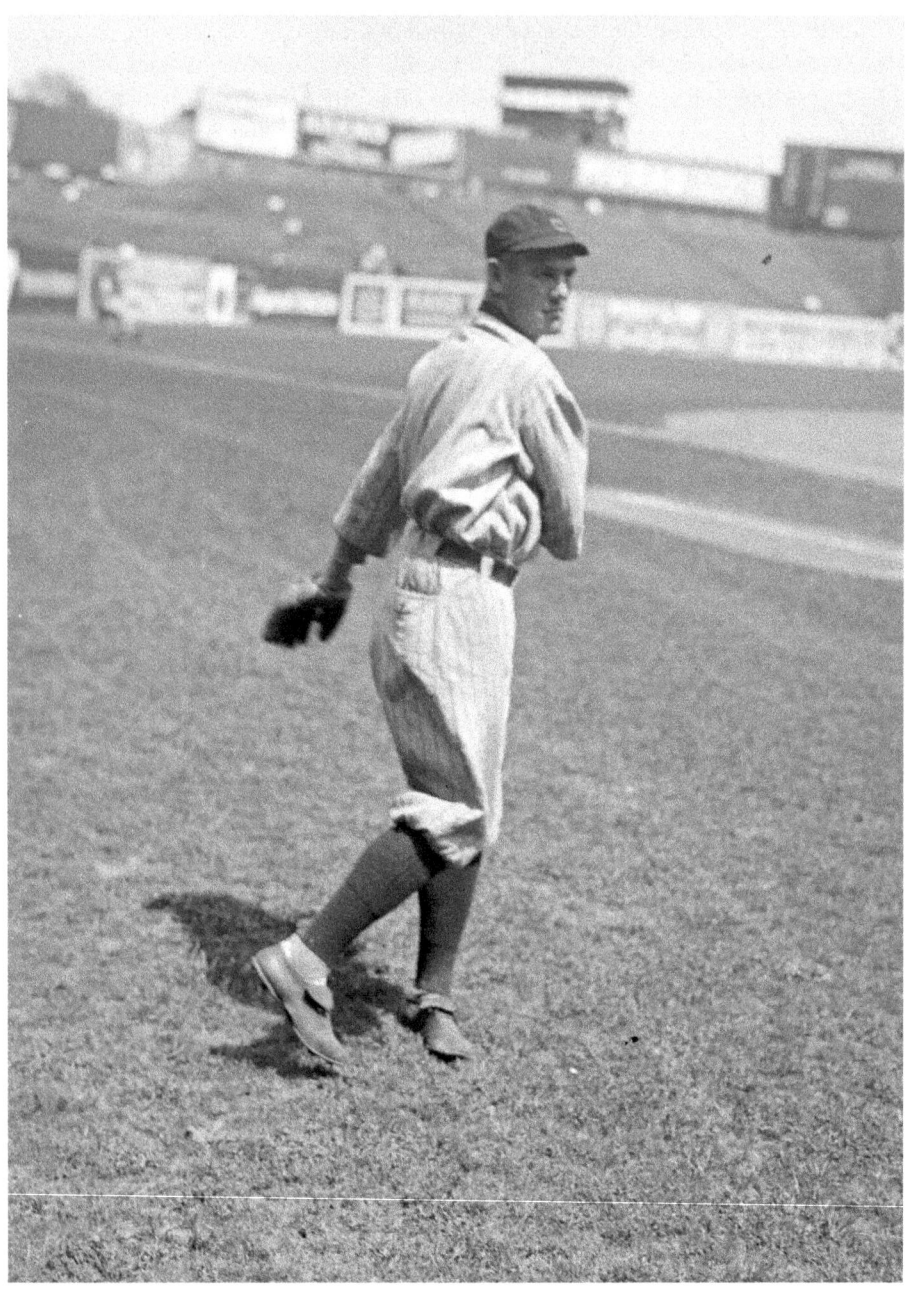

Ray Chapman was the only player ever killed when hit by a pitch in a major league game. At the age of 29 the shortstop was perhaps headed for the Hall of Fame when tragedy struck (Library of Congress).

doctors made a three-inch incision at the base of his skull and found clotted blood and a ruptured lateral sinus before removing a piece of his fractured skull. His wife, pregnant with the couple's first child, was summoned to New York but did not arrive in time to see her husband alive.

One of the teammates who helped carry Chapman to the clubhouse was Jack Graney, who stayed with Chappie until the ambulance came. Graney stated that Ray was conscious, looked up at him and tried to speak but could not get the words out. According to Russell Schneider, Graney said: "I knew by the look in his eyes that he desperately wanted to tell me something, so I got some paper and put a pencil in his hand. He made a motion to write but the pencil dropped to the floor. Paralysis was setting in. We found out later that his skull had been fractured on one side, there was a concussion on the other side and his neck was broken."[68]

Meanwhile, Mays remained in the game, showed the ball to Connolly, and told him the pitch had sailed because a rough spot on the ball caused it to move further inside than he had intended. The game continued, with the Indians winning, 4–3. That evening Miller Huggins, the Yankee manager, and Mays went to the nearest police station to report the incident.[69] Later Mays was exonerated of any wrongdoing by the district attorney, Manager Speaker and American League officials, but not by the public. The outcry against the pitcher was fierce and protracted. It has been incorrectly reported many times that the spitball was outlawed as a result of Chapman's beaning. Actually, the spitball was banned six months before the tragedy.[70]

Ray Chapman died at 4:30 on the morning of August 17. The game between the Yankees and the Indians scheduled for that afternoon was cancelled, but the Indians went on to win the American League pennant and defeat the Brooklyn Dodgers in the memorable 1920 World Series. Chappie's body was taken back to Cleveland for a funeral at St. John's Cathedral on August 20. A local bank had coordinated a "Flower from a Fan" campaign, in which fans were invited to contribute ten cents each for a floral tribute at the funeral, resulting in the display of a blanket of 20,000 blossoms.[71] Flags in the city were flown at half-staff as citizens mourned the loss of one of their favorite Clevelanders. Ray was buried in Lake View Cemetery in Cleveland. A bronze plaque was designed in his honor and is hung in Heritage Park, an exhibit of Indians history at Progressive Field.

Among the many tributes to Chapman, three stand out. In the *Cleveland News* Ed Bang wrote that Chapman was the greatest shortstop ever to wear the Cleveland uniform, "...considering all-around ability, batting, throwing, base running, bunting, fielding and ground covering ability, to mention nothing of his fight, spirit and conscientiousness." Bang went on to commend Ray for being "clean cut, high minded, honest, and straightforward."[72] The 1921 *Spalding Guide* said, "Chapman was not only the idol of Cleveland and thousands of fans in other cities, but was one of the most popular and beloved of players.... His rare personality, in addition to his brilliant ability, had won him the friendship of all who knew him."[73] Baseball guru Bill James wrote that Chapman was probably destined for the Hall of Fame had he lived and presented statistical data in support of his contention.[74]

Tragedy continued to stalk Ray's family after his death. His wife Kathleen never attended another game. She gave birth to a daughter, Rae-Marie, on February 27, 1921. Two years later Kathleen remarried, but on April 21, 1928, she died after swallowing a poisonous fluid. Rae-Marie went to live with her grandparents but died a year later during a measles epidemic.

His major league record: **Bold** face indicates league leader

Year	Age	Club	G	AB	R	H	HR	RBI	BA	OBP
1912	21	Cleveland AL	31	109	29	34	0	19	.312	.375
1913	22	Cleveland AL	141	508	78	131	3	39	.258	.322
1914	23	Cleveland AL	106	375	59	103	2	42	.275	.358
1915	24	Cleveland AL	**154**	570	101	154	3	67	.270	.353
1916	25	Cleveland AL	109	346	50	80	0	57	.231	.330
1917	26	Cleveland AL	**156**	563	98	170	2	36	.302	.370
1918	27	Cleveland AL	128	446	**84**	119	2	32	.267	.390
1919	28	Cleveland AL	115	433	75	130	3	53	.300	.351
1920	29	Cleveland AL	111	435	97	132	3	49	.303	.380
TOTAL			1051	3785	671	1053	17	364	.278	.358

The Faber System ranks Chapman seventh among all players who played their last major league game at the age of thirty or younger. *Total Baseball* places him in the fourth position. James ranks him as the best shortstop.

CARLOS MAY

For the young White Sox outfielder, the summer of 1969 got off to a great start. He was named to the American League All-Star team and was considered the leading candidate for the circuit's Rookie of the Year award. By early August he had already hit more home runs than his older brother, the star first baseman of the Cincinnati Reds, had hit in his entire rookie season. But his season ended on August 11, and it appeared that his major league baseball career might be over just as it was getting started. While on duty as a marine corps reserve in a two-week summer training exercise at Camp Pendleton, it was his job to clean out the mortars after they had been fired. On that fateful day, the slugger had part of his right thumb blown away when a mortar unit misfired. He was rushed to the military hospital where a team of doctors operated on the remaining portion of the thumb, which had been jammed into his wrist. Doctors feared they might have to amputate the thumb, but the youngster refused to give up. He suffered through several painful skin graft operations and began physical therapy.[75] By spring training in 1970, Carlos May was ready and able to resume his baseball career.

Carlos May was born May 17, 1948, in Birmingham, Alabama, the younger brother of Lee May. A star at Parker High School in his hometown, he was selected in the first round of the 1966 amateur draft by the Chicago White Sox, the eighteenth pick overall. After some seasoning in the minors, he made his major league debut on September 6, 1968. He appeared in 17 games that fall, not enough to render him ineligible for rookie consideration in 1969. He quickly established himself as a promising candidate for stardom. He was one of only a few rookies to appear in the 1969 All-Star game. Pinch-hitting for Johnny Roseboro against Phil Niekro with two out in the bottom of the ninth inning, he struck out to end the game as the American League went down to its seventh straight defeat in the Mid-summer Classic. Both May brothers were in the game, as Lee was a late replacement for Willie McCovey at first base for the NL.

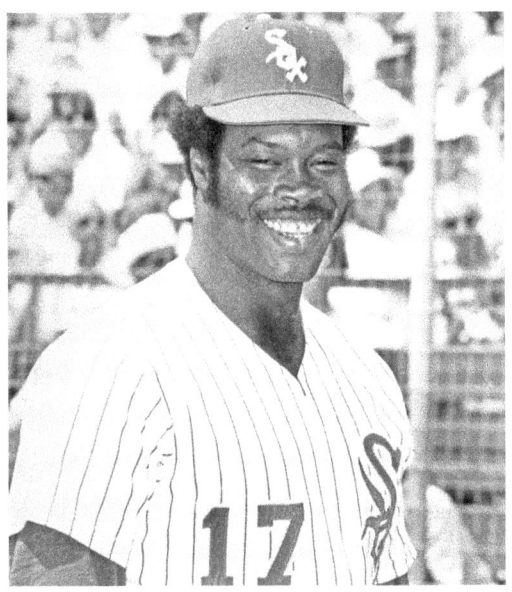

While serving in the Marine Corps reserve, Carlos May had part of his right thumb blown off in a mortar accident. Despite the injury he was the American League Rookie of the Year in 1969 and starred for the Chicago White Sox for several years (National Baseball Hall of Fame Library, Cooperstown, New York).

After his injury ended his 1969 season prematurely, May lost out in the Rookie of the Year voting by the baseball writers, finishing third behind Kansas City outfielder Lou Piniella and Red Sox pitcher Mike Nagy. Despite playing in many fewer games than Sweet Lou, May outperformed Piniella in almost every statistical category, which led some to find the selection of Piniella puzzling. On the other hand, *The Sporting News* named May its American League Rookie of the Year.

After recovering from his thumb injury, May became a mainstay of the White Sox outfield for several years. His best season was the 1972 campaign. He gave a hint of things to come on April 21, when he hit a grand slam against the Texas Rangers, the first bases-loaded jack ever delivered at Arlington Stadium.[76] For the season he finished among the top five hitters in the AL in batting average, on-base percentage, hits, bases on balls, and times hit by pitch. In addition he ranked in the top ten in on-base plus slugging, runs scored, total bases, and stolen bases. Quite a season! The Faber System identified him as the best left fielder in the American League that year.[77] Again he was named to the AL All-Star team but did not get into the game. His brother Lee played the entire game for the National League, as the senior circuit won for the ninth time in the last ten contests, this time on a single by Joe Morgan in the tenth inning.

Following his outstanding 1972 season, May played five more years in the big leagues. During most of his years with the White Sox, May wore his name and his uniform number on his back, as did most major league players. What made Carlos unique was that his number was 17, so on the back of his uniform appeared May 17, which was his birthday. He said he wore his birthday on his back.

Bill James wrote that Carlos had more talent than his brother, Lee. "He was as strong as Lee, but he could also run and he could throw a little bit. He was a natural hitter, a lefty, and he knew the strike zone. When he was 21 years old, he looked like the second coming of Willie Mays. Carlos blew off his thumb in a military training accident, which cost him a lot, but there was another problem. He played baseball as if he didn't give a ____."[78] That seems a surprising comment, considering the tremendous determination and effort May exerted in rehabilitating after the 1969 accident. However, Richard Lindberg reported that May was sometimes criticized in Chicago for his lackadaisical outfield play.[79] James also includes a rambling discourse on the reasons he thinks younger brothers don't match the motivation of their elders. Be that as it may, the May brothers rank sixth on the list of most career home runs hit by two siblings, with 444. The list is headed, of course, by the Aaron brothers, Hank and Tommie.

On May 18, 1976, May was traded to the New York Yankees for pitcher Ken Brett and outfielder Rich Coggins. The Bronx Bombers won the 1976 AL pennant, and Carlos played in his only World Series. He said, "For me, the playoffs were a greater thrill than the Series. We played Kansas City and it went five games with Chris Chambliss winning it for us with a home run. That was an exciting moment. It was pandemonium.... The World Series was not as thrilling because we were swept in four games by the Big Red

Machine."[80] Another reason he may have found the World Series less than thrilling is the fact that he was hitless in nine at-bats during the Fall Classic.

May's stay with the Yankees was short. On September 16, 1977, he was purchased by the California Angels but played only 11 games for the Angels toward the end of the season. On October 2, 1977, at the age of 29, he logged his final major league contest.

His major league record:

Year	Age	Club	G	AB	R	H	HR	RBI	BA	OBP
1968	19	Chicago AL	17	67	4	12	0	1	.179	.214
1969	20	Chicago AL	100	367	62	103	18	62	.281	.385
1970	21	Chicago AL	150	555	83	158	12	68	.285	.373
1971	22	Chicago AL	141	500	64	147	7	70	.294	.375
1972	23	Chicago AL	148	523	83	161	12	68	.308	.405
1973	24	Chicago AL	149	553	62	148	20	96	.268	.334
1974	25	Chicago AL	149	551	66	137	8	58	.249	.306
1975	26	Chicago AL	128	454	55	123	8	53	.271	.373
1976	27	Chi/NY AL	107	351	45	91	3	43	.259	.344
1977	28	NY/Cal AL	76	199	21	47	2	17	.236	.311
TOTAL			1165	4120	545	1127	90	536	.274	.357

His post-season record:

		G	AB	R	H	HR	RBI	BA	OBP
1976 ALCS	New York AL	3	10	1	2	0	0	.200	.273
World Series	New York AL	4	9	0	0	0	0	.000	.000

After his major league career ended, May played four years in Japan for the Nankai Hawks. His Japanese League record:

Year	Age	Club	G	AB	R	Hits	HR	RBI	BA
1978	29	Nankai	na	414	51	129	12	80	.312
1979	30	Nankai	na	398	59	122	26	75	.307
1980	31	Nankai	na	423	66	138	27	75	.326
1981	32	Nankai	Statistical data for 1981 not available						

Upon returning from Japan, May settled in the Chicago suburb of Park Forest. In 2002 he was serving as a hitting instructor for the Cook County Cheetahs, an independent professional team on Chicago's South Side, making public appearances for the White Sox in the club's community relations department, and playing golf whenever his schedule permitted it.[81] His main post-baseball employment, however, was with the United States Postal Service, where by 2002 he had spent 18 years as a clerk.

For a man who nearly lost a thumb in a mortar accident, Carlos May had considerable success in the game of baseball. The Faber System ranks him eighth among position players who left the big leagues by the age of thirty. *Total Baseball* regards his accomplishments in a much lower light, placing him thirty-seventh. On the other hand, James ranks him first among left fielders.

HAPPY FELSCH

During the summer of 1920 the star center fielder of the Chicago White Sox was enjoying the finest of his six major league seasons. At 29 years of age he was in the prime of his baseball life. By early September he was hitting .338 and had established personal highs with 14 home runs and 115 runs batted in. His White Sox were in the pennant race, chasing their third flag in the last four years. Charlie Comiskey, owner of the Sox, had surprised him with a $3000 raise, nearly doubling his previous high salary of $3750 annually. For the first time in his life he felt he was not underpaid. He invested in a new $1800 Hupmobile automobile. Life was good, despite rumors about crookedness in the 1919 World Series. During the offseason Comiskey had hired a detective to look into the private lives of his players, but found nothing amiss in the outfielder's lifestyle. On September 7, 1920, a Chicago grand jury was impaneled to investigate the possible fix of a Cubs-Phillies game. The grand jury soon turned its attention to the 1919 World Series. On September 27 it issued indictments against the accused Sox players. On the same day Comiskey suspended the tainted players. Later Baseball commissioner Kenesaw Mountain Landis banned the players for life from Organized Baseball. The major league career of Happy Felsch was over.

Oscar Emil Felsch was born on April 7, 1891, in Milwaukee, the son of German immigrants Maria and Charles Felsch, a carpenter. The lad was nicknamed "Happy" by his family because of his sunny disposition. His father said the boy was born laughing.[82] His easygoing nature and quick smile made the nickname an excellent fit. Newspapers had adopted the sobriquet as early as 1912.[83]

The youngster dropped out of school after completing the sixth grade. This lack of formal education may have contributed to his later problems. The teenager went to work as a factory laborer for ten dollars a week. He joined a Turners[84] club in Milwaukee. At the gymnasium he became a wrestling champion and at one point contemplated becoming a professional wrestler, but he decided he preferred life on a baseball diamond to one on a wrestling mat.

By 1911 the youth was employed as a shingler and started making a name for himself in local semi-pro baseball circles, playing mainly shortstop or third base. In 1912 he played with four different teams in the Badger State, moving up to higher level clubs as the season progressed.

On April 30, 1913, Felsch made his professional debut, and a spectacular debut it was. Playing for the Milwaukee Cream in the Class C Wisconsin-Illinois League, he went five-for-five, including a grand slam in the first inning, and a total of seven runs batted in. It was unusual for a minor league city to support two clubs in different leagues in the same year, and the Cream found it difficult to compete with the higher-ranking Milwaukee Brewers. On June 28 the Cream moved to Fond du Lac and became the Fond du Lac Molls. After the move, Happy continued his impressive hitting. With the Cream and Molls combined he had a .319 batting average, hit 18 home runs, and stole 16 bases. By early August he was promoted to the Brewers in the American Association. He played infrequently for the Brewers, hitting only .183 with two home runs in 26 games. However, he polished his skills in the outfield, where he was moved after years of sometimes sensational but often erratic play in the infield.

In 1914 Felsch really came into his own as a pro. He set home run distance records at home in Milwaukee and on the road in Kansas City. He hit .304, stole 19 bases, and led the American Association with 19 home runs. In the outfield he showed great range and a strong arm. On August 8 the White Sox acquired Felsch for $12,000 plus two players. To the delight of the Brewers, the Sox allowed the young star to remain in Milwaukee for the remainder of the 1914 season. Felsch signed a two-year contract with Chicago for $2500 a year. He made his major league debut at the age of 23 on April 14, 1915, against the St. Louis Browns. He collected two singles, stole one base, and made one error in his opening contest. Early in the season he suffered a nagging leg injury, which hampered his rookie year performance.

In his sophomore season Felsch batted .300, hit seven home runs, which tied for third in the American League during that dead-ball season, and led AL outfielders with a .981 fielding percentage. His nineteen assists helped him earn a reputation for having one of the strongest throwing arms in the game. The next year was even better. Happy led all outfielders in putouts, had the fifth-best batting average at .308, and tied for second with 102 runs batted in, the first White Sox player ever to top 100 ribbies in a season.

The White Sox won the World Series in 1917, defeating John McGraw's Giants, four games to two, as spitballer Red Faber racked up three victories for the Pale Hose. Felsch was one of the heroes of the Series as his long home run in the first game of the Fall Classic was one of the decisive blows in the Chicago win. He also made some sensational defensive plays in the outfield. Happy continued his timely hitting and outstanding fielding throughout the

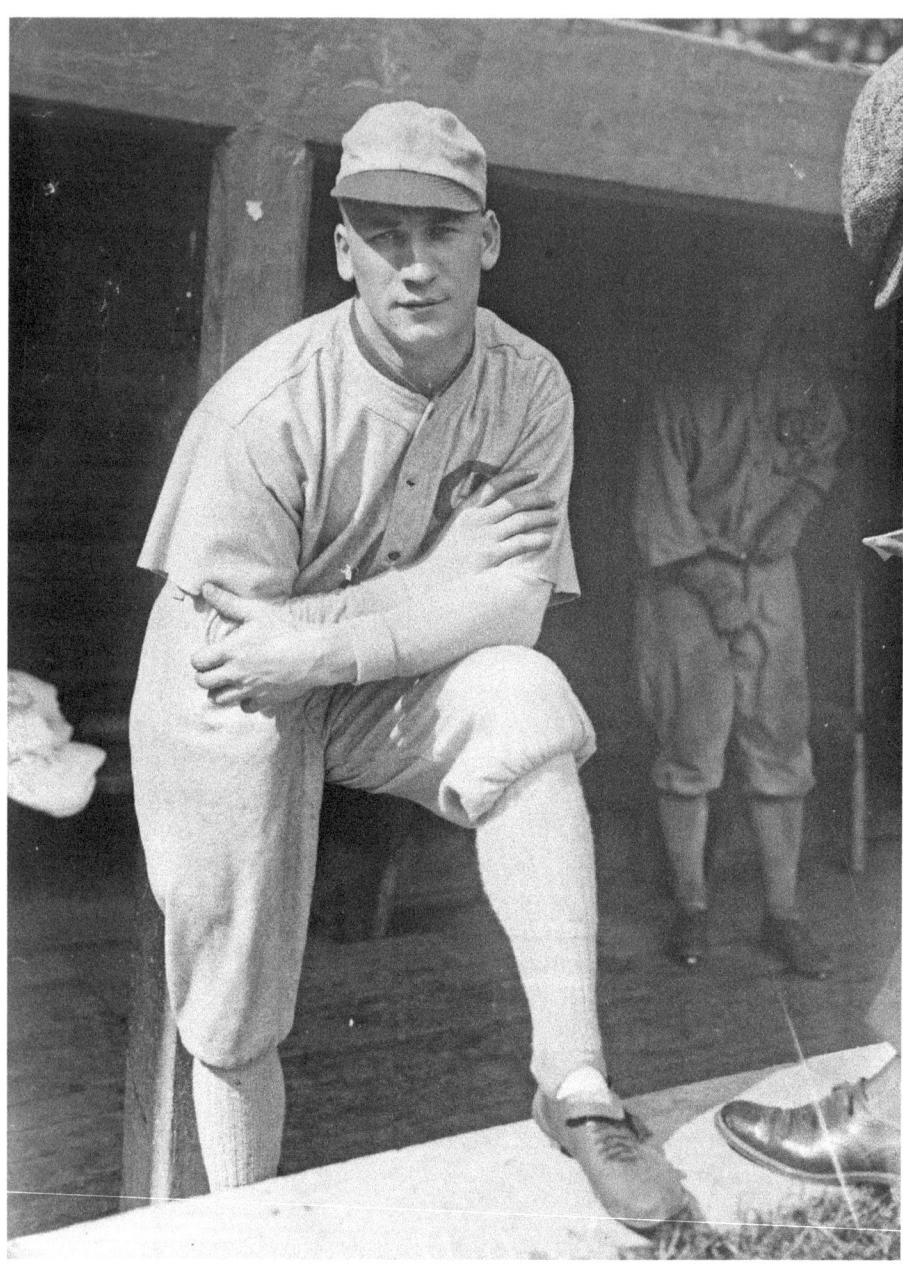

At the age of 29 Happy Felsch was enjoying his greatest year in baseball in 1920 when he was indicted for his complicity in the Black Sox scandal of 1919. Although the jury acquitted the ballplayers, Commissioner Landis banned Felsch and his tainted teammates for life (Library of Congress).

Series. His exploits were wildly cheered in his hometown of Milwaukee, as thousands followed the games on electric scoreboards in theaters and on blackboards in restaurants and other businesses.[85]

The United States had entered World War I on April 6, 1917, but the war had little effect on the 1917 season. Although all men ages 21–30 were required to register for the first universal draft in U.S. history in June, very few major leaguers were drafted that year. However, the next season was different. Married men and those with dependents were exempt, but it was estimated that 200 major league ballplayers were eligible for the draft.[86] By Opening Day of 1918, all clubs had at least one man in the armed services. On May 23 the government issued its "work or fight" order, making it mandatory for men to get into essential work by July 1 or face induction. Baseball was declared a nonessential industry. However, Secretary of War Newton Baker allowed the major leagues a two-month extension to enable them to complete an abbreviated schedule of about 125 games. The leagues played through Labor Day, and Baker granted an additional two-week extension for the two clubs that qualified for the World Series.

Red Faber enlisted in the navy on June 7. Teammate Eddie Collins joined the marines in August. However, Joe Jackson, Lefty Williams and Byrd Lynn chose to go to work in a shipyard upon receiving their notices. On July 1 Happy Felsch announced he was taking a war-effort job at the Milwaukee Gas Company for $125 a month, plus what he could earn by playing semipro ball on weekends.[87] Many players took exempt jobs in shipyards, steel mills, and war-production factories, working for companies that had industrial league teams. This practice led to some of them being derided as slackers. Among the vocal critics was Comiskey, who said, "I don't consider them fit to play on my ball club. I would gladly lose my whole team if my players wished to do their duty for the country, as hundreds of thousands of other young men are doing."[88]

Decimated by loss of players and by internal strife, the White Sox slipped to sixth place in 1918. They came roaring back in 1919, winning the pennant despite still suffering from internal dissension. Players joined warring cliques. One group, headed by Collins and including Faber, Ray Schalk, and Dickie Kerr, was considered pro-management and recipients of favored treatment from Comiskey. Collins, with a private school background and a degree from an Ivy League college, was resented by some of his teammates who had come up through the school of hard knocks. The star second sacker received $15,000 a year, more than twice the stipend of most of his colleagues and more than Chick Gandil, Joe Jackson, and Felsch combined. Furthermore, some of the players considered Collins a snob who looked down on his less-privileged teammates.

The other clique more or less coalesced around Gandil, who has been described as an angry malcontent.[89] Gandil and Collins were not on speaking terms. Among Gandil's followers were Eddie Cicotte, a great pitcher with a reputation as a surly troublemaker, and the unhappy Happy Felsch. Players who had been castigated as slackers by their owner, such as Jackson and Williams, tended to fall into Gandil's group. Adding to the discontent among the troops was the belief that Comiskey had promised them a cash bonus for winning the 1917 World Series but had delivered only a barrel of champagne instead. Many players believed, perhaps mistakenly, that the Sox minions were underpaid in comparison to their counterparts on other teams. Although it is commonly believed that the Black Sox appellation refers to the World Series scandal, some say that it was applied originally because the Sox played in dirty socks when Comiskey made them pay for laundering their uniforms.[90]

Dissension among teammates and antipathy toward their owner were certainly contributing factors to the debacle of 1919, but a stronger influence was the force exerted by gamblers. Gambling had long been an unsavory aspect of baseball. As early as 1882 umpire Dick Higham had been banished from baseball for influencing the outcome of games at the behest of gamblers. According to Harvey Frommer, the suspension of horse racing by the government during World War I led to increased activity by gamblers in baseball. "With racetracks closed down, gamblers seeking another outlet to ply their trade turned their attention to the national pastime. The lobbies of hotels where major league teams stayed became conspicuous congregating places for gamblers and their assorted retinue. And they vied with each other for the bragging rights to which games and which players they had been able to fix."[91]

The sordid tale of the 1919 fix and the subsequent trials is too well known to bear repeating at length here. In summary, eight players were indicted on September 28, 1920. Immediately after the indictments, Comiskey suspended the implicated players. Felsch and some of his teammates began a fight for reinstatement. Meanwhile, the state brought charges against the players for conspiring to defraud the public and injuring the businesses of Comiskey and the American League. The trial took place in Chicago from July 18 to August 2, 1921. After less than three hours of deliberation the jury acquitted the ballplayers. The next day, Commissioner Landis issued his edict. None of the accused players would ever again play a game of professional baseball.

Happy Felsch played his last game of major league baseball just five days after his 29th birthday, on September 27, 1920, the day before the indictments were handed down. His last season in the majors was statistically one of the best final years of any player in the history of baseball. Not yet 30 years old, and with changes in rules benefiting hitters, he looked forward to even bigger numbers in the years ahead. But it was not to be. He recognized that immediately, telling a Chicago reporter:

> Well the beans are all spilled and I think that I am through with baseball. I got my $5000 and I suppose the others got theirs too. If you say anything about me, don't make it appear that I'm trying to put up an alibi. I'm not. I'm as guilty as the rest of them. We were in it alike. I don't know what I'm going to do now.... I wish I hadn't gone into it. I guess we all do.... And now I'm out of baseball — the only profession I know anything about, and a lot of gamblers have gotten rich.[92]

His major league record:

Year	Age	Club	G	AB	R	H	HR	RBI	BA	OBP
1915	23	Chicago AL	121	427	65	106	3	53	.248	.334
1916	24	Chicago AL	146	546	73	164	7	70	.300	.341
1917	25	Chicago AL	152	575	75	177	6	102	.308	.352
1918	26	Chicago AL	53	206	16	52	1	20	.252	.306
1919	27	Chicago AL	135	502	68	138	7	86	.275	.336
1920	28	Chicago AL	142	556	88	188	14	115	.338	.384
TOTAL			749	2812	385	825	38	446	.293	.347

Despite being found not guilty in a court of law, Felsch was forced to go outside Organized Baseball if he wanted to continue playing the game he loved. He sued the White Sox for $100,000 for depriving him of his livelihood. Felsch was charged with perjury. While the lawsuits dragged on for years, Felsch and other suspended Sox formed barnstorming teams and played baseball throughout the Chicago area and Wisconsin. Back in 1915 Happy had married a 22-year-old Milwaukee woman named Marie Wagner. By 1923 the young couple had a family. In order to supplement the income from barnstorming, Happy and Marie opened a grocery story in Milwaukee. Eventually the Sox paid Felsch about $1500 in an out-of-court settlement. The perjury count was dropped, but Happy was sentenced to one year probation for false swearing.[93]

With the lawsuits out of the way, Felsch was free to travel far and wide playing baseball, which he found preferable to selling groceries. In June 1925 he and Swede Risberg joined a semi-pro team in Sibley, Montana, where they received $600 a month, plus expenses. Happy went home to Milwaukee during the offseason each year and then returned to Montana in the summers. He played for and managed a team in Regina, Saskatchewan, in 1928 and spent part of 1930 as a headliner with the American-Canadian Clown team, but mostly he was based in Montana for half a dozen years, although his teams traveled widely through the Prairie Provinces, the Dakotas, and the Upper Midwest. After 1930 he quit his traveling, and played sandlot baseball in Milwaukee. Even though he was well past his prime, Felsch was the best player on his hometown sandlots while in his forties.[94]

During the Prohibition year of 1932 the Felsch family opened a soft drink parlor. When repeal came they operated taverns for ten years. Then Happy worked as an assembler and watchman for six years. In 1949 he changed occupations for the last time to become a crane operator for the George Meyer Company.

When Eliot Asinof began research for his definitive book on the Black Sox scandal, *Eight Men Out*, only four of the disgraced players were still alive. Cicotte, Gandil, and Risberg either refused to talk to the author or were unhelpful. Reluctant at first, Felsch opened up and became the writer's chief source. Regarding the scandal he told Asinof, "It was a crazy time. I don't know how it happened, but it did all right. God damn, I was dumb, all right. Old Gandil was smart and the rest of us was dumb."[95]

In trying to assess what Felsch had been like in 1919, Asinof wrote, "Felsch was a smiling, easy going, badly educated boy from Milwaukee, constantly seeking raucus pleasure and adventure."[96] Asinof's book was highly acclaimed and made into a movie in 1988, in which Charlie Sheen portrayed Happy Felsch.

Felsch died on August 17, 1964, at St. Francis Hospital in Milwaukee of a coronary blood clot caused by arteriosclerosis. He had suffered from a variety of ailments for years, including varicose veins and a leg abscess. His health had also been compromised by diabetes, a liver ailment, and a pancreatic tumor. He was buried at Wisconsin Memorial Park in the Milwaukee suburb of Brookfield. He was survived by his wife Marie, son Oscar, two daughters, and eleven grandchildren.

How good a ballplayer was Happy Felsch? The testimony of his contemporaries is that he was a great defensive player.[97]

Connie Mack: "The greatest all around fielder in the country today, not barring Tris Speaker and Ty Cobb."

Ty Cobb: "Hap Felsch was a wonder."

Babe Ruth: "I would rate Hap Felsch of the old White Sox and Tris Speaker far superior to Cobb on defense."

A writer for *Leslie's Illustrated Weekly* penned: "Not only is Felsch a heavy and consistent batter, but he is one of the best fielders in the big show, and as a defensive gardener ranks close to Speaker."

According to the Faber System, Felsch is ninth best among all players who left the major leagues before their 31st birthday. *Total Baseball* ranks him twenty-third. James places him second among center fielders.

Part Two

Leading Pitchers

Among the 197 players discussed in this book, 90 are pitchers who meet the eligibility requirements of compiling 15 or more decisions in each of at least five seasons and appearing in their final major league game before their 31st birthday. All of these hurlers were exceptionally talented individuals. However, half a dozen of them stand out above the rest as six of the very best pitchers of all time. In Part Two biographical sketches of this special sextet are presented in the order in which the pitchers are ranked by the Faber System.[1] Of the top six, two pitched professionally only in the nineteenth century, three spanned the turn of the century, and one pitched exclusively in the twentieth century.

All six of the top pitchers according to the Faber System are also ranked highly by *Total Baseball*.[2] Four of them are ranked by Bill James.[3] The rankings among eligible pitchers by each source are as follows:

	Faber System	*Total Baseball*	*James*
Amos Rusie	1	1	2
Sandy Koufax	2	3	1
Sadie McMahon	3	7	-
Addie Joss	4	5	3
Bobby Caruthers	5	2	4
Win Mercer	6	15	-

The other pitchers included by *Total Baseball* among the big six are Silver King at fourth and Noodles Hahn in sixth place. The Faber System ranks King eleventh and Hahn ninth. This demonstrates considerable similarity in results using two drastically different rating systems. On the other hand, James ranks Tommy Bond in fifth place. Bond is ranked 25th in the Faber System and 38th in *Total Baseball*. Almost certainly he would have ranked higher in both systems had he been able to pitch until he was thirty. Unfortunately, his last full season in the National League came when he was 25, although he did pitch without much success in the Union Association at the age of 28. Of course, the age of 28 makes Bond seem like an elder statesman compared to Willie McGill, who made his major league debut at the age of 16 and was out of the big leagues at the tender age of 22.

AMOS RUSIE

At the age of 16 he dropped out of school and took a job in an Indianapolis factory.[4] While playing the outfield for a semi-pro team one day, he was called upon to replace a struggling pitcher. That move changed the life and career of Amos Rusie, as he went on to become a Hall of Fame pitcher in professional baseball. He was also partly — some say mainly — responsible for changing the face of baseball forever.[5] For it was Rusie's intimidating fastball that spurred the change in the distance of the place from which a pitcher must deliver a pitch, the last major alteration in the configuration of the baseball diamond.

Amos Wilson Rusie was born in Mooresville, Indiana, a small town in Morgan County, just a few miles southwest of Indianapolis. As a child he moved with his parents, Mary Donovan and William Asbury Rusie, a brick mason, to the capital city. While in his late teens, among other jobs, he worked in an Indianapolis furniture store as a varnisher and played baseball whenever he could. After his first start as a pitcher the youngster's reputation quickly grew. In exhibition games he shut out two National League teams — Boston and Washington — while pitching for an Indianapolis team called the Sturm Avenue Never Sweats.[6] John T. Brush, the owner of the National League's Indianapolis Hoosiers, signed the 17-year-old fastballer to a professional contract, but he turned 18 very early in the season. After a few games with the Burlington (Iowa) Babies of the Central Inter-State League, he was promoted to the big leagues. The Indianapolis team folded after the 1889 season and the league assigned Rusie to the New York Giants.

Rusie's minor league record:

Year	Age	Club	W	L	Pct	G	IP	SO	ERA
1889	18	Burlington	2	2	.500	4	36	27	n.a.

Amos was an instant sensation in the Big Apple. Restaurants named drinks after him, and vaudevillians included skits about Rusie in their acts. It was reported that Lillian Russell, the most famous Broadway star of the day, clamored to meet him.[7] The young man lived it up. He enjoyed drinking and carousing in the big city, but the night life apparently did not interfere with his pitching. Sportswriter Sam Crane wrote, "Rusie went through his active pitching days as though on a continuous joy ride. He broke training whenever he felt like it and never looked upon life as a serious matter."[8]

New York scribes frequently referred to Rusie as an Indiana farmer.[9] Of course, he had never been a farmer, but to some New Yorkers all midwesterners were farmers. They also gave him nicknames, such as "Mr. Giant" and the "Colossus of Coogan's Bluff."[10] The name that stuck, however, was the "Hoosier Thunderbolt," and it was well deserved. He was reputed to throw the fastest pitch ever seen (or not seen) in the game of baseball. His catcher, Dick Buckley, tried inserting into his glove a sheet of lead, covered with a handkerchief and a sponge to cushion the impact of the fastball.[11] Chicago Cubs outfielder Jimmy Ryan said: "Words really fail to describe the speed with which Rusie sent the ball.... The giant simply drove the ball at you with the force of a cannon. It was like a white streak tearing past you."[12] The legendary John McGraw of the Baltimore Orioles famously said, "You can't hit 'em if you can't see 'em."[13]

Not surprisingly, Rusie led the National League in strikeouts year after year. In two consecutive years—1890 and 1891—he recorded 341 and 337 strikeouts, respectively, the highest and

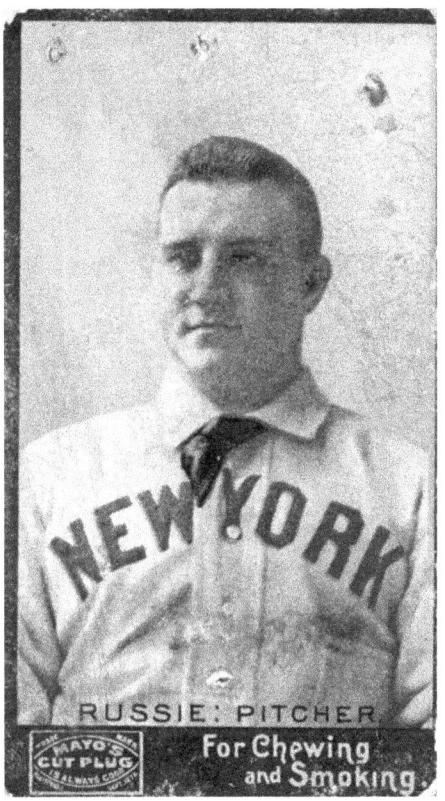

Amos Rusie, "the Hoosier Thunderbolt," had the fastest fastball of any of the nineteenth-century pitchers. His catcher tried inserting into his glove a sheet of lead, covered with a handkerchief and a sponge, to cushion the impact of the fastball. Time after time he led the National League in strikeouts, shutouts, earned run average, and other pitching categories. Four times he won more than 30 games in a season, earning him a place in the National Baseball Hall of Fame (Library of Congress).

second-highest numbers rung up in the decade. Amos said it was not easy. "It took a lot of pitchin' to strike a man out in those days. The foul strike rule hadn't come in. A guy had to miss three of 'em clean before he was out."[14] The problem was that Rusie had control problems. The ball did not always go where he wanted. His wildness plus his speed made it dangerous for a hitter to dig in at the plate. The Hoosier Thunderbolt's blinding fastball thrown from just fifty feet away so terrified batters that players agitated for a rule change. In 1893 both the National League and the American Association moved the distance from the pitching rubber to the plate to a somewhat-safer 60 feet six inches, where it has remained ever since. Of course, Rusie was not solely responsible for this change — there were other fastball pitchers, as well — but he is usually assigned major responsibility.[15]

After the end of the 1893 season, William Temple, president of the Pittsburgh Pirates, proposed that a post-season series be played between the teams that finished first and second in the National League pennant race. He donated an $800 cup to be awarded to the winner of the best-of-seven series. In 1894 the Baltimore Orioles took the flag, and the New York Giants finished second. In the ensuing Temple Cup series the Giants swept the Orioles in four straight games. The Baltimores were no match for Rusie. As one reporter wrote, "The alleged mighty hitters of the league's pennant winners are but putty in the hands of Rusie and Meekin."[16] Rusie pitched two complete-game wins, while giving up only one earned run for an ERA of 0.50. Several of the Baltimore players had not wanted to participate in the series, and there was suspicion that they did not try their hardest.

In the games played at the Polo Grounds, which had no center-field fence, large crowds ringed the outfield, with a rope strung between posts to separate them from the playing field. Some fans sat in horse-drawn carriages, getting a view of the game by looking over the heads of the standees.[17] Other horse-drawn vehicles were left unattended on Eighth Avenue below the field. With Rusie enjoying a 4–1 lead during the seventh inning of the third game, one of the horses bolted, climbed up the embankment, smashed the buggy to smithereens, and charged into the people crowded around the rope. The horse galloped through the throng, jumped over the ropes like a steeplechaser, and charged onto the playing field. He headed straight across the field, seemingly bound for left fielder Eddie Burke. A reporter noted that "Burke had shown the Polo Grounds patrons some pretty fast running in his time, but he never equaled the sprint he made to get under the left field bleachers."[18] The runaway horse was caught, Rusie resumed pitching, and the Giants triumphed, 4–1.

The change in pitching distance did not reduce Rusie's effectiveness. He continued to lead the league in strikeouts, albeit with a smaller total. In 1894 he achieved what later was called the pitcher's Triple Crown, leading the circuit in wins, strikeouts, and earned run average. He also led the loop in shutouts that season. *Total Baseball* rated Rusie's 1894 season as the best year by a pitcher in the entire history of baseball.[19] Altogether his league-leading seasons document his worthiness for the Baseball Hall of Fame: five times in strikeouts; four times in shutouts; four times in fewest hits allowed per nine innings; twice in earned run average; and once each in games pitched, complete games, wins, weighted average, and Faber System points. On the negative side, he once led the league in losses, once in wild pitches, and five consecutive years in bases on balls. His 289 walks allowed in 1890 remains an all-time major league record.

In 1898 at the age of 27 the Hoosier Thunderbolt won his last game, the 245th victory of his major league career, accomplished in only nine seasons. This is far more games than any other pitcher has ever won in a nine-year career. No one else is even close to that mark. This was achieved despite missing a full season in his prime. Problems between Rusie and the New York management led to the lost year. Rusie sat out the entire 1895 season because of a contract dispute with Andrew Freedman, owner of the Giants. Amos had been fined $200, a substantial portion of his $2500 salary, for allegedly missing curfew several times during the 1895 season. He refused to sign his 1896 contract unless the fines were refunded, as he claimed he had been in his room on the nights in question. The Hoosier went back to Indianapolis, hired Hall of Famer Monte Ward as his attorney, and brought suit for $5000 damages and his release from the Giants, claiming the reserve clause violated his constitutional rights. Both parties refused to compromise. Other National League owners, fearful of what the courts might do with the reserve clause, collected money for recoupment of the lost wages and a $5000 settlement.[20] Although challenged from time to time, the reserve clause survived for nearly a hundred years.[21] Rusie exulted, "That $5000 I received for not playing was almost $2000 more than I would have been paid for playing all season."[22] The Thunderbolt signed with the Giants for $3000 and returned to the fold in time for the 1897 season.

Late in the 1897 season Rusie tried to pick the league's base-stealing champion, Bill Lange, off first base with a sudden throw. He tore muscles in his shoulder and missed five weeks of the season. After 1897 he never pitched another game for the Giants, but the team still held ownership of the hurler. John T. Brush, who had signed the Indianapolis semi-pro to his first professional contract in 1889, owned the Cincinnati Reds, and was planning to gain controlling interest in the Giants. So on December 15, 1900, he traded Christy Mathewson to the Giants for the washed-up Rusie. When Brush took control of the Giants, Matty was there waiting for him. Rusie never won a game for the Reds. Mathewson went on to win a National League record 373 games in a Hall of Fame career.

Rusie's major league record: **Bold** face indicates he was the league leader.

Year	Age	Club	W	L	Pct.	ERA	G	IP	Sh	SO
1889	18	Indianapolis NL	12	10	.545	5.32	33	225	1	109
1890	19	New York NL	29	34	.460	2.56	67	548.2	4	**341**
1891	20	New York NL	33	20	.623	2.55	61	500.1	6	337
1892	21	New York NL	32	31	.508	2.84	65	541	2	304
1893	22	New York NL	33	21	.611	3.23	**56**	482	4	**208**
1894	23	New York NL	**36**	13	.735	**2.78**	54	444	3	**195**
1895	24	New York NL	23	23	.500	3.73	49	393.1	4	**201**
1897	26	New York NL	28	10	.737	**2.54**	38	322.1	2	135
1898	27	New York NL	20	11	.645	3.03	37	300	4	114
1901	30	Cincinnati NL	0	1	.000	8.59	3	22	0	12
TOTAL			246	174	.586	3.07	463	2410.2	30	1950

After retiring from baseball at the age of 30, Rusie went back to Indiana, where he worked at various jobs. He worked in a paper and pulp mill in Muncie and did some freshwater pearling in Vincennes. From 1911 to 1921 he was a steamfitter at a shipyard in Seattle. From 1921 to 1929 he returned to the New York Giants, where John McGraw gave him a position as superintendent of grounds at the Polo Grounds. In 1930 he again went to Washington state. That year's census shows him living with his wife, Susie, at the home of his daughter, Jeannette, and her husband, Clarence Spaulding.

Amos had married Susie May Sloan in Delaware County, Indiana, on November 8, 1890. Within a few years they were divorced. However, they remarried in Grant County, Indiana, on July 31, 1900.

The Great Depression of the 1930s exacted a toll on Rusie, as well as on millions of others. Amos worked in a paper mill that closed. He bought a chicken farm in Auburn, Washington, but it failed. In July 1934 he was injured in an automobile accident that left him with a brain concussion and several broken bones. He never fully recovered. On December 6, 1942, he died at the age of 71. His wife had died two months earlier. The great pitcher was buried in Acacia Cemetery in Seattle with a simple stone to mark the spot. Among the tributes written to the veteran fireballer is this one published as an editorial in an Ohio newspaper: "Anybody who thinks hero worship is a modern trend might delve into yellowed files and read the stories of Amos Rusie, one of baseball's greatest pitchers.... Fifty years ago little boys considered him their idol, prominent persons lavished gifts upon him and sports writers vied with one another in singing his praises. The blinding speed of the ball he threw is given as the reason for moving back the pitcher's box."[23]

In 1977 the Veterans Committee elected Amos Rusie to the National Baseball Hall of Fame in Cooperstown — a well-deserved honor. Among pitchers who departed the major leagues at the age 30 or younger, Rusie is ranked first by both the Faber System and *Total Baseball* and second by Bill James.

SANDY KOUFAX

The young man was frustrated — very frustrated. He was so frustrated, in fact, that he threw his gloves and spikes into the trash and considered devoting himself full-time to the electronics business. This was after the final game of the 1960 season. He had sacrificed so much for baseball, yet his career seemed to be going nowhere. Five years earlier he had given up his basketball scholarship and architecture classes at the University of Cincinnati to sign with his hometown Brooklyn Dodgers. He had enrolled in night classes in architecture at Columbia University, just in case his baseball career did not work out. In 1958 the Dodgers moved to Los Angeles, and he left his hometown to follow the team west. Despite a blazing fastball, he was little used by the Dodgers, sitting on the bench for long stretches without getting into a game. He asked to be traded but was refused. So he thought he would leave the game, but he found that the electronics business was not for him. That winter he worked hard, got himself in shape, and decided to give baseball one more try. When he walked into the spring training camp at Vero Beach in the spring of 1961, the clubhouse man, Nobe Kawano, handed him the gear he had rescued from the garbage. His career revived, Sandy Koufax was on his way to the Baseball Hall of Fame.

Sanford Braun was born in Brooklyn on December 30, 1935, the son of Evelyn and Jack Braun, an accountant and a salesman, respectively. When Sandy was three years old his parents divorced. Six years later his mother married Irving Koufax, an attorney. Jack Braun stopped calling his son and paying child support. Irving encouraged the lad in all his pursuits, and Sandy took his stepfather's surname. The family moved to nearby Rockville Centre, Long Island, for a while but returned to the city before Sandy reached tenth grade. Because the city teachers were refusing to supervise extracurricular activities without extra pay, Lafayette High School had no sports teams that year. Basketball was the boy's favorite sport, and he spent most of his free time playing hoops at the Jewish Community Center. He had played some baseball on the sandlots, mostly as a first baseman. At the age of 15 he tried pitching for the first time with a local youth baseball league known as the Ice Cream League. When sports were restored at Lafayette, Sandy became the school's basketball star. He also played first base on the baseball team. His high school coach tried to recruit him for the football team, but the lad demurred. The summer

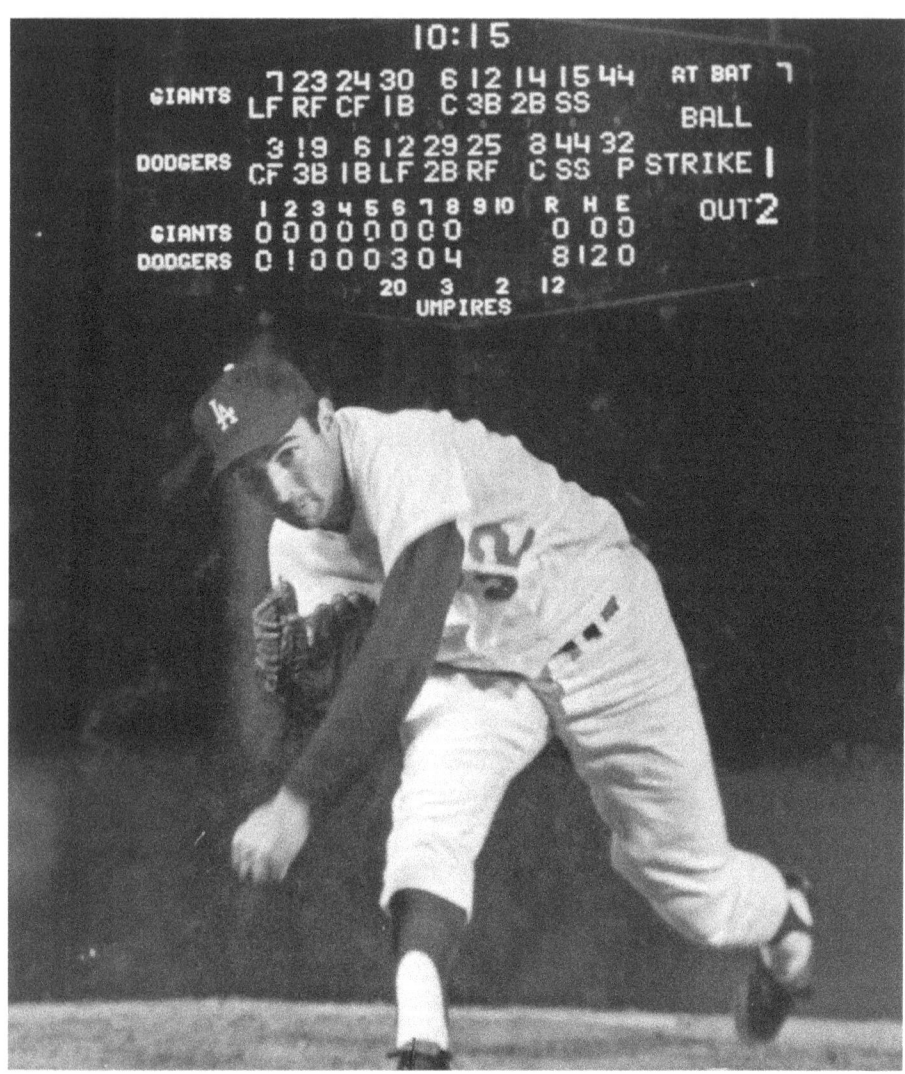

With two outs in the ninth inning, Sandy Koufax works on a no-hit game. He induces Harvey Kuenn to ground back to the mound and throws to first base to complete the second of his National League record four no-hitters. Severe arthritis forced Koufax to retire at the height of his career, but he had already established Hall of Fame credentials (National Baseball Hall of Fame Library, Cooperstown, New York).

that he was 17 he pitched in the Coney Island Sports League, where he caught the attention of professional baseball scouts.

Upon graduation from Lafayette High School, Sandy accepted a basketball scholarship to the University of Cincinnati. In the spring of 1954 he made the college baseball varsity squad, going 3–1 with 51 strikeouts and 30 walks in 31 innings. Baseball scouts intensified their pursuit of the young lefty. He tried out with the New York Giants, the Pittsburgh Pirates, and the Dodgers. The Pirates offered him a contract but by then he had already committed to Brooklyn. The Dodgers gave him a $14,000 signing bonus, making him what was at the time known as a "bonus baby" and ineligible to be sent to the minors until after two full years on the major league roster. He planned to use the money as tuition to finish his college education in the event he was unable to make it in baseball.[24]

Dodger scout Al Campanis said, "There are two times in my life the hair on my arms has stood up: the first time I saw the ceiling of the Sistine Chapel and the first time I saw Sandy Koufax throw a fastball."[25]

Koufax had an overpowering fastball and he eventually developed one of the best curveballs in the game, but he had control problems. In his first two seasons he had nearly as many bases on balls as strikeouts, but when he could get the ball over the plate he was devastating. In 1955, his first season, he won only two games; both were complete-game shutouts. He pitched only three more shutouts in the next five years combined. Again in 1956 he won only two games, and he notched only five wins in 1957. In his first six years with the Dodgers, he reached double digits in victories only once (with 11 wins in 1958). On August 31, 1959, he set a National League record with 18 strikeouts in a game, but he won only eight games that year. When he almost gave up the game after the 1960 season, he had 36 wins and 40 losses to show for six years in the big leagues. It is understandable why the Dodgers were reluctant to give him more starts.

Sandy turned his career around in 1961. His catcher, Norm Sherry, convinced him to ease up on the fastball. By not throwing it so hard, he could control the pitch better. Sherry also helped him develop a strong curve and start working on a change-up.[26] From a part-time starter and bench warmer, Koufax suddenly emerged as the best pitcher in baseball. From 1962 through the end of his career in 1966, he led the league in earned run average each and every season. In the entire history of baseball, he is the only pitcher to lead his league in ERA more than four consecutive years. Few other pitchers have ever approached the dominance that Sandy demonstrated from 1961 through 1966. During these six years he led the league in wins three times, in won-lost percentage twice, in strikeouts four times, in WHIP (fewest walks plus hits per innings pitched) five times, in shutouts three times, in strikeouts per nine innings pitched five times, and in strikeouts-to-walks ratio three times. In every season that he did not rank number one in any of the above categories, he was close to the top spot. His 382 strikeouts in 1965 is a modern NL record. His 11 shutouts in 1963 represent the most in a season by any major league left-hander since 1893. Over his career he allowed the fewest hits per nine innings given up by any southpaw in major league history.

Koufax is one of the two pitchers to win the National League's mythical Triple Crown for pitchers — leading the league in wins, strikeouts, and earned run average the same season — three times in a row. (Grover Cleveland Alexander is the other.) His other awards are legion. He was named to the NL All-Star team six years in a row, won three Cy Young awards, and won *The Sporting News* Pitcher of the Year award four times. In 1963 he was named the National League's Most Valuable Player. Bill James named him Pitcher of the Year in 1963, 1965, and 1966.[27] The Faber System recognized him as the NL Pitcher of the Year in 1965.[28]

He holds the National League record for the most no-hit games with four. His first came against the New York Mets in 1962. Sandy's second no-hitter came against the San Francisco Giants. In 1964 he threw a no-no in Philadelphia against the Phillies. Three no-hitters in three years was a record, but he went it one better in 1965, when he tossed a perfect game against the Chicago Cubs. In this contest Bob Hendley of the Cubs pitched a one-hitter, making this the only game in major league history in which the two teams combined for only one hit. The Dodgers won the game, 1–0, on an unearned run when Lou Johnson walked, reached second on a sacrifice bunt, stole third, and scored on an error.

During his best years Koufax frequently pitched in pain. As early as 1962 he developed circulatory problems in his pitching arm after being hit by a pitch. The ball hit the bat just above his left hand, breaking an artery in the fleshy part of the hand. His finger was numb when he threw his no-hitter against the Mets on June 30. Three starts later he was virtually finished for the season. The loss of his index finger was threatened because he had suffered a condition called Reynaud's Phenomenon. Circulation into the left index finger was so restricted that when he pressed the finger, it turned white. The finger began to get gangrenous. Drugs and intravenous injections dissolved the clots.[29] In mid–September he tried to resume pitching but was knocked out in three starts.

In 1964 he suffered two setbacks. On April 22 he felt something amiss and had to get cortisone shots in his elbow and missed three starts. In August he jammed his pitching arm while diving back into second base to beat a pick-off attempt. Soon thereafter he could not straighten his arm. The arm soreness and throbbing that he had experienced after every game became more severe. "I had to drag my arm out of bed like a log," he said. "That's what it looked like — a log. A water-logged log. Where it had been swollen outside the joint before, it was now swollen all the way from the shoulder down to the wrist."[30] He could neither straighten the arm nor bend it. The Dodgers' team doctor, Robert Kerlan, diagnosed him with traumatic arthritis, and Sandy did not pitch again that season.

During spring training in 1965 Koufax's entire left arm turned black and blue from hemorrhaging. He got through the season by taking codeine for pain and Butazolidin for inflammation, applied Capsolin ointment before each game, and soaked his arm in a tub of ice afterwards.[31] He not only got through the season, he was the best pitcher in baseball, winning the Triple Crown again, another Cy Young Award, and finishing second in the MVP voting, while leading the Dodgers to another pennant. He received a lot of criticism and much praise for refusing to pitch in the first game of the World Series because it fell on Yom Kippur, a Jewish high holy day. He pitched and lost the second game of the classic, but came back to win Games Five and Seven. In the clinching game he had such intense arthritic pain that he could not throw the curveball. Relying almost entirely on fastballs, he threw a three-hit shutout to win his second World Series MVP award.

In contract talks before the 1966 season began, Koufax and fellow pitcher Don Drysdale discovered that the Dodger GM was using the men against each other in the negotiations. As a result, the two decided to negotiate together and hired a lawyer to represent them, an unusual move in an era when players were not normally represented by an agent. They held out until the last week of spring training before signing for somewhat less than they had demanded. In April Dr. Kerlan told Sandy it was time to retire. The physician thought the arm could not take another season. Koufax ignored the advice, pitched in pain and won 27 games with a 1.73 ERA. Since then no major league pitcher has won more games in a season or posted a lower ERA.

After the 1966 World Series, which the Dodgers lost to the Baltimore Orioles in four straight games, Koufax retired. The arthritis was too bad for him to continue. "I've had a few too many shots and too many pills because of arm trouble," he said. "I didn't want to take the chance of disabling myself. I'm young. I want to live a lot of years after this and I don't want to become bitter because I pitched one year too many. I've got a lot of years left after baseball and I would like to live them with the complete use of my body."[32] He left the game at the peak of his career at the age of 30. It is unlikely that any pitcher ever had a better final year in the sport than Sandy Koufax had in 1966.

Koufax's major league record. **Bold** type indicates he was the league leader.

Year	Age	Club	W	L	Pct.	ERA	G	IP	Sh	SO
1955	19	Brooklyn NL	2	2	.500	3.02	12	42	2	30
1956	20	Brooklyn NL	2	4	.333	4.91	16	59	0	30
1957	21	Brooklyn NL	5	4	.556	3.88	34	104	0	122
1958	22	Los Angeles NL	11	11	.500	4.48	40	159	0	131
1959	23	Los Angeles NL	8	6	.571	4.05	35	153	1	173
1960	24	Los Angeles NL	8	13	.381	3.91	37	175	2	197
1961	25	Los Angeles NL	18	13	.581	3.52	42	256	2	**269**
1962	26	Los Angeles NL	14	7	.667	**2.54**	28	184	2	216
1963	27	Los Angeles NL	**25**	5	.833	**1.88**	40	311	**11**	**306**
1964	28	Los Angeles NL	19	5	.792	**1.74**	29	223	7	223
1965	29	Los Angeles NL	**26**	8	**.765**	2.04	43	**336**	8	**382**
1966	30	Los Angeles NL	**27**	9	.750	**1.73**	41	**323**	5	**317**
TOTAL			165	87	.655	2.76	397	2324	40	2396

World Series Record

Year	Age	Opponent	W	L	Pct.	ERA	G	IP	Sh	SO
1959	23	Chicago AL	0	1	.000	1.00	2	9	0	7
1963	27	New York AL	2	0	1.000	1.50	2	18	0	23
1965	29	Minnesota AL	2	1	.667	0.38	3	24	1	29
1966	30	Baltimore AL	0	1	.000	1.50	1	6	0	2
TOTAL			4	3	.571	0.95	8	57	1	61

Upon retirement from active play, in 1967 Koufax signed a one million dollar contract with NBC-TV to broadcast games on the *Saturday Game of the Week*. Not comfortable in front of the camera, he quit before the start of the 1973 season. For several years he served as a pitching coach for various teams during spring training. From 1979 to 1990 he worked for the Dodgers as a roving minor league instructor in their farm system. He has continued in various capacities with the Dodgers most of the time since then. In 2003 he severed the relationship for a year when the *New York Post* (which like the Dodgers was part of Rupert Murdoch's business empire) published rumors about his sexual orientation, but he resumed his association with the club when they acquired a new owner. Koufax tries to guard his privacy, but given his celebrity status, it is hard to do. Sandy has been married twice. His marriage on New Year's Day 1969 to Anne Widmark, daughter of movie actor Richard Widmark, and their subsequent divorce were widely reported. However, he managed to keep his second marriage and divorce out of the headlines. In 2008 he was back in the news as a victim of Bernie Madoff's Ponzi scheme.

Baseball has not forgotten Sandy Koufax. In 1972, in his first year of eligibility, he was elected to the National Baseball Hall of Fame. At 36 he was the youngest man ever enshrined in Cooperstown. The Dodgers retired his uniform number the same year. In 1999 *The Sporting News* placed him at number 26 on its list of "The 100 Greatest Baseball Players." In the same year he had the second-most votes behind Nolan Ryan on balloting for the "Master Card All-Century Team."

The brevity of his tenure in the major leagues has affected his ranking by baseball analysts. Bill James ranks Koufax tenth all-time, but other systems rank him lower. The Faber System ranks him 104th among all pitchers, but 13th in points per season. *Total Baseball* places him 76th. Among pitchers featured in this book, those who ended their career at age 30 or younger, the Faber System ranks Koufax second, behind Amos Rusie, while *Total Baseball* places him third, and James has him number one.

SADIE MCMAHON

He grew up in the Henry Clay Village area of Wilmington, Delaware, on Brandywine Creek, near the Experimental Station of the E. I. du Pont de Nemours Company, manufacturers of dynamite, gunpowder, and other explosives. The products blew up occasionally, so the area may not have been a pleasant residential community. As a youngster he ran with an Irish street gang before his magic right arm got him off the street. He started pitching for various amateur, semi-pro, and professional baseball teams in northern Delaware and southeastern Pennsylvania. His success came to the attention of the Athletics of Philadelphia and he advanced to the big leagues. Sadie McMahon was on his way to becoming one of the biggest stars of nineteenth-century baseball.

John McMahon was born in Wilmington on September 19, 1867, the son of Irish immigrants. How he acquired the nickname "Sadie" is a matter of dispute. It was strictly a baseball cognomen. All baseball reference books call him Sadie; all non-baseball sources refer to him as John. The dichotomy is complete. He was pitching for Norristown in 1889 when the Athletics signed him in midseason. He made his major league debut on July 5 and won 15 games during the remainder of the season. In 1890 he was by far the A's best pitcher and had won 20 games by the Fourth of July, but the Philadelphia club was running into financial problems and sold him along with catcher Wilbert Robinson and outfielder Curt Welch to Baltimore in September. His combined record with the two teams was 36 wins and 21 losses. He set a major league record with 18,851 weighted rating points, a mark that has stood for well over 100 years.[33] He was the Faber System Pitcher of the Year for 1890.[34] He led the American Association in wins, games pitched, innings, and strikeouts. Both McMahon and Robinson were rather plump, leading to their being dubbed the "Dumpling Battery."

When the American Association folded after the 1891 season, the Baltimore club joined the National League, where as the Baltimore Orioles they became one of the legendary teams in the history of baseball. The Orioles gained their fame not only because their three straight pennants made them one of the best teams of the era (some say one of the best of all time), but because of their reputation as the dirtiest team ever. Tripping, shoving, and blocking base runners occurred frequently, and infielder John McGraw introduced the art of impeding a runner's progress around the bases by grabbing his belt and holding on. When running the bases the Orioles slid into the bags with their spikes flashing. They attempted, with some success, to intimidate both their opponents and the umpires.[35] John Heydler, who was an umpire at the time and later president of the National League, told a sportswriter, "The Orioles were mean, vicious, ready at any time to maim a rival player or an umpire.... The things they would say to an umpire were unbelievably vile."[36]

McMahon fit right in with this crew, perhaps not in viciousness but certainly in rowdiness. He was reputed to be a heavy drinker and a carouser. Robert L. Thiemann wrote that Sadie was something of a hell-raiser, especially on the road.[37] In 1892 he was suspended for the final month of the season for missing a game and then cussing out his manager and owner in an argument over his fine for being absent. He continued to pitch well, winning more than 20 games each year from 1892 through 1894. In 1894 he was having one of his best seasons, with a 25–8 record, when he was sidelined by a shoulder injury at the end of August. The Orioles won the pennant anyway but lost the post-season Temple Cup matches to the runner-up New York Giants.

As the shoulder was slow to heal, Sadie decided to sit out the next season. Meanwhile, the Orioles and the Cleveland Spiders were fighting for the 1895 pennant. During the summer the two teams alternated in first place. Led by first baseman–manager Patsy Tebeau, who was reputed to be a brawler and a bully, the Spiders were giving the O's a run for their money, not only in the pennant chase but also in the rowdiness department. At one point Baltimore had fallen to third place and its championship hopes looked dim.

About this time Baltimore manager Ned Hanlon ran into Sadie on a downtown street corner. Burt Solomon reconstructed the ensuing conversation as going something like this[38]:

"What's the matter, Ed. You look downhearted."

"I am, Mac. I'm afraid they've got us licked."

"Don't worry. I'm ready to go now and I'll win you that championship."

The pitcher was true to his word. On August 1 he rejoined the club and pitched his first game of the year, a dramatic 1–0 victory, the first of eight straight wins. The magic was back in his arm. The curveballs and changes of pace were working. The Orioles won 14 straight and had grabbed a two-game lead by the middle of September when they faced the Spiders in a crucial four-game series. The teams split the first two games. Hanlon said Charley Esper would probably pitch the all-important third game. In the clubhouse before the game the manager was again asked who would pitch. "The best man we've got," he replied. "This is very important, and we need it."

From the corner of the clubhouse McMahon asked, "Want me to pitch?"

"Yes, if you feel like it," replied the skipper.

"Well, then I'll pitch," said Mac.[39]

And pitch he did — a one-hitter, virtually wrapping up the pennant for Baltimore. In those last few weeks of the season the right-hander won 10 of 13 decisions.

In some years the post-season Temple Cup series between the league champion and runner-up was greeted with massive apathy by fans and players alike. But 1895 was different. Cleveland fans were fired up by hearing allegations that other western clubs had purposely lost games to the Spiders in a vain attempt to help the latter win the pennant. Baltimore players were eager to make amends for losing the previous year's cup to the Giants. Players and fans from both clubs were annoyed at their opponents for alleged dirty play during the season.

The series opened in Cleveland. Ruffians pelted the Orioles with potatoes and stones. At least three Baltimore players were hit in the head with vegetables or minerals. With Sadie McMahon going for the O's against Cy Young of Cleveland, Baltimore had a one-run lead in the eighth inning. With Patsy Tebeau on second base, a Cleveland batter lofted a fly ball to Joe Kelley in the outfield. A dozen fans rushed onto the field straight at Kelley, but he caught the ball. The fans then surrounded him and threw their coats in his face to prevent him from throwing the ball to the infield. Tebeau tagged up and ran all the way home with what he thought was the tying run before the umpire sent him back to second base. He scored later as McMahon weakened. The Spiders won that game and the next two to go up three games to none.

The series moved to Baltimore. Crowds met the Spiders at the train station and pelted them with eggs and rotten apples.[40] Ugly behavior worsened as the series went on. The Orioles were unable to overtake their rivals and lost the Temple Cup for the second year in a row. In 1896 Baltimore got revenge by taking the cup from Cleveland and won it for the second time against Boston in 1897, but by then interest in the series had waned.

Sadie pitched for the Orioles on Opening Day in 1896, but had won only 10 games when he was shelved by stomach trouble during a July road trip. When he tried to return to action, his shoulder injury flared up again.[41] He won only one more game in the big leagues. The Orioles released him after the season. He signed with Brooklyn but was unable to win a single game in 1897. He made his last major league appearance on July 12, 1897, at the age of 29.

During his career he led his league twice in wins, complete games, and shutouts and once in strikeouts. He finished as high as second in won-lost percentage and in strikeouts-to-walks ratio. He ranked fourth one year in earned run average and fourth one time in WHIP (walks plus hits per innings pitched).

His major league record. **Bold** face indicates league leader.

Year	Age	Club	W	L	Pct.	ERA	G	IP	Sh	SO
1889	21	Philadelphia AA	14	12	.538	3.53	28	242	2	117
1890	22	Philadelphia AA	29	18	.617	3.34	48	410	0	225
		Baltimore AA	7	3	.700	3.00	12	99	1	66
Year		Phil/Balt	36	21	.632	3.27	**60**	509	1	**291**
1891	23	Baltimore AA	35	24	.593	2.81	61	**503**	5	219
1892	24	Baltimore NL	19	25	.432	3.24	48	397	2	118
1893	25	Baltimore NL	23	18	.561	4.37	43	346	0	79
1894	26	Baltimore NL	25	8	.758	4.21	35	276	0	60
1895	27	Baltimore NL	10	4	.714	2.94	15	122	4	37
1896	28	Baltimore NL	11	9	.550	3.48	22	176	0	33
1897	29	Brooklyn NL	0	6	.000	5.86	7	63	0	13
TOTAL			173	127	.577	3.51	321	2634	14	967

McMahon retired to Delaware City and pitched in local leagues. His last game in Organized Baseball came in 1903 when he went to Baltimore to visit his old teammates Hughie Jennings and Wilbert Robinson, who were co-managers of the Orioles, now in the Eastern League. He volunteered to pitch and hurled a complete game, defeating the Newark Sailors.[42] From 1911 to 1925 he was a scout on the payroll of another former Oriole teammate, John McGraw, then managing the New York Giants. The skipper said that in addition to being a great pitcher, Sadie was a great judge of ballplayers and a close student of the game.[43] McMahon accepted the scouting assignment with these words, " I may not find a good one, but I won't dig up any bad ones. It's my idea that too much time and money are wasted on bad players just for the sake of trying them out."[44] Months went by before the manager heard anything from his scout. When at last he reported, he said, "Mac, I have covered the whole United States and I have found but one ballplayer who looks good. I'll bet on him."[45] That one good ballplayer was George Burns. McMahon found him playing for Utica in the New York State League; the Giants signed him, and he helped them win five pennants during a distinguished 15-year major league career.

The 1920 census showed John McMahon and his wife, Nora, as live-in servants in the household of Bessie du Pont, ex-wife of the gunpowder tycoon, Alfred du Pont. Nora was identified as a housemaid and John as a house man. It may be difficult to envision the rough and rowdy Sadie McMahon living in the home of a society matron, but there he was. In the 1930 census Mac was listed as a house carpenter.

John McMahon died in Wilmington on February 20, 1954, at the age of 86. He is buried in the Brandywine Church Cemetery.

Sadie was inducted into the Delaware Sports Museum Hall of Fame in 1979. The two men who have won more games than any other managers in the history of baseball both had high praise for McMahon. Connie Mack called him "the one-man pitching staff of the greatest team in baseball."[46] John McGraw picked Sadie as one of the six pitchers on his all-time baseball team, describing the right-hander as "one of the greatest hurlers who ever lived, whose best quality was his nerve and coolness under fire; one of the earliest money pitchers."[47] Among pitchers whose major league careers ended at the age of 30 or younger, the Faber System ranks him third and *Total Baseball* pegs him in the seventh position.

ADDIE JOSS

That April afternoon the tall, slender young man strode to the mound in St. Louis to make his major league debut. What a debut it was! Just up from Toledo in the Western Association, the rookie had curly, dark brown hair and unusually long arms, which made his frame seem even more elongated and thinner than it was. His new teammates had already dubbed him "the Human Slat." In the first inning he retired all three batters in order, fooling them with sharp curveballs. In the second the rookie unveiled his fast ball, striking out the side on just ten pitches. In the third inning the Browns unleashed their bench jockeys in an effort to unnerve the neophyte. From one coaching box Jack O'Connor yelled across the diamond, "So you're the guy who came up from Toledo to teach us how to play ball, are you Jack?" From the other box, Jesse Burkett hollered back, "Yes, I'm it. I broke the Inter-State all to pieces. And I thought I'd come up and show you mugs how to pitch." Back and forth the hectoring went. "Well, you long-legged toothpick, if you don't stop working so hard you'll lose your bonnet." "Oh, no, I won't. It's pinned to my curly locks." Unfazed by the heckling, the rookie held the Browns hitless in the third inning and again in the fourth and fifth innings. So far he had allowed no hits and no runs. Burkett led off the sixth inning by hitting a pop fly to short right field. The outfielder raced in and caught the ball off his shoe tops. However, the umpire ruled that the ball had hit the ground, depriving Addie Joss of a no-hitter in his first major league start. Nevertheless, Joss won the game and was on his way to Cooperstown, pitching two official no-hitters along the way.[48]

Adrian Joss was born April 12, 1880, in Woodland, a tiny hamlet in southern Wisconsin, the only child of Theresa Staudenmeyer and Jacob Joss. A native of Switzerland, Jacob had immigrated to Wisconsin during the Civil War and started manufacturing cheese and buying land for dairy farms. He made a fortune in the cheese business and entered politics, but his fortune declined. He died at the age of 37 of liver disease, brought on by alcoholism. In order to support herself and ten-year-old Addie, Theresa Joss opened a millinery shop and sewing school in Juneau, the county seat of Dodge County. By the time Addie reached high school he towered over his classmates. He played tackle on the football team and second base on the diamond.

At the age of 16 Addie graduated from high school, passed an examination for a teaching certificate and started teaching the next fall at a rural school in Herman Township, Dodge County. He spent his summers playing baseball for the Juneau town team. The baseball coach of Wayland Academy recruited him to pitch for the school the next spring. The following year Sacred Heart College gave him a scholarship to represent that institution. During the summers he pitched for various semi-pro teams in Juneau, Oshkosh, and Manitowoc. His success with the latter club won him his professional contract, with the Toledo Mud Hens of the Inter-State League. In 1900 Joss had a 19–16 record. In 1901 Toledo joined the Western Association. Addie dominated the new league; he won 27 games, recorded four shutouts and 210 strikeouts, and issued only 67 walks.

This performance attracted the attention of major league scouts, who began wooing the young right-hander. Toledo owner Charles Strobel did not want to lose the young moundsman and gave him a $150 advance toward his 1902 salary, but Addie did not sign a contract. Instead, he signed with the Cleveland Bluebirds of the fledgling American League. He returned $100 to Strobel, but not the entire amount. Shortly before Addie's major league debut, Strobel brought charges against Joss, on the grounds that the hurler had accepted the owner's advance under false pretenses, a felony punishable by jail time. However, a grand jury refused to indict Joss, citing a lack of evidence.

His minor league record:

Year	Age	Club	W	L	Pct	ERA	IP	Sh	SO
1900	19	Toledo Inter-State League	19	16	.543	n.a	n.a.	n.a.	n.a.
1901	20	Toledo Western Association	27	18	.600	2.84	370	4	210
TOTAL			46	34	.575	n.a.	n.a.	n.a.	n.a.

With his deceptive sidearmed, corkscrew pitching motion, his superb control, great speed, and fast-breaking curve, Addie Joss was one of the most dominant pitchers of the early twentieth century. In one six-year stretch he posted an earned run average of less than 2.00 five times. His perfect game against Ed Walsh in 1908 has been called the greatest game ever pitched. The Baseball Hall of Fame waived its ten years in the majors eligibility rule so he could be awarded his well-deserved plaque in Cooperstown (Library of Congress).

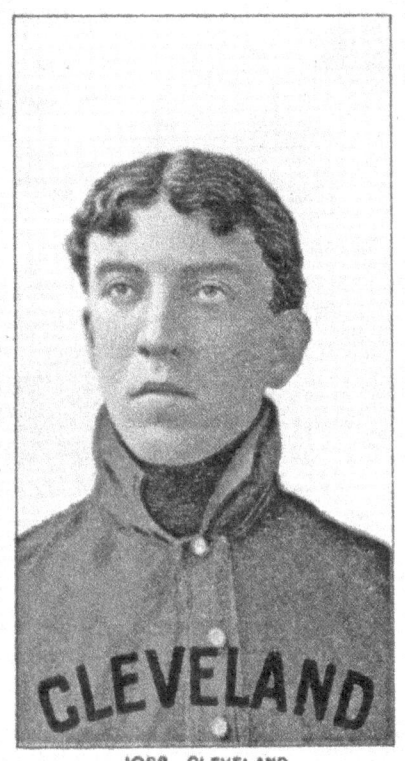

JOSS, CLEVELAND

Addie was no ruffian. Affable, easygoing, articulate, educated, and noted for good sportsmanship, Joss was the antithesis of the hard-drinking, illiterate brawler who was the stereotypical ballplayer of the era.

Following his auspicious debut in 1901, Addie continued to pitch outstanding ball. He won 17 games in 1902 and 18 in 1903. Illness in 1904 limited his number of starts, so he won only 14 games but posted a league-leading 1.59 earned run average. In 1905 he hurled the first of four consecutive 20-win seasons — 20 victories in 1905, 21 in 1906, a league-leading 27 in 1907, and 24 in 1907. His earned run average was amazing. Five times in six years he allowed fewer than two earned runs per game, highlighted by a 1.16 mark in 1908, which set an American League record that has been bested only twice in the ensuing 100-plus years. His "bad" year during that stretch was 1905, when his ERA was 2.01.

From 1902 through 1909 Addie Joss pitched eight seasons for Cleveland. During those eight years he was among the American League's top ten pitchers every season in ERA, WHIP, and strikeouts-to-bases on balls ratio. He was in the top ten in wins six times, in won-lost percentage six times, in fewest hits allowed per nine innings six times, in complete games six times, in fewest bases on balls per nine innings seven times, and in shutouts seven times. Not only was he in the top ten all those years, but often he was in the top five. In those nine categories he ranked in the top five a combined 42 times in eight seasons.

On October 2, 1908, Addie Joss and Ed Walsh of the Chicago White Sox hooked up in what Bill James called perhaps the greatest pitcher's duel in the history of the game.[49] Few, if any, baseball historians would disagree with that assessment. The White Sox, Detroit, and Cleveland were locked up in one of the tightest pennant races ever. Going into the game the Tigers had a half-game lead over the Naps. (During Addie's stay with the club Cleveland's unofficial nickname had morphed from the Bluebirds, to the Blues, to the Broncos, and finally to the Naps, in honor of their manager and great second baseman Napoleon Lajoie.) Cleveland had a one-game edge over the Sox. With his deceptive sidearmed, corkscrew pitching motion, his superb control, great speed, and fast-breaking curve, Joss was at the height of his game. Big Ed Walsh, possibly the greatest spitball pitcher of all time, was on his way to the last 40-win season ever achieved in the major leagues.

In the first inning Addie sat the side down in order. Walsh did the same for the Sox. In the first three innings Joss retired all nine men he faced. In the home half of the third, Joe Birmingham got the game's first hit, stole second, and went to third on an error. The next batter bounced out to short. Addie, next up, tried to bunt but struck out. The next batter, Wilbur Goode, also struck out, but the catcher could not handle the third strike and Birmingham came home with the game's first run. Trying to make that one run stand up, Joss really bore down. He gave up no hits in the fourth, fifth, or sixth inning. Big Ed matched him pitch for pitch. By the seventh frame the huge crowd began to realize that no Chicago runner had reached base. With one out in the seventh, Chicago player-manager Fielder Jones stepped to the plate, determined to end the perfect game. He worked the count to three and two. Addie zipped a sidearm curve under his wrists. The umpire called it strike three. Jones argued vehemently but to no avail. Joss retired the side in order in the eighth. In the bottom of the inning, Walsh gave up another hit, the fourth of the game, but he gave up no runs, and registered his 15th strikeout, a new AL record. In the ninth inning, with three outs to go, the White Sox sent up three straight pinch-hitters. Addie got the first one on an infield grounder and struck out the second, leaving just one more out to get. The veteran John Anderson was the manager's choice to pinch-hit. Anderson hit the ball down toward the third base bag. Bill Bradley, who was guarding the line, made the stop and a long throw across the diamond. The throw was low, but George Stovall scooped the ball out of the dirt for the final out of the game. Addie Joss had pitched a perfect game. Ed Walsh had lost, 1–0, on a wild-pitch strikeout.

The Naps had put a little distance between themselves and the White Sox. Unfortunately for Cleveland, Detroit kept winning and claimed the pennant. The Naps and Tigers both finished the season with 90 wins, but Cleveland had 64 losses to 63 for Detroit. Under present rules, Detroit would have had to play a make-up game, but according to the 1908 rules the Tigers won the championship by a half-game margin over the Naps. Addie Joss never got to pitch in a World Series.

During the offseasons Joss kept busy. After the 1906 campaign he wrote a Sunday sports column for the *Toledo New Bee*. He became known as an extremely talented and popular sportswriter.[50] In the 1908 and 1909 offseasons he brushed up on the civil engineering that he had studied at Sacred Heart and designed an electric scoreboard that would allow fans to keep track of balls and strikes. He sold the device to the Cleveland management, and it was installed in League Park.[51]

In 1910 he pitched his second no-hitter; he became the second American Leaguer to accomplish that feat. Only Cy Young had done it previously. His 1908 perfect game was the second one pitched in the junior circuit. Who had pitched one before him? Cy Young, of course. The 1910 no-hitter was Addie's last great performance. A torn ligament in his right elbow foreshadowed an early end to his major league career. He pitched his final game on July 25 at the age of 30. At the time he did not know his career was over. Although he had arm trouble during spring training in 1911, he expected to be able to return to action. On April 3, however, before an exhibition game in Chattanooga, he fainted on the field. He went home to Toledo, where his physician diagnosed an attack of pleurisy. Just a few days later, on April 14, Joss died suddenly of tubercular meningitis. It was two days after his 31st birthday.

His major league record: **Bold** type indicates he led the league.

Year	Age	Club	W	L	Pct.	ERA	G	IP	Sh	SO
1902	21	Cleveland AL	17	13	.567	2.77	32	269	5	106
1903	22	Cleveland AL	18	13	.581	2.19	32	284	3	120
1904	23	Cleveland AL	14	10	.583	**1.59**	24	192	5	83
1905	24	Cleveland AL	20	12	.625	2.01	33	286	3	132
1906	25	Cleveland AL	21	9	.700	1.72	34	282	9	106
1907	26	Cleveland AL	27	11	.711	1.83	42	339	6	127
1908	27	Cleveland AL	24	11	.686	**1.16**	42	325	9	130
1909	28	Cleveland AL	14	13	.519	1.71	33	243	4	67
1910	29	Cleveland AL	5	5	.500	2.26	13	107	1	49
TOTAL			160	97	.623	1.89	286	2327	45	920

The funeral for Adrian Joss was held in Toledo on April 17. The Naps were scheduled to play that day, and American League president Ban Johnson ruled that the game must go on. All of Addie's teammates insisted on attending the funeral. George Stovall, the team captain, declared his team on strike.[52] Finally, Johnson relented, and the game was postponed. Joss was buried in

Woodlawn Cemetery in Toledo. Two months later a group of American League all-stars played the Naps in an exhibition game to benefit Addie's widow, Lillian (née Shinavar), and their two children. More than 15,000 fans attended the game, which raised nearly $13,000 for the family.[53] At least seven future Hall of Famers participated in the game.

Time has not dimmed the luster of Addie's accomplishments. He allowed his opponents the lowest on-base percentage of any twentieth century pitcher. He has the second lowest ERA of all pitchers, all time, behind only Ed Walsh. He is tied for 28th with 45 lifetime shutouts, but every pitcher who ranks ahead of him in that category pitched more years than Joss. The Faber System ranks him as the fourth-best pitcher whose career ended at the age of 30 or younger. *Total Baseball* ranks him fifth, and James places him third. In 1978 the Veterans Committee of the Baseball Hall of Fame persuaded the Board of Directors to waive the ten-year rule so they could award him his well-deserved plaque in Cooperstown.

BOB CARUTHERS

The frail young boy was undersized for his age and sickly. His doctor recommended outdoor exercise. Although he certainly did not look like an athlete, the lad took up baseball, despite the objections of his overprotective mother. When the family moved from Memphis to Chicago the boy, now a teenager, continued playing baseball. Still smaller than his teammates (as an adult he stood 5'7" and weighed 140 pounds), he developed a muscular physique and compensated with his brain for what he lacked in brawn. As a pitcher he developed an ability to size up opposing batters and capitalize on their weaknesses. Fast on his feet, he was an excellent fielder and a good hitter. Soon he became a well-known performer on Chicago's amateur teams. At the age of 19 he signed a professional contract, and Bob Caruthers, the once-sickly lad, was on his way to big league stardom.

Robert Lee Caruthers was born in Memphis, Tennessee, on January 5, 1864, the son of a successful attorney. In 1883 he began his professional career as an outfielder with the Grand Rapids Rippers of the Northwestern League. The next year he pitched and played right field for Minneapolis in the same circuit. Late in the season he joined the St. Louis Browns in the American Association and made his major league debut on September 7, 1884, as a twenty-year-old pitcher and outfielder. In the 1880s it was not unusual for a pitcher to play another position in the field when he was not pitching, but Caruthers probably did it more than anyone else. In his ten major league seasons, he pitched in 340 games, played in the outfield in 366 games, and made 13 appearances at first base and nine at second base.

In 1885 Bob Caruthers turned in an amazing performance. He won 40 games, accounting for more than half of his team's victories, as he pitched the Browns to their first major league pennant. He led the league in wins, won-lost percentage, and earned run average that season. The editors of the *Baseball Encyclopedia* honored him with the first of two ex post facto Cy Young awards and also the first of two consecutive AA Most Valuable Player awards that year.[54] During the offseason Bob and his teammate, Doc Bushong, vacationed in France. While overseas Caruthers engaged in lengthy contract negotiations via transatlantic cable, earning the nickname "Parisian Bob."

In 1886 the right-hander won 30 games, as the Browns took their second consecutive AA pennant. He also played 43 games in right field, alternating with fellow pitcher-outfielder Dave Foutz at the two positions. Bob's exploits at the plate nearly matched his performance in the pitcher's box, as he hit .334 and led the league in on-base percentage with .448. This earned him the *Baseball Encyclopedia*'s MVP honors. On August 16 he hit two home runs, a double, and a triple for 13 total bases in one game. He is one of only a handful of pitchers to smash four extra-base hits in one game. An umpire's call on a close play at first base deprived him of a chance to become the first pitcher to hit for the cycle.[55]

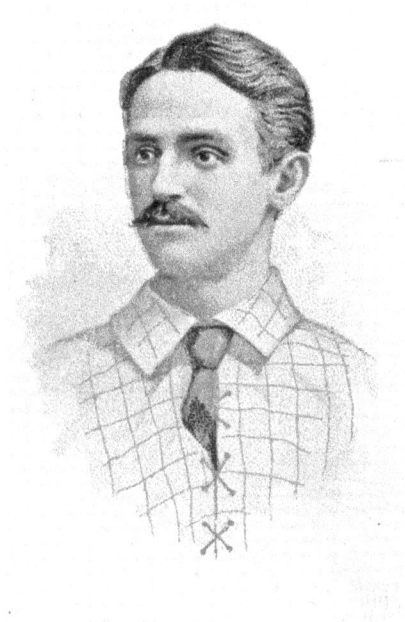

·R. L. CARUTHERS.
ALLEN & GINTER'S
RICHMOND. Cigarettes. VIRGINIA.

Bob Caruthers was not only a great pitcher but also a hard-hitting batsman. In 1885 he won 40 games, more than half his team's total victories, as he led the St. Louis Browns to their first pennant. In that season he led the league in wins, won-lost percentage, and earned run average. From 1885 through 1889 he averaged more than 33 wins per year. A sore arm suffered at the age of 27 brought his pitching career to a premature end and has thus far prevented him from entering the Baseball Hall of Fame (Library of Congress).

For a third straight year Caruthers led the Browns to a pennant in 1887, winning 29 games against nine losses for a league-best .763 winning percentage. He also allowed the circuit's fewest walks plus hits per nine innings and played 54 games in the outfield. He hit .357 and had an on-base percentage of .463, reinforcing his reputation as one of baseball's best hitting pitchers ever.

In 1887, as they had each year since 1882, the champions of the American Association faced the National League titleholders in a post-season series. Billed as the World's Championship Series, the contests were viewed as mere exhibition games by some of the players and with good reason. For example, the 1887 series consisted of 15 games between the Browns and the NL champion Detroit Wolverines, played in several different cities. One day the teams played a morning game in Washington and an afternoon encounter in Baltimore.[56] In order to relieve the monotony of the travel and the meaningless (to them) games, some of the St. Louis players engaged in recreational activities that may have taken precedence over their preparations for baseball. At least that was the opinion of Chris von der Ahe, owner of the Browns. As Caruthers was an expert billiards and poker player as well as something of a carouser, the owner placed the onus on Parisian Bob for the loss of the series, 10 games to 5. He put Caruthers on the market.

Two years earlier in 1885, King Kelly had been sold by Chicago to Boston for the unheard-of price of $10,000. The sale of Caruthers pushed the Kelly deal to second place. A report out of Chicago on December 15, 1887, explained the transaction:

> It has finally been decided that Bob Caruthers will go to Brooklyn. The great pitcher met Joe Pritchard and C. H. Byrne at the Clifton house yesterday, and affixed his signature to a Brooklyn club contract. Monday night Pritchard and Byrne called on Mrs. Caruthers, Bob's mother, and in a lengthy interview, did their best to overcome her objection to her boy going to Brooklyn. The real work of negotiating with and signing Caruthers was left to Joe Pritchard of St. Louis, but when it became necessary to obtain Mrs. Caruthers' consent Byrne was detailed to do the talking. When Pritchard and Byrne went to their hotel Monday night they were not exactly certain as to the result of their endeavors, though they were confident, for Bob, after a quiet talk with his mother, had promised to meet them. He kept his appointment, and as soon as he arrived at the hotel, he agreed to sign. After he had made glad the hearts of the Brooklynites by this feat, he and Pritchard talked about the deal, but were very reticent about it.
>
> When asked about the terms of the contract and the salary he was to receive, Caruthers said, "I will get a larger salary than any ball player has ever received, but I can't say what it is. My mouth is closed."
>
> "It lays the Kelly deal entirely in the shade," said Pritchard, "and that is all I want to say about it." ... Byrne was more communicative. "As for Caruthers his Association contract calls for $2000, but we will give him more money than ever has been or ever will be paid any other player."[57]

Newspapers estimated that St. Louis would receive $8250 and Caruthers would get $4000 in salary plus $2000 in bonuses for a total cost to Brooklyn of $14,250. More than 20 years later another newspaper reported that the sum of $14,250 "is still unique in baseball lore."[58]

Before the start of the 1888 baseball season Bob married Mary "Mamie" Danks, who had been born in Kentucky in the late 1860s. They received wedding gifts worth $4000,[59] at a time when the average worker in the United States earned less than $500 per year.[60] Several Brooklyn players tied the knot that winter, so many, in fact, that sportswriters took to calling the team the Bridegrooms. Caruthers had a good year in 1888, winning 29 games. He was even better in 1889, winning 40 games for the second time in his career, and leading the league in both victories and winning percentage as he helped Brooklyn claim its first-ever AA pennant. The diminutive hurler notched his second ex post facto Cy Young Award from the *Baseball Encyclopedia*. The Faber System named him the AA Pitcher of the Year.[61] He helped the Bridegrooms set a major league attendance record.

The Brooklyn club jumped to the National League in 1890 and won the championship of the senior circuit. Caruthers won 23 games, the last time he was to post 20 or more victories in a season. In 1891 he won 18 in his final season in Brooklyn. That was his final campaign in the Borough of Churches. He resurfaced in St. Louis in 1892, but his arm was nearly dead and he won only two games that season. However, he played more than 100 games in the outfield for the Cardinals (as the St. Louis club was now called.) The Cardinals released him in March 1893 and he played a few games for Chicago and Cincinnati that season before going back to Grand Rapids, where he had started his professional career 10 years earlier. Some writers have suggested that he was unable to adjust to the new 60′6″ pitching distance that was introduced in 1893, but he was finished as a pitcher before that occurred.

His major league record, both pitching and hitting. **Bold** indicates league leader.

			Pitching							*Batting*						
Year	Age	Club	W	L	Pct.	ERA	Sh	SO	G	AB	R	H	HR	RBI	BA	OBP
1884	20	St. Louis AA	7	2	.778	2.61	0	58	23	82	15	22	2	0	.268	.302
1885	21	St. Louis AA	**40**	13	.755	**2.07**	6	190	60	222	37	50	1	12	.225	.289
1886	22	St. Louis AA	30	14	.682	2.32	2	166	87	317	91	106	4	61	.334	**.448**
1887	23	St. Louis AA	29	9	.763	3.30	2	74	98	364	102	130	8	73	.357	.463
1888	24	Brooklyn AA	29	15	.659	2.39	4	140	94	335	58	77	5	53	.230	.328
1889	25	Brooklyn AA	**40**	11	**.784**	3.13	7	118	59	172	45	43	2	31	.250	.408
1890	26	Brooklyn NL	23	11	.676	3.09	1	64	71	238	46	63	1	29	.265	.397
1891	27	Brooklyn NL	18	14	.563	3.12	2	69	56	171	24	48	2	23	.281	.372
1892	28	St. Louis NL	2	10	.167	5.84	0	21	143	513	76	142	3	69	.272	.386
1893	29	Chicago NL							1	3	0	0	0	0	.000	.000

			Pitching						Batting					
Year	Age	Club	W	L	Pct.	ERA	Sh	SO	G	AB	R	H	HR	RBI	BA	OBP
1893		Cincinnati NL							13	48	14	14	1	8	.292	.477
TOTAL			218	99	.688	2.83	24	900	705	1492	508	695	29	359	.282	.391

Although his pitching arm was shot, Caruthers was able to play a few more years in the minor leagues, mainly at first base, where it was not necessary to make many strong throws. He wound up his playing career with the Burlington, Iowa, Colts at the age of 33.

His minor league record:

Year	Age	Club	W	L	.Pct	G	R	H	BA
1883	19	Grand Rapids NWL				50	51	63	.288
1884	20	Minneapolis NWL	17	15	.531	51	31	41	.218
1894	30	Grand Rapids WL				133	166	181	.331
1895	31	Jacksonville WA				92	100	119	.319
1896	32	Burlington WA				52	45	56	.292
1897	33	Burlington WA				3	1	4	.400

After his playing days were over, Caruthers tried his hand at umpiring. His record as an umpire was not nearly so distinguished as his accomplishments as a pitcher or hitter. He umpired in the American League in 1902 and 1903, in the Western League in 1904, and later in the Three-I League, moving from the majors to Class A to Class B circuits. Often he was involved in controversies. Being involved in a controversy is not unusual for an umpire; it goes with the job. However, some of the disputes involving Parisian Bob were noteworthy.

In an American League game between Boston and New York in 1903, Highlander pitcher Jesse Tannehill was upset when Caruthers called a ball on a pitch the hurler thought should have been a strike. When Tannehill confronted the ump at the plate, Caruthers ejected him from the game. The New York players lost their cool. Second baseman Jimmy Williams joined the argument, grabbed Caruthers by the collar of his shirt, pulled him close, and screamed in his face. The umpire tossed him out of the game and ordered both Tannehill and Williams off the field. The players refused to leave and continued hurling insults from the bench. Caruthers calmly took a watch from his pocket and set a deadline for their departure. Only after a teammate pleaded with them to leave did the two men depart, allowing the game to resume. This incident perhaps marked the beginning of the long rivalry between the teams now known as the Red Sox and the Yankees. "The tone was set. No New York–Boston game would ever be meaningless, despite what the standings sometimes said."[62]

Waterloo fans and at least one sportswriter were incensed at calls by Caruthers in a 1910 Three-I League contest between the homestanding Boosters and the Springfield Senators. The scribe wrote: "Robert Caruthers, he of big league fame known throughout the universe, was still in our midst before the game opened and still there when it ended, but Robert was indeed fortunate. Had this same Robert pulled off these stunts in most any other park, his friends would be looking down on him with tears in their eyes, but the Waterloo fans are different. They thought of his wife and family and let him off by telling him the truth about his ability as an umpire."[63]

The writer was even more critical of Caruthers' post-game conduct than he was of the officiating during the game. It seems that a young man said the umpire was rotten. Overhearing the remark, Caruthers confronted the youth and upbraided him in a profanity-laced tirade and even threatened to "get him" before he left the city. The reporter wrote: "Umpire Caruthers showed his caliber last evening.... If a ball player or a fan would resort to the language that Caruthers used he would forever be barred from the park."[64]

What the scribe did not know was that Caruthers was probably a very sick man at the time. He was to suffer a nervous collapse in 1911. Less than a year after the Waterloo incident another newspaper reported, "Pale and emaciated, Robert Caruthers, once an idol of the baseball world — a star pitcher — was sentenced to twenty days in the workhouse, the result of drink."[65] Caruthers never served his twenty-day sentence, for he did not have that many days left in his life. On August 5, 1911, only two weeks after his arrest, he died at St. Francis Hospital in Peoria, the city where he and Mamie were living with her parents. Neither the obituary nor the newspaper accounts of his passing reported the cause of his death. The obituary said he had been ill for more than a month. Bill James quoted the 1912 *Reach Guide* as saying Caruthers died of a nervous breakdown.[66] Robert Lee Caruthers was 47 years old when his life ended.

At present Caruthers is remembered not for his unfortunate final years but for the magnificent accomplishments of his youth. Among all the pitchers in the history of major league baseball who won 200 or more games, only one — Whitey Ford — had a higher winning percentage than Caruthers. The Yankee lefty edged Parisian Bob .690 to .688. Among the pitchers whose careers ended at the age of 30 or younger, *Total Baseball* ranked him second, behind only Amos Rusie, James listed him in fourth place and the Faber System put him fifth. In the first decade of the twenty-first century, there was a movement which tried, thus far unsuccessfully, to get Bob Caruthers into the Baseball Hall of Fame.

WIN MERCER

In 1902 the bromide "Washington—first in war, first in peace, last in the American League" was not yet in vogue, but with a couple of slight changes it would have been apropos. The Gay Nineties had not been a happy time for baseball fans in the nation's capital. When a certain handsome young pitcher made his debut with Washington in 1894, the Senators finished 11th in the 12-team National League. They remained a second-division club during his entire stay with them. By 1902 the slightly built right-hander had pitched nine seasons in the majors, never with a contender, not once for a team that won as many games as it lost. Pitching for a new club in a new league in 1902, there appeared to be a chance for his fortunes to improve. He won 15 games for Detroit that year. After the season ended, he organized a team of American League all-stars that played a team of National League standouts for a three-month barnstorming tour. The Tigers announced that the hurler would be the Detroit manager in 1903. The future appeared bright for the popular 28-year-old pitcher. However, as another adage has it, appearances can be deceiving. One January day in 1903, a San Francisco hotel watchman smelled the odor of gas coming from a room, broke down the door, and found Win Mercer in bed with a tube running from the gas jet into his mouth.

George Barclay Mercer was born June 20, 1874, in Chester in the extreme northernmost part of West Virginia's panhandle, just across the Ohio River from East Liverpool, Ohio. During his childhood the family moved first to Wheeling, then to East Liverpool. As a teenaged pitcher he won so many games for semi-pro teams sponsored by pottery factory teams that he acquired the nickname "Winner," which soon became "Winnie" or simply "Win." At the age of 18 he started his professional career with the Dover, New Hampshire, club in the New England League. After only one season in the minors, Win advanced to the big time.

His minor league record:

Year	Age	Club	League	W	L	Pct.	ERA
1893	18	Dover	New England	20	13	.606	2.05

Win Mercer made his major league debut about the time that the big league career of Bob Caruthers was winding down. There were two striking similarities shared by the two men. Both were of exceptionally small stature for baseball stars. Their measurements were identical—5'7" and 140 pounds. Both were excellent hitters who played several different positions on the diamond. There were also pronounced differences between the two. Caruthers was born into a family of wealth and privilege; Mercer was not. If Bob perhaps was a mama's boy, Win most definitely was a ladies man. More importantly, Caruthers pitched mostly for championship-caliber teams, whereas Mercer hurled for clubs mired in the second division. Had the two moundsmen been of equal ability, Caruthers would surely have posted a better record, simply because of the level of support he received from his team. They were not of equal ability, of course. Parisian Bob was a more talented pitcher, but they were not as far apart as their records indicate.

In his rookie season Mercer led the Washington club in wins with 17, but he also led them in losses with 23. In 1895 he again led the Senators in both categories, but in 1896 he had a breakthrough year with 25 wins while ranking third among the team's pitchers in losses. In 1897 he had a 20–20 season, 20 wins and 20 losses. It was the fourth consecutive year in which he led the team in wins. After that his pitching skills declined somewhat, and he played more often at other positions, particularly at third base, although he also participated in some games at first base, second base, shortstop, and all three outfield spots — every position except catcher. In 1899 he was the club's regular third sacker and hit .299 with a .360 on-base percentage. For his career he had a .285 average and thrice hit .300 or better.

Young and handsome with piercing dark eyes and an outgoing personality, Mercer quickly became a fan favorite in Washington.[67] According to Nash and Zullo, women in particular were attracted to Mercer and he loved the ladies. Washington's ownership designated Tuesdays and Fridays as Ladies Days and arranged for the star attraction to pitch on those days. In 1897 one Ladies Day game ended in shambles when umpire Bill Carpenter ejected the fan favorite. The writers reported, "An army of angry females poured out of the stands. They surrounded Carpenter, shoved him to the ground and ripped his clothing. Finally police brought the situation under control."[68]

After the 1899 season the National League reorganized, dropping Washington and three other clubs to become an eight-team circuit. Mercer was assigned to the New York Giants. He pitched only one season in Gotham. Evidently he liked Washington, for in 1901 he jumped to the new Washington club in the American League. However, the Senators sold him to Detroit. Apparently the move was good for him. He had his best year since 1897, leading the Tigers with 15 wins and posting a career-best ERA of 3.04. His four shutouts were second in the AL to Addie Joss. He played his last game on September 27, 1902, at the age of 28. Of course, no one knew at the time that it was to be his final major league appearance.

Mercer's major league record: **Bold** type indicates league leader.

			Pitching					Batting							
Year	Age	Club	W	L	Pct.	ERA	Sh	SO	G	AB	R	H	HR	RBI	BA	OBP
1894	19	Washington NL	17	23	.425	3.85	0	72	53	165	29	48	2	29	.291	.328
1895	20	Washington NL	13	23	.361	4.46	0	84	63	196	26	50	1	26	.255	.308
1896	21	Washington NL	25	18	.581	4.13	2	94	49	156	23	38	1	14	.244	.302
1897	22	Washington NL	20	20	.500	3.24	3	88	50	139	23	44	0	19	.317	.354
1898	23	Washington NL	12	18	.400	4.81	0	52	80	249	38	80	2	25	.321	.369
1899	24	Washington NL	7	14	.333	4.60	0	28	108	375	73	112	1	35	.299	.360
1900	25	New York NL	13	17	.433	3.86	1	39	76	248	32	73	0	27	.294	.366
1901	26	Washington AL	9	13	.409	4.56	1	31	51	140	26	42	0	16	.300	.402
1902	27	Detroit AL	15	18	.455	3.04	4	40	35	100	8	18	0	6	.180	.226
TOTAL			131	164	.444	3.99	11	528	565	1768	278	505	7	197	.286	.344

After the season Detroit announced that Win would be its manager the next year at a hefty salary of $3800.

During the offseason Mercer and Tip O'Neill, the old-time batting champion of the St. Louis Browns, organized a three-month barnstorming tour of the American West. With Mercer handling the American Leaguers and O'Neill managing the National League stars, the two teams played in cities from Chicago to Los Angeles. In California they played against various local clubs. The plan was to end the tour with a three-game series in San Francisco in the middle of January.

Exactly what happened in San Francisco and why it happened are still matters of dispute more than 100 years later. What we do know is that on January 13, 1903, Mercer left his team at the Langham Hotel and went to the Occidental Hotel, where he registered as George Murray of Philadelphia. After writing several notes, he ran a tube from the gas jet into his mouth and asphyxiated himself. What we do not know for certain is what led him to that action. One note stated, "A word to friends: beware of women and a game of chance."[69] Historians have focused more on the reference to gambling than on the one about women. Although it seems possible that an encounter with a female could have contributed to his suicide, that possibility is ignored in most speculations about his death.

Among the papers found in the room after Win's death were notes to some of his teammates, to his sweetheart, and to his widowed mother, Maggie Mercer, in East Liverpool. The message to his mother read

Darling, Mother:
I do not want to break your heart, but I am afraid I will by committing the act that I am now about to commit. I think I am doing the right thing, dear mother, so please forgive me. Women have got the best of me, but I forgive them, even though they are my downfall. God bless them.
From Winnie."[70]

In this note Mercer again blamed women for his act, but commentators on his death tend to overlook it.

Back in East Liverpool, Win's mother and some of his close friends believed the young man's death was not a suicide but a murder. After consultation with officials of baseball clubs on which Mercer had played, they composed a telegram to the San Francisco police chief, asking him to make a close investigation. They claimed the letters were not written by Mercer, who never signed himself "Winnie." The writers of the telegram further stated that the recent attempt to rob Mercer showed that desperate men were after him. As for the reported shortage in funds, they claimed he had property and hundreds of friends who would have backed him for any amount.[71]

The San Francisco police replied that there was no indication that Mercer was murdered. They insisted it was a plain case of suicide. All of his farewell letters were positively identified. The druggist from whom Mercer purchased the rubber hose identified both Mercer and the hose.[72]

At one time William E. Akin wrote that Mercer had lost heavily at a Los Angeles horse racing track the day before his suicide. Akin surmised that Win's losses had included not just his own money, but also funds from the barnstorming teams.[73] In his later writings Akin downplayed that possibility. In his article for the SABR Biography Project, Akin quoted Fred Lieb's denial that Mercer had lost the players' money.[74] He further cited the statement of Scott Longert, Addie Joss's biographer, that Joss had received his full share of the proceeds, some $600.[75] Had Mercer gambled away the players' money, Joss would have received nothing, Akin surmised.

Longert related another strange incident. A few days before the scheduled departure, a man identifying himself as a messenger for Win gave a note to the front desk clerk at the Langham Hotel. The note asked for a large envelope in the hotel safe be handed over so it could be taken to a field where some of the players were working out. Without asking for any identification, the clerk complied with the request. A few minutes later the messenger reappeared, saying he had been given the wrong envelope. He needed the one containing the team receipts. As the receipts came to about $15,000, the clerk became suspicious and excused himself for a few minutes. He found a ballplayer, Jack Chesbro, who had stayed behind in the lobby, and asked him to go down to the park and ask Mercer about the messenger. When Chesbro returned with news that the messenger was a phony, the man ran from the lobby and disappeared.[76]

Longert wrote that speculation ran rampant that Mercer's suicide was somehow related to the attempt by the fake messenger to abscond with the gate receipts. Rumors persisted that Win had lost money to gamblers. Others suggested that Mercer suffered from heart disease, which caused him to become despondent.[77] Tom Deveaux wrote that Mercer was "given to bouts of depression."[78]

After Mercer's death there was conjecture that the final three games of the barnstorming tour would be cancelled. However, it was decided to play out the schedule. An additional contest was added as a benefit game, with the proceeds to go to Win's mother. A newspaper reported, "Not that she is in need, but as a token of the regard in which her son is held."[79] Addie Joss accompanied the body of his friend back to East Liverpool, where relatives waited to make funeral arrangements. George Barclay Mercer was buried in Riverview Cemetery in East Liverpool, just across the river from his birthplace in Chester, West Virginia.

Win Mercer's statistics suffered from the fact that he had the misfortune of always pitching for losing teams. Nevertheless, he racked up some impressive wins. Among pitchers whose careers ended at the age of 30 or younger, Mercer is ranked sixth by the Faber System and fifteenth by *Total Baseball*.

Part Three
All Position Players

Part Three contains biographical information and essential baseball statistical data about all 107 position players who are eligible for inclusion in this book; that is, those who were regularly in a major league lineup for at least five years and ended their big league playing career at the age of thirty or younger. Terms such as early leavers, premature departures, or early exits are sometimes used in referring to these individuals.

The biographical sketches are arranged alphabetically within position groupings, starting with first basemen. A standard format is followed, starting with birth name, date, and place of birth. Debut refers to the date the first major league game was played. Last game means the date of the final appearance as a player in a major league contest. The listing of clubs is confined to major league teams. Any information about minor league play or major league appearances in a non-playing role is confined to the body of the text.

Biographical sketches by other writers are noted if they appear in any of these five sources: *Baseball's First Stars*; *Deadball Stars of the American League*; *Deadball Stars of the National League*; *Nineteenth Century Stars*; or the SABR Biography Project.

Rankings are provided based upon the Faber System, *Total Baseball*, and Bill James's analyses.[1] The Faber System rates all eligible players, *Total Baseball* rates virtually every player who ever appeared in a major league game, and James ranks the top 125 at each position. None of the three sources segregates early leavers from other players, but rankings of those with short careers can be derived from the ratings given. The number of players included whose careers ended by age thirty is Faber System 107, *Total Baseball* 107, and James 26. Unless otherwise specified, all rankings given in the biographical sketches below refer to the player's rank among players at the particular position who made a premature departure from big league play.

FIRST BASEMEN

Player	G	R	H	HR	RBI	BA	OBP	Faber System Bat	Field	Total
Willie Aikens	774	301	675	110	415	.271	.354	437	117	554
Jack Burns	890	541	980	44	417	.279	.391	183	342	525
Nate Colbert	1004	481	833	173	520	.243	.322	439	242	681
Nick Esasky	810	336	677	122	427	.250	.329	257	104	361
Brad Fullmer	807	395	778	114	442	.279	.336	215	21	236
Dick Hoblitzell	1318	591	1310	27	593	.278	.341	499	349	848
Don Hurst	905	510	976	115	610	.298	.375	562	251	813
Mike Ivie	857	309	727	81	411	.269	.324	281	101	382
Dalton Jones	907	268	548	41	237	.239	.295	42	-44	-2
Pete LaCock	715	214	444	27	224	.257	.326	-6	57	51
Vic Saier	865	455	775	55	395	.263	.351	369	191	560
Phil Todt	957	372	880	57	453	.258	.305	-57	420	363

Willie Aikens

Born: Willie Mays Aikens, October 14, 1954, Seneca, SC
Debut: May 17, 1977; age 22
Last Game: April 27, 1985; age 30
Clubs: California AL; Kansas City AL; Toronto AL

Willie Mays Aikens bore little resemblance to his famous namesake. Although he hit with some power, he was slow afoot, a poor fielder, and far from a role model. Willie played baseball at South Carolina State University in 1973–74, but the school dropped the sport after the 1974 season in favor of women's softball in order to comply with the gender equity provisions of Title IX. He was selected in the first round (second pick overall) by the California Angels in the 1975 amateur draft. He rose quickly through the organization. Starting with Quad Cities of the Midwest League in 1975, he was promoted to El Paso of the Texas League in 1976 and Salt Lake City of the PCL in 1977, before being called up to the majors. He was traded to Kansas City in 1980. In the World Series that fall he became the first player ever to have two multi-homer games in the same Fall Classic. Following the 1983 season he was arrested for attempting to possess cocaine and was sentenced to 90 days in federal prison. Commissioner Bowie Kuhn suspended him for a year, but the suspension was reduced by an arbitrator and Aikens was reinstated in May 1984. He was traded to Toronto but failed to perform well for the Blue Jays and was sent down to Syracuse and Tidewater in the International League in 1985. In 1986 he made an amazing comeback with Puebla in the

Mexican League, leading the Class AAA league with some incredible numbers. His batting average of .454 was not only a record for that circuit, but the second highest ever recorded in the history of the National Association of Professional Baseball Leagues. Willie also set Mexican League records with 154 RBIs, 87 extra-base hits, and 384 total bases. In 1989 he was still in the Mexican League, playing for the Leon Braves. He led the loop in batting average at .395, in runs scored with 108, and in RBIs with 131. In his middle thirties, he appeared to have a lot of baseball left in him. However, his career came to a crashing halt three years later. In 1992 he was arrested on drug charges and sentenced to 20 years in the federal prison in Atlanta.

Ranking: Faber System fifth; *Total Baseball* second.

Jack Burns

Born: John Irving Burns, August 31, 1907, Cambridge, MA
Debut: September 17, 1930; age 23
Last Game: September 27, 1936; age 29
Clubs: St. Louis AL; Detroit AL

Jack Burns spent most of his adult life in baseball. His professional playing career began at the age of 20 in 1928 in the New England League. Playing for Tulsa, he led the Western League in home runs with 36 in 1929. While playing for Wichita Falls in 1930, he made the Texas League all-star team. Late that season he reached the big leagues with the St. Louis Browns. In the majors he never showed the home run power he had exhibited with Tulsa, but he hit for a decent average and displayed speed on the bases. In 1932 he scored 111 runs. In 1935 he led the AL with 20 sacrifices. It was in the field, however, where he excelled. He twice led AL first basemen in assists and three times in double plays. After his playing career ended, he managed the Toronto Maple Leafs in the International League in 1938 and 1939. In 1949 he joined the Boston Red Sox system and spent the rest of his life with the organization. He managed Red Sox affiliates at Scranton and Albany in the Eastern League from 1949 to 1954, winning a pennant with the Albany Senators in 1952. From 1955 through 1959 he was with the big club in Boston as third base coach. From 1960 until his death he scouted for the Sox. He was at his home in the Brighton section of Boston on April 18, 1975, dressing to go to Fenway Park when he died, suddenly and unexpectedly, probably of a heart attack. He was 67.

Ranking: Faber System sixth; *Total Baseball* twelfth.

Nate Colbert

Born: Nathan Colbert, April 9, 1946, St. Louis, MO
Debut: April 14, 1966; age 20
Last Game: October 1, 1976; age 30
Clubs: Houston NL; San Diego NL; Detroit AL; Montreal NL; Oakland AL

As an amateur free agent, 17-year-old Nate turned down the Yankees to sign for less money with his hometown St. Louis Cardinals. He spent two years in the Cardinals farm system and was left unprotected in the 1965 Rule 5 draft. Selected by Houston, he spent most of 1966 to 1968 in the minors, playing only a few games in the majors. When San Diego entered the National League after the 1968 season, the Padres selected Colbert as their ninth pick in the expansion draft. In the early 1970s Colbert became the Padres' greatest star, leading the club in home runs each of his first four years. He also became an excellent first baseman, twice leading the league in assists at that position. He was named to the NL all-star team three times. On August 1, 1972, Nate tied Stan Musial's record of five home runs in a doubleheader and set a major league record with 13 RBIs in the twin-bill. His 111 RBIs that season set a record for driving in the highest percentage of his team's runs. After the 1974 season Colbert was traded to Detroit. From there he went to Montreal and Oakland, playing only a few games each year because of a chronic back problem. He returned to the Padres, serving as team chaplain and as a hitting instructor in the San Diego system from 1987 to 1990.

In 1991 Colbert was convicted of lying on bank documents used to secure more than $138,000 in loans. Despite expressing remorse and promising restitution, he was sentenced to a year in prison. After his release, he and his wife became co-owners of a company that provides advice and counseling to amateur athletes considering careers at the professional level.

Ranking: Faber System third; *Total Baseball* third; James second.

Nick Esasky

Born: Nicholas Andrew Esasky, February 24, 1960, Hialeah, FL
Debut: June 19, 1983; age 23
Last Game: April 21, 1990; age 30
Clubs: Cincinnati NL; Boston AL; Atlanta NL

Nick was drafted out of Carol City (Florida) High School by the Cincinnati Reds as the 17th pick in the first round of the 1978 amateur draft. The young man spent more than five years in the Reds' farm system at Billings, Tampa, Waterbury, and Indianapolis before joining the parent club in midseason 1983. He had fair success in Cincinnati, playing third base, first base, and in the outfield. After the 1988 season he was traded to the Boston Red Sox. He had his best year in 1989, hitting 30 home runs and getting 108 RBIs for the BoSox. At the end of the season, he opted for free agency and signed a three-year, $5.6 million contract with the Atlanta Braves. In return for those millions he played a total of nine games for Atlanta. In April 1990 he got off to a terrible start, committing five errors in the nine games he played. Although he did not know it at the time, his major league career ended one night in April when he sprained his right shoulder as he fell trying to field a grounder off the bat of Barry Larkin. He was placed on the 15-day disabled list, then transferred to the 60-day DL when he suffered dizziness and blurred vision. His problem was diagnosed as vertigo, perhaps caused by an inner-ear infection and exacerbated by Lyme disease. Treatment for the infection and Lyme disease did not cure the vertigo. The Braves kept him on the roster throughout the 1990 and 1991 seasons, hoping he could make a comeback. He worked out with the club during spring training in 1992 but did not get into a game. In June he was sent to Richmond of the International League on a rehabilitation assignment. After the rehab he agreed to accept an outright assignment to Richmond. He played well enough that he thought he deserved another shot at the big leagues, but the Braves did not have room for him on their roster. He gave them an ultimatum to either call him up or release him. The Braves released him. He had hit .278 with five home runs and 14 RBIs in 30 games on the farm, but no other club wanted to take a chance on him because of his medical history. He bought a home in suburban Atlanta and was living a comfortable life when his teenage daughter developed a serious methamphetamine addiction. Eventually he placed his daughter into inpatient rehab and received legal custody of her baby, his granddaughter. He and his wife later started a non-profit organization, called K.I.M. Foundation for "Kids in Meth."

Ranking: Faber System ninth; *Total Baseball* eighth.

Brad Fullmer

Born: Bradley Ryan Fullmer, January 17, 1975, Chatsworth, CA
Debut: September 2, 1997; age 22
Last Game: July 24, 2004; age 29
Clubs: Montreal NL; Toronto AL; Anaheim AL; Texas AL

Brad was drafted out of Montclair College Preparatory School in Van Nuys by the Montreal Expos in the second round of the 1973 amateur draft. His prep school teammate, Russ Ortiz, also reached the big leagues. Brad played for Harrisburg in the Eastern League and Ottawa of the International League before being promoted to the majors in September 1997. In his first major league at-bat he hit a pinch-hit home run. Although he played first base for the Expos, he was used mainly as a designated hitter after being traded to the American League. His best year came in 2000 when he hit .295 with 32 home runs and 104 RBIs for the Toronto Blue Jays. In 2002 he appeared in twelve post-season games for Anaheim, including five World Series contests. In the twelve games he averaged .294, hit one homer, scored six runs, and batted in five. The Angels released him after the 2003 season, and he signed as a free agent with Texas. In mid-season 2004 he injured his knee and was placed on the disabled list for the remainder of the year. The Rangers released him at the end of the season. Waiting for the knee to heal, he was out of baseball in 2005. The Chicago White Sox signed him as a free agent in July and assigned him to the Charlotte Knights, their farm club in the International League, but he never played for the team. The knee never became sound enough for him to resume his baseball career.

Ranking: Faber System tenth; *Total Baseball* sixth.

Dick Hoblitzell

Born: Richard Carleton Hoblitzell, October 26, 1888, Waverly, WV
Debut: September 5, 1908; age 19
Last Game: June 7, 1918; age 29
Clubs: Cincinnati NL; Boston AL

In high school and college Dick was a football star. The captain of the football team during both his freshman and sophomore years at Parkersburg High School, the lad finished his prep schooling at Marietta Academy. After graduation he starred at halfback at Marietta College for two years, and then transferred to a collegiate powerhouse, the Western University of Pennsylvania (now the University of Pittsburgh), where he played end. In the early 1900s professional football was not a viable option, so Hoblitzell turned to baseball for his livelihood. He started his professional baseball career while still in college, playing for Clarksburg in the Western Pennsylvania League in 1907 under the assumed name of Hollister in order to protect his amateur status. In 1908 he played for Wheeling in the Central League, which led to considerable confusion about his status. Clarksburg sold him to the Cincinnati Reds, but the manager of the St. Louis Cardinals went to Wheeling and took the young first baseman back to St. Louis with him. The National Commission ruled that as Clarksburg had allowed Hoblitzell to play for Wheeling on the condition that it retained the right to sell him to another club, the sale to Cincinnati

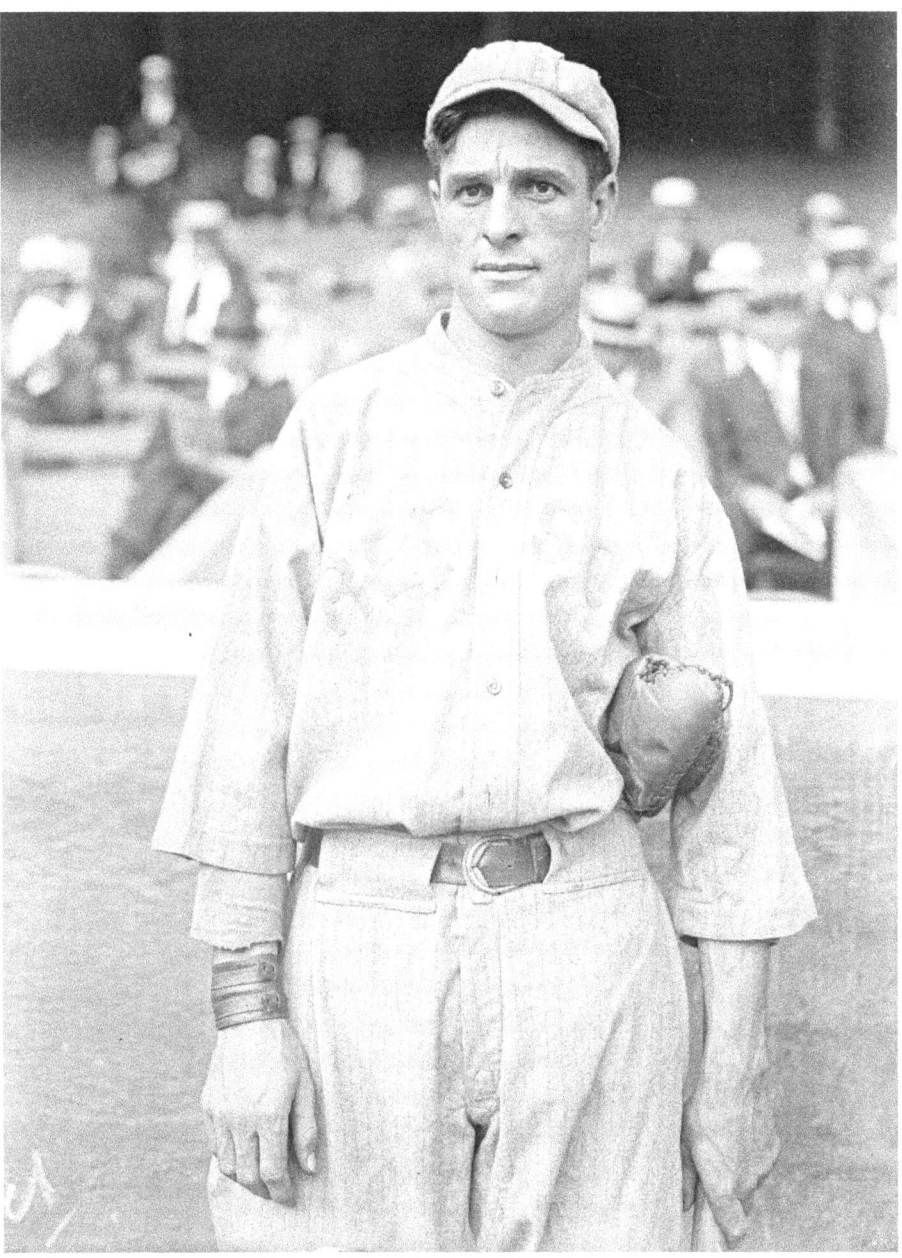

Dick Hoblitzell was generally considered one of the top first basemen of the Deadball Era, both as a hitter and as a fielder. During World War I he entered the United States Army Dental Corps and never returned to major league baseball (Library of Congress).

was valid. The fact that Garry Herrmann was president of both the Reds and the National Commission raises the possibility of a conflict of interest. Nevertheless, Dick became a Red and stayed with the club until a slump in 1914 led the team to place him on waivers. He was claimed by the Boston Red Sox, recovered his batting stroke, and helped Boston win two pennants and two World Series titles in the next three years.

During offseasons while with the Reds, Hoblitzell studied dentistry at the Ohio College of Dental Surgery. This led to his being nicknamed "Doc" and indirectly to his exit from major league baseball. In March 1918 he passed an examination for the United States Army Dental Corps. Hampered by a sore toe, he played only 25 games that spring before going on active duty as a first lieutenant. The Red Sox again won the World Series that fall and gave their ex-teammate a partial share of $300 from the proceeds. While stationed in El Paso, Doc contacted influenza and nearly died from the Spanish flu pandemic that swept the nation. After his recovery he was assigned to West Point as the baseball coach for the military academy. After his discharge from the army in 1920, Hoblitzell spent eight years in the minor leagues, usually as a playing manager. From 1925 through 1928 he was out of baseball, working full-time in the real estate business. He returned as a player and/or manager for three more years before leaving the game for good in 1931.

Following the 1931 season Dick moved back to West Virginia to farm, host a sports radio show, write a column for the *Parkersburg News*, and umpire baseball games. Active in community affairs, he served at various times as county treasurer, sheriff, and Sunday school superintendent. An excellent marksman, he enjoyed quail hunting. Although he never officially practiced dentistry, he set up a dental chair in his home and filled cavities for his neighbors, without charge or Novocaine. Hoblitzell died in Parkersburg on September 14, 1962.

Although he seldom led the league in any important category, he was generally considered one of the top first basemen of the Deadball Era, both as a hitter and as a fielder. He is profiled in *Deadball Stars of the National League* and in SABR's *Baseball Biography Project*.

Ranking: Faber System first; *Total Baseball* fourth; James first.

Don Hurst

Born: Frank O'Donnell Hurst, August 12, 1905, Maysville, KY
Debut: May 13, 1928; age 22
Last Game: September 20, 1934; age 29
Clubs: Philadelphia NL; Chicago NL

Although he was born in Kentucky, Don grew up in Ohio, in Norwood, a suburb of Cincinnati. In 1923 he enrolled at Ohio State University, where he played freshman football and perhaps a little baseball before dropping out in the spring of 1924 to pursue a career in professional baseball. His first summer was with the Paris Bourbons, where he led the Blue Grass League with a .382 average and 20 home runs. By 1926 he had made it up to the International League, where manager Burt Shotton of the Syracuse Stars converted him from an outfielder to a first baseman. He made the IL all-star team that year. During the 1927 offseason, St. Louis and Philadelphia negotiated a complicated deal, whereby Hurst remained in the Cardinals' farm system until the Phillies called him up to the big leagues in the spring of 1928. A big (6', 215 pounds) power hitter, Don established himself as one of the National League's premier sluggers. Playing in an era of a lively ball and in the home run friendly Baker Bowl, Don hit higher than .300 and slugged better than .500 in his first six years with the Phillies. He hit 31 home runs in 1929, twice scored more than 100 runs in a season, and twice had 125 or more RBIs. In 1932 he led the league with 143 RBIs. He was one of four Phillies to knock in more than 100 runs in 1929. Only the 1936 Yankees have had more teammates accomplish that feat. He was traded to the Chicago Cubs for Dolph Camilli during the 1934 season. Camilli went on to become a star, while Hurst was out of the majors at the end of the year. He was purchased by the Columbus Red Birds in 1935 and later finished his career with the Los Angeles Angels of the Pacific Coast League. For several years he was employed in a managerial capacity at the Veterans Memorial Auditorium in Culver City, California. After an illness of several months he died en route to a Los Angeles hospital on December 6, 1952, at the age of 47.

Ranking: Faber System second; *Total Baseball* fifth.

Mike Ivie

Born: Michael Wilson Ivie, August 8, 1952, Atlanta, GA
Debut: September 4, 1971; age 19
Last Game: May 7, 1983; age 30
Clubs: San Diego NL; San Francisco NL; Houston NL; Detroit AL

As a teenager in suburban Atlanta, Mike put up some outstanding numbers for Decatur's Walker High School. He hit .465 as a sophomore, .565 as a junior, and slumped to around .245 his senior year. His performance caught the attention of scouts around the country, and the San Diego Padres selected him as the first pick in the first round of the 1970 amateur draft. The 17 year old was thrilled. "I feel like a little kid at Christmas," he said. "I've never wanted anything except to be a big league catcher since I was six years old. It feels great to be No. 1. This is a dream come true."[2] Within a few years the dream of being a great catcher turned into a nightmare. He had a clause inserted into his 1978 contract stating that he would not be asked to catch again.

Ivie's professional career got off to a good start in the minors with teams such as Tri-City, Lodi, Alexandria, and Hawaii. He came up to the majors in September 1971 and hit .471 in six games. He made it back to the big time to stay in 1974, but mainly as a first baseman. As a catcher he was having trouble throwing the ball back to the pitcher. A sports psychologist said such problems usually start as physical errors, and then become mental blocks for fear the error will be repeated. Ivie is not the only major leaguer to have this problem. Dale Murphy had the same difficulty, but was converted to an outfielder and had a stellar career. Rick Ankiel had to give up pitching and become an outfielder because he lost the ability to throw the ball over the plate. However, some critics were not sympathetic. Rick Monday said, "Mike Ivie is a forty-million-dollar airport with a thirty-dollar control tower."[3] Without citing any evidence to support his view, one sportswriter said that Ivie imploded due to anxiety brought on by a domineering father. Some claimed he had an attitude problem.

Management usually (but not always) tried to accommodate him. San Diego used him almost exclusively at first base or third base. In 1978 the Padres traded him to San Francisco, where he hit .308 for his best major league average and tied a major league record by belting two pinch-hit home runs. In 1979 the Giants played him in the outfield and at second base in addition to first and third. He responded by hitting a career-high 27 home runs. Things were looking up for the young man, but during the offseason he sliced part of his pinky finger off with a hunting knife and was unable to play well during the 1980 season. The Giants traded him to Houston the next spring. At his request the Astros released him so he could sign with Detroit. He continued to struggle with the Tigers and was released during the 1983 season. He retired from baseball at the age of 30. For the man who had been considered the best prospect in baseball as a teenager, it was a disappointing career. Yet he was in the major leagues for eleven seasons, was a better than average big league hitter, and fielded adequately at several positions.

Ranking: Faber System and *Total Baseball* both seventh.

Dalton Jones

Born: James Dalton Jones, December 10, 1943, McComb, MS
Debut: April 17, 1964; age 20

Last Game: October 4, 1972; age 28
Clubs: Boston AL; Detroit AL; Texas AL

Growing up in Baton Rouge, Dalton got his start in baseball at an early age. His father, a former professional player, coached him in Little League and American Legion ball. A star shortstop, Jones led his Istrouma High School team to the Louisiana state championship game. In 1961 the Boston Red Sox signed him as an amateur free agent for a $60,000 bonus. He played that year for the Alpine (Texas) Cowboys in the Sophomore League. The next season he was promoted to York of the Eastern League. After hitting higher than .300 in his first two seasons, he moved up to the Seattle Rainiers of the Pacific Coast League and was switched to second base. He made the big club the next spring. Although he hit fairly well for the Sox, he had difficulty in the field, leading to a shift to third base. In 1969 he was tried at the other infield position — first base — where he fielded better. However, his offensive production continued to slide. Even so, he set the Red Sox record for career pinch-hits. During the offseason he was traded to Detroit. After two lackluster years with the Tigers, he was traded to Texas and concluded his career with the Rangers. In 1973 Jones was back in the minors for an unproductive stint with the Peninsula Whips in the International League. After baseball, Jones tried several different lines of work, mainly in financial services. At last report, he was retired and living in Liberty, Mississippi.

Dalton Jones is profiled in SABR's *Baseball Biography Project*. Although he played more games at second and third, Jones was most successful at first base.

Ranking: Faber System twelfth; *Total Baseball* tenth.

Pete LaCock

Born: Ralph Pierre LaCock, Jr., January 17, 1952, Burbank, CA
Debut: September 6, 1972; age 20
Last Game: October 5, 1980; age 28
Clubs: Chicago NL; Kansas City AL

At Taft High School in Los Angeles, Pete was an outstanding football player. A tackle on both offense and defense, he was offered several college football scholarships. The Toreadors baseball coach talked him into joining the baseball team. The left-handed-hitting first baseman showed so much promise that the Chicago Cubs selected him in the first round (twentieth pick overall) of the 1970 amateur draft. The Cubs brought him along slowly. In 1970 he played for Caldwell in the Rookie League and Quincy in the Midwest League; in 1971 and 1972 he was in the Texas League with Midland and San

Antonio; in 1973 and 1974 he prepped with Wichita in the American Association. In both of his Texas League seasons he led the league in bases on balls; he also led in triples in 1972.

In the majors LaCock was never a star but he played well enough to appear in 715 games in nine seasons. The Cubs traded him to Kansas City following the 1976 season. He played in seven post-season games for the Royals, hitting .333 with a .500 OBP. Kansas City granted him free agency after the 1980 World Series and he went to Japan for the 1981 season. He was unhappy in Japan and retired temporarily from baseball after one year overseas. After some years as an account executive for a financial services company in Kansas City, he returned to baseball as a manager and hitting coach for various minor league clubs. In 2009 he was hitting coach for the Tucson Toros of the Golden Baseball League.

LaCock is the son of a famous father who used the stage name Peter Marshall as the original host of the long-running TV series *Hollywood Squares*. Ranking: Faber System eleventh; *Total Baseball* ninth.

Vic Saier

Born: Victor Sylvester Saier, May 4, 1891, Lansing, MI
Debut: May 3, 1911; age 19
Last Game: August 5, 1919; age 28
Clubs: Chicago NL; Pittsburgh NL

At St. Mary's High School in Lansing, Vic starred in both football and baseball. After graduating in 1908, the youngster enrolled in St. Mary's Business College and played for a local town team, the Oldsmobile Nine. In 1910 he played for the Lansing Senators in the Southern Michigan League, leading the circuit with 175 hits, as he batted for a .339 average and stole 42 bases. In midseason the Chicago Cubs purchased him for $1500 and promoted him to the big club in 1911. He made his major league debut the day before his 20th birthday. He had his best year in 1913, when he led the league with 21 triples, hit .289 with a .370 OBP, scored 94 runs and had 92 RBIs. He was on his way to an even better season in 1915, leading the NL in runs, RBIs, doubles, and triples when he suffered a serious leg injury while sliding into home plate. The injury kept him out of the lineup for three weeks, and after his return he never regained his former productivity. In the sixth game of the 1917 season, he tried to score from second on a single and broke his leg in a collision at home plate, sidelining him for the remainder of the year. In 1918 he was out of baseball, and worked in a defense plant. Before the 1919 season began he was sold to the Pittsburgh. He did not hit well for the Pirates and was released before the season ended.

After his baseball career was over Saier returned to Lansing, where he managed the City Club for many years. He died in East Lansing on May 14, 1967, at the age of 76. Vic Saier is profiled in *Deadball Stars of the National League*.

Ranking: Faber System fourth; *Total Baseball* first.

Phil Todt

Born: Philip Julius Todt, August 9, 1901, St. Louis, MO
Debut: April 25, 1924; age 22
Last Game: September 25, 1931; age 30
Clubs: Boston AL; Philadelphia AL

When Phil was a 16-year-old sandlot star in St. Louis, he signed a contract with the hometown Cardinals in 1917. However, his father refused to validate the contract by co-signing for the underage youngster. Three years later Phil signed a contract with the other St. Louis team, the Browns. The Cardinals cried foul, claiming the lad belonged to them. Newly hired baseball commissioner Kenesaw Landis made his first baseball decision, ruling that Phil was free to sign with the Browns. Newspapers had a field day writing about Todt as a sandlot sensation, possessing the magic of Ruth, Speaker, and Sisler. Even the fact that Phil was born in a graveyard was newsworthy. (Phil's father was caretaker at St. Peter's Cemetery and the family resided in a house on the property.) The Browns sent Phil to Tulsa, and the teenaged outfielder lived up to the hype, hitting .308 and clouting 28 home runs. The next year saw him in Columbus of the American Association. He was optioned to San Antonio of the Texas League, where he hit .333 in 1923. At the end of that season he was purchased by the Boston Red Sox. Early in 1925 the New York Yankees offered to trade Lou Gehrig for Todt, but the Red Sox turned them down. The Sox converted Phil into a first baseman, and he became an outstanding defensive player at that position. In 1926 he made 1755 putouts, the third highest ever made by a first sacker. In 1928 he led the American League in fielding percentage with .997. Despite his early success, he never hit well in the major leagues. After playing for last-place teams throughout his career in Boston, Todt was sold to the Philadelphia Athletics in 1931. Although he was primarily a substitute for the A's, he did get into the 1931 World Series and had a perfect 1.000 OBP, as he drew a base on balls in his only plate appearance.

After the A's released him, Todt played six years for St. Paul in the American Association, twice serving as interim manager. He twice led the league in fielding, setting an AA record with a .998 average in 1934. In 1938 he was with Dallas in the Texas League and Chattanooga of the Southern Association. Unable to recover completely from an injury to his knee suffered while with Dallas, Todt ended his professional career as the playing manager of Crookston of the Northern League in 1939. He ran a flower shop in St. Louis and served as an official with the St. Louis Bowling Association. In 1941 he became baseball coach at Corcordia Seminary in St. Louis. Todt died in a St. Louis hospital on November 15, 1973. He was buried in St. Peter's Cemetery, the same cemetery in which he was born.

Phil Todt is profiled in the SABR *Baseball Biography Project*. Ranking: Faber System eighth; *Total Baseball* eleventh.

SECOND BASEMEN

Player	G	R	H	HR	RBI	BA	OBP	Faber System Bat	Field	Total
Mike Andrews	893	441	803	66	316	.258	.353	506	174	680
Charley Bassett	917	392	806	15	402	.231	.285	-31	318	287
Jerry Browne	982	431	866	23	288	.271	.351	318	15	333
Hub Collins	680	653	790	11	319	.284	.365	522	149	671
Tim Cullen	700	155	387	9	134	.220	.282	-161	-89	-250
Gene DeMont	922	537	1096	17	497	.303	.340	329	139	468
Marcus Giles	792	468	813	76	333	.277	.353	371	297	668
Wilton Guerrero	678	197	473	11	127	.282	.308	-139	-28	-167
Frankie Gustine	1261	553	1214	38	480	.265	.322	198	139	337
Jim Lefebvre	922	313	756	74	404	.251	.323	205	118	323
Barry McCormick	989	433	867	15	417	.238	.297	-156	120	-36
Cass Michaels	1288	508	1142	53	501	.262	.349	214	251	465
Al Myers	833	429	788	13	359	.245	.314	43	-129	-86
Rennie Stennett	1237	500	1239	41	432	.274	.306	245	496	741
Bill Sweeney	1039	442	1004	11	389	.272	.349	329	363	692
Bump Wills	831	472	807	36	302	.266	.335	351	386	737
Steve Yerkes	711	307	676	6	254	.268	.328	120	62	182

Mike Andrews

Born: Michael Jay Andrews, July 9, 1943, Los Angeles, CA
Debut: September 18, 1966; age 23
Last Game: September 29, 1973; age 30
Clubs: Boston AL; Chicago AL; Oakland AL

A three-sport star at South Torrance High School in suburban Los Angeles, Mike chose to play football in college. After accepting a football scholarship to UCLA, he had to spend a year at a junior college to meet UCLA's foreign language requirement. Playing split end at El Camino College, he earned junior college All-American honors. When the Boston Red Sox offered him a $12,000 signing bonus, he deserted the gridiron for the diamond. He started his professional career as a shortstop with Olean in the New York–Penn League in 1962. In 1963 and 1964 he played for Red Sox farm teams in Waterloo, Winston-Salem, and Reading, hitting well but struggling with his defense. In 1965 and 1966 he was promoted to the Toronto Maple Leafs of the International League, where manager Dick Williams converted him into a second baseman. In 1967 Williams was Boston's rookie manager and Andrews was the team's rookie second baseman. They were together two years in Toronto, three years in Boston, and later for a few eventful months in Oakland. In 1968 Andrews led AL second sackers in Faber System points.[4] After the 1970 season Mike was traded to Chicago, but the White Sox released him at his request in July 1973 so he could sign as a free agent with Oakland, where Dick Williams was managing the A's toward a third straight pennant.

Once the post-season rosters were set with Mike at second base, Oakland's eccentric owner, Charlie Finley, wanted to add a highly touted late-season acquisition, Manny Trillo, to the roster, but was blocked from doing so by Commissioner Bowie Kuhn. In the second game of the World Series, the Mets had taken a one-run lead in the twelfth inning when John Milner hit a ball that took a bad hop past Andrews. The next batter, Jerry Grote, hit a grounder to Mike, who fielded it cleanly but his throw to first base pulled Gene Tenace off the bag. The two errors charged to Andrews led to three unearned runs and infuriated Finley. The owner and the team physician persuaded Mike to sign a document stating he had a shoulder injury and should be placed on the disabled list. Finley then added Trillo to the roster. This action upset Mike's teammates, his manager, and Oakland fans. Commissioner Kuhn ordered the reinstatement of Andrews. After the Series was over Mike was released and Williams resigned.

Mike played in Japan for the Kintetsu Buffaloes and then retired from baseball. He took a position as an agent with the Massachusetts Mutual Insurance Company. When he had played in Boston, Mike, along with many of his teammates, had been active in the Jimmy Fund, an organization devoted to helping cancer victims, particularly children. In 1979 Mike was invited to become an assistant director of the Fund. He soon gave up his insurance job to work full-time for the charity and became its executive director in 1984.

Mike Andrews was a fine young player who never developed to his full potential because of injuries. As a rookie he led the American League in sacrifice hits. His best season was 1969, when he hit .293 with an OBP of .390 and a slugging average of .455. For a time in 1973 he suffered from what he called the "throwing yips," the same inability to make a throw that afflicted Chuck Knoblauch, Steve Sax, Mike Ivie, and others.

Andrews is profiled in SABR's *Baseball Biography Project.* Ranking: Faber System fourth; *Total Baseball* eighth.

Charley Bassett

Born: Charles Edwin Bassett, February 9, 1863, Central Falls, RI
Debut: July 22, 1884; age 21
Last Game: October 15, 1892; age 29
Clubs: Providence NL; Kansas City NL; Indianapolis NL; New York NL; Louisville NL

In the spring of 1884, during his sophomore year at Brown University, Charley became a star third baseman, hitting third in the lineup. After the term was over, he made his professional debut with the Providence Grays. He played second base, shortstop, third base, outfield, and even caught one game, filling in wherever needed. He was a thin young man, weighing only 150 pounds, yet he never hit his weight with the Grays, batting .139 and .144 in his two years with the club. Nevertheless, Kansas City gave him a try at shortstop in 1886. Indianapolis installed him at second base in 1887 and he led the league in Faber System fielding points.[5] After three years with the Hoosiers he went to New York and again led the league in fielding in 1891, but this time at third base for the Giants.[6] He closed out his major league career with Louisville in 1892 at the age of 29. He never became a good hitter, but he fielded well enough to play in the majors nine seasons and in the minors for another five. He played for Providence in the Eastern League from 1893 through 1897. In 1899 he joined the Pawtucket police force and remained on the force until he received his pension. He later worked at the Rhode Island Hospital Trust in Providence as a security guard until 1932. He died at Memorial Hospital in Pawtucket on May 28, 1942, at the age of 80.

Ranking: Faber System twelfth; *Total Baseball* thirteenth.

Jerry Browne

Born: Jerome Austin Browne, February 13, 1966, Christiansted, Virgin Islands
Debut: September 6, 1986; age 20
Last Game: October 1, 1995; age 29
Clubs: Texas AL; Cleveland AL; Oakland AL; Florida NL

Jerry was signed as an amateur free agent by the Texas Rangers in 1983. He spent four years on the farm in the Gulf Coast, Midwest, Carolina, and Texas leagues. In 1986 he hit .303 for Tulsa and led the Texas League second basemen in fielding at .984. Near the end of the season he was called up to Arlington, the eighth player born in the Virgin Islands to reach the big leagues. He started 1987 as the Rangers' regular second baseman and set the club's record for hits by a rookie. In 1988 he slumped and was sent back down to Oklahoma City in mid-year. At the end of the season, he was traded to Cleveland, where he had his best year in the majors, hitting .299 with a .370 OBP in 1989. He could not keep this up and was released by the Indians during spring training in 1992. He signed as a free agent with Oakland and spent two years with the A's, where he led the league in sacrifice hits in 1992. After winding up his major league playing career with the Florida Marlins, he continued in baseball. In 2002 he was a minor league infield instructor for the Toronto Blue Jays. Since then he has been a coach on several clubs: the Augusta GreenJackets, the Savannah Sand Gnats, the Hagerstown Suns, and the Potomac Nationals.

Although he was primarily a second baseman, Jerry logged more than 100 games at third base and in the outfield, and appeared infrequently as a designated hitter, first baseman, and shortstop.

Ranking: Faber System tenth; *Total Baseball* fourteenth.

Hub Collins

Born: Hubert B. Collins, April 15, 1864, Louisville, KY
Debut: September 4, 1886; age 22
Last Game: May 14, 1892; age 28
Clubs: Louisville AA; Brooklyn AA; Brooklyn NL

After playing for various amateur clubs in his native Louisville, Hub signed his first professional contract with Columbus of the Southern League in 1885. He played the next season with Savannah in the same loop, until his hometown team brought him to the majors late in the season. Playing mainly in the outfield, he immediately became a star, but the Colonels, needing cash, sold him to Brooklyn near the end of the 1888 season. For the two clubs Hub hit .307, led the league with 31 doubles, and was the Faber System Hitter of the Year for 1888.[7] Batting first or second in the lineup, Collins scored more than 100 runs per year for each of his first four seasons. Fast on the base paths, he stole 60 or more bases each of those years, including the league's second-best total of 85 in 1890, after Brooklyn had moved to the National League. Never as good in the field as at the plate, he was tried at all the infield positions as well as in the outfield, but logged more games at second base than any other position. His bat helped Brooklyn win pennants in 1889 and 1890, and he hit well in post-season play, with a .344 batting average and a .432 OBP, while scoring 20 runs in 16 games. During regular-season play he ranked in the top ten in his league from one to three times in almost every offensive category except home runs. In 1891 he suffered a head injury in a collision with teammate Oyster Burns, which limited him to 107 games. The next spring he appeared to be at full strength. He was hitting .299 and had a career-best .396 OBP when on May 14 he complained of a cold and removed himself from the game. The end came quickly. Seven days later, on May 21, 1892, he was dead of typhoid fever at the age of 28.

Hub Collins is profiled in *Baseball's First Stars*.

Ranking: Faber System fifth; *Total Baseball* first.

Tim Cullen

Born: Timothy Leo Cullen, February 16, 1942, San Francisco, CA
Debut: August 8, 1966; age 24
Last Game: October 1, 1972; age 30
Clubs: Washington AL; Chicago AL; Oakland AL

Tim was a basketball and baseball star at Junipero Serra High School in San Mateo. A 1960 graduate of the private school, he was named to the school's athletic hall of fame in 1991. At Santa Clara University he starred in both sports. In 1962 he played third base in the College World Series. In the championship game he was two-for-six with three runs batted in, as the Broncos lost a 12-inning thriller to the Michigan Wolverines, 5–4. In 1964 he was drafted by the Boston Red Sox, who lost him to the Washington Senators in the first-year draft. Washington traded him to the Chicago White Sox in February 1968 in a deal involving Ron Hansen, among others. In August the Sox sent Cullen back to Washington for Hansen, making them the only two players in MLB history to be traded for each other twice in the same season. In 1972 he was released. He signed as a free agent by Oakland, and the A's sent him to their farm club in Des Moines. Called up by the A's in August, he sat on the bench during the World Series that fall. In 1973 he retired from baseball to devote full-time to his business as a stock broker. Cullen was a weak hitter but a good utility man who could fill in at several positions. Despite making three errors in one inning in a 1969 game, he was considered a good fielding second baseman, and he led the AL with a .994 average in 1970. He also played a great deal at third base and shortstop. Time spent at those positions detracted from his opportunity to make putouts and assists at second base, resulting in fewer Faber System points than he might otherwise have achieved. He finished his major league career with negative 250 points, the lowest ranking of any of the 1769 position players in the book *Baseball Ratings*.[8] In 2009

Tim was back in baseball as vice president of special projects for the Fresno Grizzlies, a San Francisco affiliate in the Class AAA Pacific Coast League.

Ranking: Faber System seventeenth; *Total Baseball* eleventh.

Gene DeMont

Born: Eugene Napoleon DeMontreville, March 26, 1874, St. Paul, MN
Debut: August 20, 1894; age 20
Last Game: April 26, 1904; age 30
Clubs: Pittsburgh NL; Washington NL; Baltimore NL; Chicago NL; Brooklyn NL; Boston NL; Washington AL; St. Louis AL

Although he never officially changed his name, it was usually shortened in newspapers and other publications to DeMont or Demont. He started playing baseball after his family moved from St. Paul to Washington. Gene commenced his professional career with Binghamton in the Eastern League in 1894, around the time of his 20th birthday. Before that first season was over, he played for Buffalo and made his major league debut with Pittsburgh. After playing only two games with the Pirates, he was back in the Eastern League at Toronto for most of the following year before making it to Washington near the end of the season. The next two years in Washington were his best years at the plate. In 1896 DeMont hit .343, scored 94 runs, batted in 77, and had an OBP of .381. His 1897 numbers were similar — a .341 batting average, 92 runs scored, 93 RBIs, and .366 OBP. However, his performance in the field left something to be desired. Playing shortstop, he led the league with 97 errors in 1896 and 78 the next year. He was then traded to Brooklyn and played mainly at second base during the remainder of his career. DeMont spent all or part of 11 seasons in the majors with eight different teams and compiled a career batting average of .303. From 1905 through 1910 he played in the minor leagues at Toledo, Birmingham, and New Orleans, where he was a playing manager. After hanging up his spikes he continued managing at New Orleans. At some point he also managed at Montreal and Meridian. Over the course of his career in the majors and minors combined, DeMont played for or managed clubs in 17 different cities.

On February 18, 1935, as manager of concessions at the Mid-South Fairgrounds in Memphis, he suffered a fatal heart attack while running to investigate a minor fire. He died at the age of 61.

Eugene DeMontreville is profiled in *Nineteenth Century Stars*. Ranking: Faber System and *Total Baseball* both rank him seventh.

Marcus Giles

Born: Marcus William Giles, May 18, 1978, San Diego, CA
Debut: April 17, 2001; age 22
Last Game: September 28, 2007; age 29
Clubs: Atlanta NL; San Diego NL

At the age of 18 Marcus was selected by the Atlanta Braves in the 53rd round of the 1996 amateur draft. He had played baseball in Little League, in Pony League, and at Granite Hills High School in El Cajon. When he was 12 years old he got an up-close view of professional ball. His older brother, Brian, who was playing for the Watertown Indians, got him a summer job as a batboy. Players gave the boy a rough initiation, sending him to look for a box of curveballs, the key to the batter's box, and left-handed fungo bats before letting him in on the joke. Brian said, "The best thing after that game, he drank a whole twelve-pack. I was so proud of him."[9] Marcus spent many of his summers with Brian, including long bus rides during minor league seasons and hanging around big league clubhouses after his older brother made it to the majors. Years later they played together for one season in San Diego. Marcus spent four years in the minors at Danville, Macon, Myrtle Beach, and Greenville before being called up to Atlanta. He split 2001 and 2002 between the Braves and Richmond.

In 2003 he became a regular for the Braves and was named to the NL squad for the All-Star game. He was unable to play in the contest, however, because he suffered a concussion in a collision on the base paths with Mark Prior about a week before the game. Nevertheless, 2003 was his best season in the majors. Marcus hit a career-high .316 with a .390 OBP. He led the NL in Faber System points at second base in fielding and in total play.[10] In 2004 he collided with center fielder Andruw Jones as both were chasing the same pop fly. A broken collarbone, a concussion, and a bruised wrist caused him to miss 52 games. After a brief rehab in Rome and Myrtle Beach, Giles was back and avoided further injury, although he was hospitalized briefly in 2006 with acid reflux. The Braves released him after the 2007 season, and he played one year for San Diego before the Padres waived him. In 2008 Marcus signed a minor league contract with Colorado but was released before the start of the season, whereupon he agreed with the Dodgers on a minor league contract but changed his mind and did not report. In January 2009 he signed a minor league contract with the Phillies but did not make the team and was released in March.

Ranking: Faber System sixth; *Total Baseball* tied for third.

Wilton Guerrero

Born: Wilton Alvaro Guerrero, October 24, 1974, Don Gregorio, Dominican Republic
Debut: September 3, 1996; age 21
Last Game: October 1, 2004; age 29
Clubs: Los Angeles NL; Montreal NL; Cincinnati NL; Kansas City AL

The 17-year-old Dominican was signed by the Los Angeles Dodgers as a free agent in the fall of 1991. He made his professional debut with the Great Falls Dodgers in 1993, moved up to Vero Beach in 1994, San Antonio in 1995, and Albuquerque in 1996, before making it to the big leagues in September of that year. He split 1997 between the Dukes and the parent club. During the season he was suspended for eight games and fined $1000 for using a corked bat. In mid-season 1998 he was traded to Montreal, where he joined his younger brother, Vladimir. In September 2000 the Guerreros became the first pair of brothers to homer in the same game four different times. At the end of that season Wilton was granted free agency and played with various clubs over the next several years, including Cincinnati, Montreal again, and Kansas City in the majors and Louisville, Omaha, Memphis, and Charlotte in the minors. After the 2005 season he returned to the Dominican Republic and resumed his career in his native land.

Wilton was a good hitter, averaging .282 in the majors and .312 in the minors. He had very little power, hitting only eleven major league home runs and getting ten round-trippers in the minors. He was an adequate fielder at second base, shortstop, or in the outfield, making him a very useful utility player. However, utility players seldom compile good statistics. Wilton never played more than 132 games or had more than 357 times at bat in a major league season. Consequently, his numbers do not do him justice.

Ranking: Faber System sixteenth; *Total Baseball* fifteenth.

Frankie Gustine

Born: Frank William Gustine, February 20, 1920, Hoopeston, IL
Debut: September 13, 1939; age 19
Last Game: May 17, 1950; age 30
Clubs: Pittsburgh NL; Chicago NL; St. Louis AL

In the summer of 1936 when Frankie was 16 years old and playing for the Union Printers, a semi-pro team on the South Side of Chicago, Hall of Fame third baseman and Pittsburgh Pirates scout Pie Traynor signed him to a minor league contract. After Frankie graduated from Parker High School the next spring, he made his professional debut with Paducah in the Kitty

League and moved up to the Hutchinson Larks of the Western Association at midseason. He started 1939 with Gadsden of the Southeastern League and, still a teenager, was called up to Pittsburgh in September. For the next nine years Gustine played for the Pirates, mostly at second base but frequently at shortstop or third base. His progress was hindered somewhat by a chronic double hernia and assorted injuries. The hernia may also have kept him out of the armed forces during World War II, when so many major leaguers were serving their country. Frankie made the National League All-Star team three consecutive years, starting in 1946. In 1947 he led NL third basemen in both putouts and assists. It was also his best year at the plate, as he hit .297 with an OBP of .364. According to the Faber System he was the league's best fielding second sacker in both 1947 and 1948.[11] After the 1948 season he was traded to Chicago. He divided 1949 between the Cubs and their farm club in Los Angeles. In the fall of 1949 he was selected off waivers by the Philadelphia A's but was traded to the St. Louis Browns before the next season began. The Browns released him in May 1950.

Gustine became part-owner of a Sheraton Inn in Pittsburgh. His co-owner, John E. Connelly, also owned a casino riverboat. Frankie was in Davenport, Iowa, for the first voyage of the boat when he suffered a heart attack and died at the age of 71 on April Fools Day, 1991.

Ranking: Faber System ninth; *Total Baseball* sixteenth.

Jim Lefebvre

Born: James Kenneth Lefebvre, January 7, 1942, Inglewood, CA
Debut: April 12, 1965; age 23
Last Game: September 19, 1972; age 30
Club: Los Angeles NL

From the age of eight Jim was groomed by his father, Benny Lefebvre, for a major league career. Benny ran a baseball camp in Catalina, and would not let his son play Little League baseball for fear the coaches would teach him bad habits. Serving as a batboy for the Los Angeles Dodgers, the lad picked up some valuable hints. At Morningside High School Jim and his brothers were stars. Playing shortstop Jim hit .450 his senior season and shared MVP honors with his twin Tip, a catcher, who hit .420. Younger brother Gil hit .351 as a third baseman that year. In 1962 Jim signed with the Dodgers for an $8000 bonus. The Angels offered considerably more but Benny thought Jim would have a better future with the Dodgers. Assigned to the Reno Silver Sox, Jim became a fan favorite. He batted .327, hit 39 home runs, and drove in 132 runs. Named to the California League all-star team, he was the club's most valuable player, and received the Helms Foundation's award as the outstanding first-year professional from Southern California. In 1963 he made the Northwest League all-star team as a member of the Salem Dodgers. Jim spent some time in the army but was discharged in time to play for Spokane in the Pacific Coast League late in the 1964 season. That winter he starred in the Arizona Rookie League. He was called up to the big club in 1965 and spent his entire major league playing career with the Dodgers, mainly as a second baseman but frequently at third base. He was the NL Rookie of the Year in 1965. In the majors he never came close to his minor league stats. His best year was 1966 when he hit .274 with 24 home runs and made the NL All-Star team. While with the Dodgers Jim earned considerable notoriety for appearing on television shows, especially *Gilligan's Island* and *Batman.*

After the 1973 season Lefebvre was released by the Dodgers and went to Japan, where he played for the Lotte Orions from 1973 through 1976. After returning from Japan, Jim has served in a number of baseball capacities all over the world. He managed the Lethbridge Dodgers in the Rookie League in 1978, and then was the Dodgers' first base coach in 1979 before becoming hitting coach for the San Francisco Giants from 1980 to 1982. He was director of player development for the Giants in 1983–84 and managed the Phoenix Giants in 1985 and 1986. From 1989 to 1991 he managed the Seattle Mariners. The next two years he was manager of the Chicago Cubs. For the next several years he was a hitting coach, first for Oakland, and then for Milwaukee. In 1999 he served as interim manager of the Brewers. He spent two years conducting hitting clinics in Europe, and joined the staff of the Cincinnati Reds in 2002. From 2003 to 2006 Lefebvre managed the Chinese national team in various Asian championship games and in the 2006 World Baseball Classic. He also managed the Chinese team in the 2008 Summer Olympics. After three years as a hitting instructor in the San Diego farm system, Jim became the hitting coach for the Padres in 2009.

Ranking: Faber System eleventh; *Total Baseball* tied for third; James first.

Barry McCormick

Born: William J. McCormick, December 25, 1874, Maysville, KY
Debut: September 25, 1895; age 20
Last Game: August 30, 1904; age 29
Clubs: Louisville NL; Chicago NL; St. Louis AL; Washington AL

Barry is included here as an early leaver because he played his last major league game at the age of 29. However, he spent almost his entire adult life in the sport. He broke into the professional game with Louisville at the age of 20 and was involved almost continuously as a player, manager or umpire until he retired 41 years later. A versatile utility infielder, he was not a productive hitter but he could play second base, shortstop or third base. He did have one memorable day with the bat, however. On June 29, 1897, he went six-for-eight, with a triple, a home run, and five runs scored for Chicago in a 36–7 trouncing of Louisville. After seven years in the National League (six of them with Chicago), he jumped to the St. Louis Browns in 1902. The Browns traded him to Washington the following year. His hitting was not good enough to keep him in the majors, but he extended his career by eight years in the minors, most of them with Milwaukee in the American Association. McCormick played a short time with Minneapolis and St. Paul, then finished his playing career as a second baseman in 1912 in the Ohio State League, where he played for and managed the Newark and Mansfield clubs. In 1913 he managed Peoria in the Three-I League. He umpired in the National League from 1917 through 1929. He was behind the plate calling balls and strikes in the longest game in major league history, the 26-inning marathon between Brooklyn and Boston in 1920. From 1930 to 1936 Barry umpired in the International League.

Barry McCormick died of a heart ailment in Cincinnati on January 28, 1956, at the age of 81.

Ranking: Faber System fourteenth; *Total Baseball* seventeenth and last place.

Cass Michaels

Born: Casimir Eugene Kwietniewski, March 4, 1926, Detroit, MI
Debut: August 19, 1943; age 17
Last Game: August 27, 1954; age 28
Clubs: Chicago AL; Washington AL; St. Louis AL; Philadelphia AL

Although Cass was a star in Detroit's parochial high school league and hung around Nevin Field, the Tigers' ballpark, he did not sign with his hometown team. Instead, a Chicago scout convinced him to sign with the White Sox. Recognizing that his surname was hard to spell and pronounce, the 17 year old decided to change it upon entering pro ball. After rejecting Kwiet because it sounded too much like quiet or quit, he settled upon Michaels. The Sox played him two games at third base in 1943, then sent him to Little Rock in the Southern Association. After 54 games with the Travelers in 1944, Cass was hitting .356 with an OBP of .459. The Sox called him up to the parent club, and he never played in the minors again. A perforated ear drum caused him to be classified 4-F, disqualifying him for military service in World

War II. With so many big league players in the armed services, there was room for the teenager on the roster even though he did not hit well his first few years with the Sox. He played third base and shortstop before becoming Chicago's regular second baseman. His hitting improved somewhat over time. Bill James praised Michaels as one of the best second basemen in baseball in the late 1940s.[12] In 1949 Cass had his best year at the plate, hitting .308 with a .417 OBP, earning him a spot in the All-Star game. He was traded to Washington, where his performance declined, but he made the All-Star game again in 1950. After short stays in Washington, St. Louis, and Philadelphia, he was back in Chicago in 1954. In a game against Philadelphia on August 27, the Sox jumped on A's pitcher Marion Fricano in the first inning. The first five Chicago batters hit safely. Michaels was the sixth man up. Fricano did what many pitchers of his day would have done under similar circumstances. He threw a pitch high and inside, intending to brush the hitter back, maybe making him hit the dirt to get out of the way of the pitch. Cass had an unusual batting stance, standing wide over the plate with his left shoulder facing the pitcher and his jaw on his chest. This was before the time of the batting helmet. Michaels wore only a protective lining under his cap. A fastball hit him right on the temple. He fell straight down, bleeding from the mouth, nose, and ears. Taken to a hospital, Cass was in a coma for a while. Eventually, he recovered enough to go to spring training the next year, but he got dizzy and had to quit baseball. Michaels returned to the Detroit area, opening a neighborhood bar in suburban Warren. He died of what the funeral home called "natural causes" in a Grosse Pointe hospital on November 12, 1982. His obituary in the *New York Times* stated that the cause of death of the 56-year-old ex-ballplayer was not immediately known.

Ranking: Faber System eighth; *Total Baseball* ninth; James third.

Al Myers

Born: James Albert Myers, October 22, 1863, Danville, IL
Debut: September 27, 1884; age 20
Last Game: October 3, 1891; age 27
Clubs: Milwaukee UA; Philadelphia NL; Kansas City NL; Washington NL

Al broke into professional baseball at the age of 20 with Muskegan of the Northwestern League in 1884. When that club disbanded, he played for the Winona Clippers of the same circuit until he made it to the big leagues with the Milwaukee Brewers of the ill-fated Union Association that fall. After the UA collapsed, Al (or "Cod" as he was sometimes called) joined Philadelphia in the National League in 1885. The following year he was sold to the

Kansas City Cowboys. Seemingly Myers was a jinx for club owners, as the Cowboys dropped out at the end of the season, the third club in three years that had folded while Al was a member. The National League assigned Myers to Washington in 1887. During the 1889 season the Nationals sold Cod to Philadelphia and he finished his career in the City of Brotherly Love. Throughout his career he played almost exclusively at second base. Not a very good hitter, he had his best year at the plate in 1890, when he hit .277 and had an OBP of .365. His fielding was barely adequate, and he finished with a career fielding percentage of .911. After baseball Myers became a saloon-keeper, owning the Health Office Saloon and an apartment building in Terre Haute. He died in nearby Marshall, Illinois, on Christmas Eve 1927, at the age of 64.

Ranking: Faber System fifteenth; *Total Baseball* twelfth.

Rennie Stennett

Born: Renaldo Antonio Stennett, April 5, 1951, Colon, Panama
Debut: July 10, 1971; age 20
Last Game: August 24, 1981; age 30
Clubs: Pittsburgh NL; San Francisco NL

Before many major league clubs were recruiting in Latin America, scout Howie Haak discovered an 18-year-old prospect in Panama and signed Rennie Stennett to a Pittsburgh Pirates contract. The teenager started his professional career as an outfielder with Gastonia in the Western Carolinas League in 1969, moved to Salem in the Carolina League the next year, and played one game for Columbus in the International League at the tail end of the season. In 1971 the Pirates moved their IL affiliate to Charleston and the Charlies converted the outfielder into a second baseman. The switch to the keystone proved to be a good one for Stennett, as Pittsburgh's regular second sacker, Dave Cash, was called for active military duty in July, and Rennie was brought up to replace him. He spent the next nine years with Pittsburgh, occasionally playing other positions but keeping the second base job even when Cash returned from service. According to the Faber System, Stennett was the top fielding second baseman in the NL for three straight years, from 1974 through 1976.[13] He led NL second sackers in both putouts and total chances per game in 1974 and again in 1976, once handling 418 consecutive chances without an error.

Although he was not a great hitter, Stennett had one fantastic day at the plate. On September 16, 1975, he became the only hitter in the twentieth century to collect seven hits in one nine-inning game. Included were five singles, one double, and a triple. He also scored five runs. In 1976 he was well on his way to his best season in the majors, hitting at a .336 clip, second in the league. However, on August 21, he broke his ankle sliding into second base, ending his season prematurely. Although he never quit trying, he could not regain his former prowess. He never hit as high as .250 in his remaining years in the majors. After San Francisco released him in 1982, he signed with Montreal and was assigned to the Expos' farm club at Wichita. Although he hit .309 for the Aeros, the Expos did not bring him back to the majors. He was disappointed about his treatment by both the Giants and Montreal, but he held onto his dream of returning to the big leagues. Since breaking his ankle, he could not move as he once did, severely reducing his range. He thought the Giants did not give him a fair chance to play himself back into shape. He did not understand why the Expos released him after he hit over .300 at Wichita, ignoring the fact that he fielded at a .828 clip while there.

To keep his name noticed, he played in old-timers games, participated in autograph sessions, and was drafted by the St. Petersburg club in a fledgling Seniors Professional Baseball Association in 1989. However, a better opportunity came along. While serving as an instructor in a fantasy camp run by the Pirates in January, he showed flashes of his former range and hitting ability. He signed a contract and was invited to the Bucs' spring training camp, hoping to become the first player in the history of baseball to become an everyday player five years after retiring from the sport. He expected to start the season with the Pirates' minor league club in Buffalo. Although he hit well in the camp, Stennett did not make the team. In releasing him, Pittsburgh's director of minor league operations said, "Rennie is one of those people who will think he can hit forever. We felt like his speed, his arm, and his defensive skills had diminished."[14]

Still hopeful, Stennett crossed the Pacific to play in a Japan–United States senior all-star game in 1991. Later in the same year he crossed another ocean to participate in an Ambassadors of Baseball tour in Europe, proudly wearing his huge World Series rings from the 1971 and 1979 classics during autograph sessions. Time finally caught up with him. At last report Rennie was living in Florida and enjoying his days on the golf course.

Ranking: Faber System number one; *Total Baseball* sixth; James second.

Bill Sweeney

Born: William John Sweeney, March 6, 1886, Covington, KY
Debut: June 14, 1907; age 21
Last Game: October 5, 1914; age 28
Clubs: Chicago NL; Boston NL

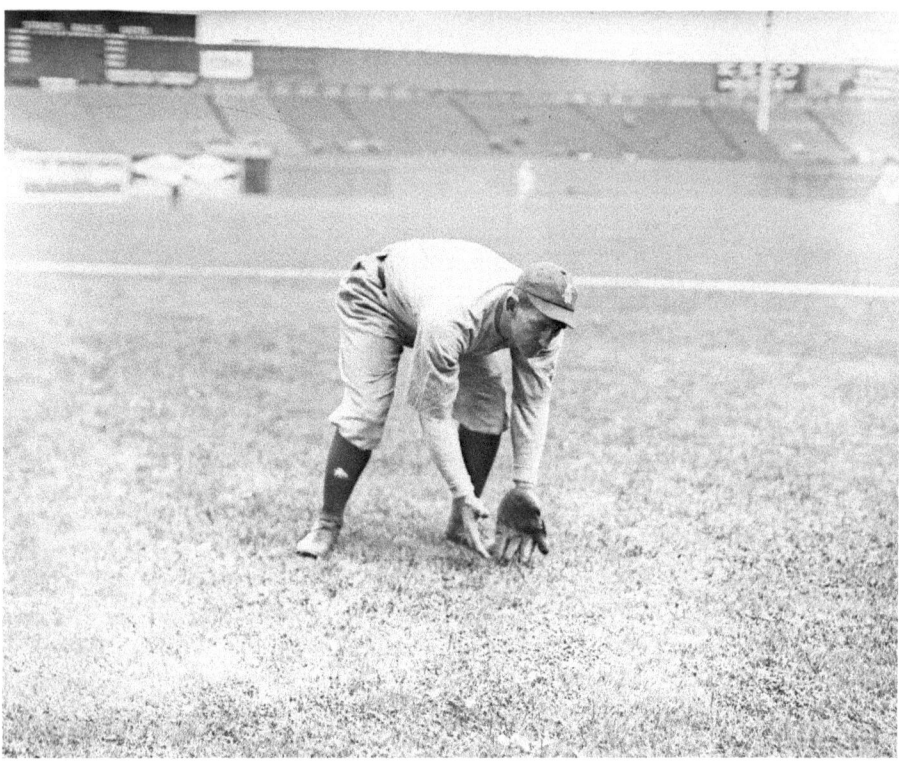

Bill Sweeney was an error-prone shortstop until he was moved to second base, where he became the National League's best second sacker in 1911 and again in 1912. In the latter year he led the league in fielding average, assists, and double plays, and set a record for putouts that stood for 21 years. In addition, he ranked near the top of the loop in nearly every batting category. However, in 1913 he suffered injuries to his wrist and throwing hand from which he never fully recovered, ending his career prematurely (Library of Congress).

Born in Covington, Bill grew up in adjacent Newport, and played shortstop in Cincinnati at Xavier (either the college or a prep school attached to the college). At the age of 18 he made his professional debut with Toledo in the American Association but did not hit well for the Mud Hens and was demoted to Rock Island of the Three-I League. With the Islanders his play improved. In 1905 he was named team captain, but in September of that year he was sold to Portland of the Pacific Coast League. At the end of the 1906 season he was drafted by the National League champion Chicago Cubs. During the offseason Bill injured his feet by lacing his roller skates too tightly and cutting off circulation. The injury made it impossible for him to break into the Cubs infield, featuring the famous double-play combination of Tinker to

Evers to Chance, plus Harry Steinfeldt at third base. Sweeney got his chance in June when Tinker suffered a Charley horse, and Bill was inserted at shortstop. Bill made six errors in three games, and the Cubs promptly traded him to Boston. Sweeney lost out on a chance to play in the World Series, as the Cubs won pennants in 1907 and 1908 and the Doves languished in the second division. In the field the young man had good range but an unusual sidearm throwing motion that caused him to lead the league in errors at his position — whether third base, shortstop, or second base — five straight years. He could make the shorter throws from second more accurately, and he was installed permanently at the keystone position. At the plate he had outstanding seasons in 1911 and 1912. In both those years his hitting and fielding enabled him to garner more Faber System points than any other NL second sacker.[15] In 1912 he was the NL Player of the Year.[16] He hit .344 with an OBP of .416, led the league in singles and times on base, was second in runs batted in, and finished in the top ten in bases on balls, doubles, triples, total bases, batting average, on-base percentage, and on-base plus slugging percentage. To top it off he led second basemen in fielding as well, setting a record for putouts that stood for 21 years, and leading the league in assists and double plays.

A few more years like that and he would have been Hall of Fame material. However, in 1913 he suffered nagging injuries to his wrist and throwing hand. In 1914 Boston traded Sweeney back to the Cubs. That was the year the Miracle Braves came from last place to win the pennant, so Sweeney lost out on another chance to play in the World Series. Bill did not hit well for the Cubs. Chicago released him in the offseason, enabling him to go to spring training with the Red Sox in 1915. However, he failed to make the team and for the third time missed out on a World Series opportunity as Boston won the classic in 1915.

In 1913 Bill had set up an insurance business in the Boston suburb of Cambridge. In 1916 he sold the Braves a $500,000 accident insurance policy from which his premium was said to amount to more than a year's salary in baseball. That same year he coached the Boston College baseball team, then retired from the sport to devote full-time to his insurance business and his family. He died in Cambridge on May 26, 1948, at the age of 64.

Biographical sketches of Bill Sweeney appear in *Deadball Stars of the National League* and in SABR's *Baseball Biography Project*. The Faber System ranks him third; *Total Baseball* has him fifth.

Bump Wills

Born: Elliott Taylor Wills, July 27, 1952, Washington, DC
Debut: April 7, 1977; age 24

Last Game: October 3, 1982; age 30
Clubs: Texas AL; Chicago NL

Being the son of a famous father may be difficult for a young man wishing to establish his own identity. It is almost impossible to find an article about Bump Wills that does not refer to him, usually in the opening sentence, as the son of Maury Wills. Bump handled the situation well. He was proud of his father, looked up to him, and even played for a team Maury managed in the Mexican League. After Maury mentioned an incident in his 1991 autobiography that Bump felt should have been kept private, relations between father and son became somewhat strained.

Nicknamed "Bump" for his childhood tendency to bump into things, the boy grew up in Los Angeles, where his father starred for the Dodgers. In 1972 and 1973 Bump helped Arizona State to the runner-up spot in the College World Series. Playing left field in 1972, he made the all-tournament team. In 1973 he was the shortstop as the Sun Devils again fell to USC in the finals. In his senior year he suffered a minor injury that caused his major league prospects to decline. He played for his father in Mexico that summer and was drafted by the Texas Rangers in the first round (sixth overall pick) in the secondary phase of the 1975 amateur draft. A switch-hitter, he hit .307 for Pittsfield and .324 for Sacramento before being called up to the majors at the beginning of the 1977 season. As a rookie he hit .287, a figure he never reached again in the big leagues. In 1978 he stole 52 bases, his career-high in that category. In the field he played almost exclusively at second base, and led AL fielders at that position twice in putouts, assists, and total chances per game. He led in Faber System fielding points in 1977, 1978, and 1981, and topped all AL second sackers in total points (hitting plus fielding) in his rookie year.[17] He lost the Rookie of the Year award to future Hall of Famer Eddie Murray.

In 1982 Bump was traded to the Chicago Cubs, who granted him free agency at the end of the season. Wills then went to Japan and played two years for the Hankyu Braves. Returning home after the 1984 season, he worked as a security guard in Arlington, Texas, before rejoining the Rangers four years later as a minor league manager. He managed in the minors for ten seasons but never made it to the big leagues. However, he never left the game of baseball. He moved to Spokane, where he gave private baseball lessons, taught at camps, and managed clinics. In 2004 he began working as an instructor with a non-profit organization called Sports USA, which built a large sports complex in the city. In 2009 he was coaching at Central Valley High School in suburban Spokane.

Bump Wills is ranked second by both the Faber System and *Total Baseball*.

Steve Yerkes

Born: Stephen Douglas Yerkes, May 15, 1888, Hatboro, PA
Debut: September 29, 1909; age 21
Last Game: October 1, 1916; age 28
Clubs: Boston AL; Pittsburgh FL; Chicago NL

Steve first made a name for himself in baseball by playing shortstop for the University of Pennsylvania in 1906. He started his professional career with Worcester in the New England League and played for Wilson in the Eastern Carolina League before getting a brief trial with the Boston Red Sox in 1909. He returned to the minors, first with Worcester again and then to Chattanooga of the Southern Association before making it back to the big club in 1911. His most memorable time with the Red Sox came during the 1912 World Series. In the first game his seventh-inning single drove in the winning run. The second game was called after eleven innings on account of darkness and ended in a tie. The Giants and the Sox split the next two contests. In the fifth game Harry Hooper hit a triple; Yerkes knocked him in with a triple of his own, and scored the deciding run on a sacrifice fly as the Sox won, 2–1, and took a three-to-one lead in Series wins. The Giants won the next two bouts to even the Series at three games apiece.

The eighth and deciding contest has been called the most exciting World Series game of the Deadball Era. With Christy Mathewson on the mound for the Giants and Smoky Joe Wood in relief of Hugh Bedient, the Giants took a 1–0 lead in the top of the tenth. In the bottom of the frame, pinch-hitter Clyde Engle led off by lifting a routine fly to Fred Snodgrass in center field. Snodgrass dropped the ball and Engle slid safely into second base. Hooper hit a liner to center, which Snodgrass corralled with a spectacular catch. Engle tagged up and advanced to third. Yerkes was up next and worked Matty for a walk. Tris Speaker, Boston's best hitter, came to the plate to face the great Giant hurler. He hit a foul popup; Mathewson, first baseman Fred Merkle, and catcher Chief Meyers circled under the ball, which dropped untouched. Given another chance Spoke spanked the ball into right field, driving in Engle with the tying run. Yerkes went to third and Speaker to second as the right fielder threw to the plate. Matty intentionally walked Duffy Lewis, setting up a force play at every base. Larry Gardner lifted a long fly to outfielder Josh Devore, who made the catch easily and threw home, but Yerkes outran the ball and scored the winning run. Yerkes had knocked in the winning run once and scored the winning tally twice as Boston won the World Series.

Two years after his heroics in 1912, Steve jumped to Pittsburgh in the Federal League. In 1915 he led the loop's second sackers in Faber System fielding points.[18] When that loop folded, he wound up his major league career by playing 44 games for the Chicago Cubs in 1916. After leaving the majors, Yerkes spent many years in the minors as a player and manager. He played for Indianapolis in the American Association from 1917 to 1923. In 1924 he managed Harrisburg in the New York–Pennsylvania League. In 1932 he skippered the Norristown/St. Clair Saints in the Interstate League. He managed in the Canadian-American League from 1936 through 1940, winning two consecutive league championships at Perth and Perth-Cornwall in 1936 and 1937, respectively. In 1947 he handled the Ogdensburg Maples of the Border League. At one time he coached the freshman team at Yale University. Wherever his baseball career took him, he maintained his residence in Pennsylvania. The 1930 census listed him as the proprietor of a bowling alley in his native Montgomery County.

Steve Yerkes died in Lansdale, Pennsylvania, in the county of his birth, on January 31, 1971, at the age of 82. Ranking: Faber System thirteenth; *Total Baseball* tenth.

SHORTSTOPS

	G	R	H	HR	RBI	BA	OBP	Faber System Hit	Field	Total
Don Buddin	711	342	551	41	225	.241	.358	142	210	352
Ray Chapman	1051	671	1053	17	364	.278	.358	608	394	1002
Frank Fennelly	786	609	781	34	408	.257	.345	453	44	497
Shorty Fuller	964	652	867	6	350	.236	.323	35	53	88
Bill Gleason	798	613	907	7	298	.267	.313	494	-296	198
Enzo Hernandez	714	241	522	2	113	.224	.283	-111	147	36
Sonny Jackson	936	396	767	7	162	.251	.308	61	-60	1
Buddy Kerr	1067	378	903	31	333	.249	.312	12	637	649
Tony Kubek	1092	522	1109	57	373	.266	.303	201	394	595
Manny Lee	922	304	686	19	249	.255	.305	14	222	236
Kevin Stocker	846	340	703	23	248	.254	.338	-101	302	201
Buck Weaver	1254	623	1308	21	420	.272	.307	291	244	535

Don Buddin

Born: Donald Thomas Buddin, May 5, 1934, Turbeville, SC
Debut: April 17, 1956; age 21
Last Game: September 25, 1961; age 27
Clubs: Boston AL; Houston NL; Detroit AL

Don Buddin first made the sports pages as a 13-year-old pitcher/infielder with American Legion teams in his native South Carolina. At Olanta High

School he earned all-star honors in baseball, basketball, and football. He hit .612 his senior year as Olanta won the state baseball championship. In an all-star football game, the Pee Dee Tobacco Bowl, he was "head over shoulders the best offensive and defensive back on the field."[19] During his freshman year at Wofford College Don played football, intramural basketball, and starred on the baseball team. Scout Mace Brown signed him to a contract with the Boston Red Sox for a $50,000 bonus, saying, "He's the best major league prospect I've ever scouted."[20] The Sox assigned him to Roanoke in the Piedmont League and then promoted him to Greensboro, where he made the Carolina League all-star team and led the loop with 123 RBIs in 1953. Buddin made the leap to the International League in 1954, playing two years with the Louisville Colonels. The Red Sox sent him to Venezuela for winter ball in 1954–55. After his rookie year in Boston, he missed the entire 1957 season while serving in the army. He managed the Third Army baseball team at Fort McPherson and spent some time in Korea. In five years with the Sox, Don never hit up to expectations and became the target of boos from the fans because of his erratic fielding. Although he had good range and could go well both to his right and left, he had trouble fielding balls hit directly at him. In 1958 and again in 1959 he led AL shortstops in errors. He also led the circuit in double plays both years. After the 1961 season the Red Sox traded him to Houston. The next year the Colt .45s sold him to Detroit. He did not hit well for either of those clubs and was sent to the minors. He played for Syracuse in 1962, Richmond in 1963, Rochester in 1964, and finally for Knoxville in 1965. After retiring from baseball, Buddin returned to South Carolina, where he has managed a liquor store, sold insurance, and served as the general manager of a local newspaper.

The Faber System and *Total Baseball* both rank him sixth.

Ray Chapman

Born: Raymond Johnson Chapman, January 15, 1891, Beaver Dam, KY
Debut: August 30, 1912; age 21
Last Game: August 16, 1920; age 29
Club: Cleveland AL

See entry on Ray Chapman in Part One of this book. Chapman is profiled in *Deadball Stars of the American League* and in SABR's *Biography Project*. The Faber System, *Total Baseball,* and Bill James all agree in placing him first among shortstops making a premature exit.

Frank Fennelly

Born: Francis John Fennelly, February 18, 1860, Fall River, MA
Debut: May 1, 1884; age 24
Last Game: June 18, 1890; age 30
Clubs: Washington AA; Cincinnati AA; Philadelphia AA; Brooklyn AA

Frank first gained attention as a member of the Flints, a strong amateur team in his native Fall River. He made his pro debut with the Camden Merritts of the Inter-State League in 1882. On May 25 of that year he went six-for-six, with a double, three triples, and two home runs for 19 total bases, a record that was not matched in any professional league for more than a century. In 1883 he played for Brooklyn in the same league. He started his major league career with Washington in 1884 but was sold to Cincinnati during his rookie year for an amount variously reported as $1000 and $2500. For the next four years he was part of the era's most famous infield, joining Long John Reilly at first base, Bid McPhee at second, and Hick Carpenter at third. Fennelly was considered one of the most graceful shortstops in the game. He and McPhee were rated as the best keystone combo of the 1880s by Bill James.[21] The statistics, however, reveal that Fennelly's fielding may not have been as good as it looked. In 1886 he set an all-time American Association record with 117 errors and followed that with 99 miscues in 1887. In 1884 Frank ranked among the leaders in batting average, on-base percentage, slugging, doubles, triples, and bases on balls. He led the AA with 89 RBIs in 1885 and finished among the circuit's top ten in that category three times. He was runner-up for the home run crown in 1885. A leader on the field, Frank served as team captain both at Cincinnati and in Brooklyn. In 1890 he tore ligaments in his leg while sliding into a base, ending his major league career. However, he came back in 1893 to play for Fall River in the New England League and played a few games for Portland the following year. From 1905 to 1908 Fennelly represented Fall River in the Massachusetts legislature. Census reports show him as an insurance collector in 1900 and 1910 and as a census enumerator in 1920. He died in Fall River on August 4, 1920, at the age of 60.

Frank Fennelly is profiled in *Baseball's First Stars*. He is ranked fifth by the Faber System and second by *Total Baseball*.

Shorty Fuller

Born: William Benjamin Fuller, October 10, 1867, Cincinnati, OH
Debut: July 19, 1888; age 20
Last Game: June 2, 1896; age 28
Clubs: Washington NL; St. Louis AA; New York NL

Ben Fuller came by his nickname honestly. He was listed at 5'6" in height. At the age of 19 he broke into professional baseball with the New Orleans Pelicans of the Southern Association and was in the major leagues with the Washington Nationals the following season. Shorty got off to a terrible start with the Nats, hitting only .182 for the season and committing four errors in one inning in a game against Indianapolis on August 17. In December he was sold to the St. Louis Browns for $800. Despite a career batting average of .236 and a fielding percentage of .891, Fuller managed to stay in the major leagues for nine seasons. His best season was 1890, when he hit .278, scored 118 runs, and stole 60 bases. From 1896 through 1899 he played in the minor leagues for such teams as the Springfield Ponies of the Eastern League, the New York Metropolitans of the Atlantic Association, and the Detroit Tigers and Columbus Senators of the Western League. In 1903 he attempted a comeback with a team in Muncie but became ill with a lung condition and had to give up baseball. On April 11, 1904, Ben Fuller died at his home in Cincinnati, probably from tuberculosis. He was 36 years old.

In both the Faber System rankings and *Total Baseball*'s compilation Shorty Fuller ranks tenth.

Bill Gleason

Born: William G. Gleason, November 12, 1858, St. Louis, MO
Debut: May 2, 1882; age 23
Last Game: June 18, 1889; age 29
Clubs: St. Louis AA; Philadelphia AA; Louisville AA

As a teenager, Bill played semi-pro ball with the St. Louis Reds in 1876. During the next two years he played for teams in Minneapolis and Peoria. In 1879 he and his brother Jack played in a recognized professional league with the Dubuque Red Stockings of the Northwestern League. In 1880 the brothers returned to St. Louis and semi-pro ball with the Reds and with the Browns in 1881. The next season the Browns gained a franchise in the American Association, and Bill spent his entire major league career in that circuit. As a rookie, Bill led AA shortstops in assists and total chances per game, as well as in errors. He was considered to be an above-average fielder, but the statistics do not support his reputation. Gleason was known to give a runner a knee or a hip when one came past second base, making him disliked by opponents. One writer stated, "If some day he should break a limb or his neck, not a ballplayer in the American Association would feel the slightest regret."[22] At the plate he was a good singles hitter with little power and an ability to get on base by walks or being hit by the pitcher. In one game in 1887 he was credited with going seven-for-seven, although four of his hits were actually bases on balls. (For the only time in major league history, walks were counted as hits in 1887.) He was credited with a .336 batting average in 1887 under the scoring rules of that year, but that figure has been reduced to .288 by deleting 41 walks from his hit total. The 135 runs he scored that season were legitimate. On the base paths Gleason was aggressive, fearlessly colliding with fielders in an era when breaking up a double play was not an accepted style of play. After the 1887 season Bill was traded to the Athletics but hit poorly and was benched. He quit before attempting a comeback with Louisville in 1889 but could not make the grade. He spent two years in the minors (Washington of the Atlantic Association in 1890 and Rockford of the Three-I League in 1891) before retiring from baseball. Gleason had worked for the St. Louis fire department during the offseason for many years. In 1892 he joined the department full-time and by 1907 was promoted to captain. He was still with the firemen when he died on July 21, 1932, at the age of 73.

Bill Gleason is profiled in *Nineteenth Century Stars*. The Faber System ranks him ninth; *Total Baseball* places him eighth; Bill James has him fourth.

Enzo Hernandez

Born: Enzo Octavio Hernandez, February 12, 1949, Valle de Guanape, Venezuela
Debut: April 17, 1971; age 22
Last Game: August 19, 1978; age 29
Club: San Diego NL

Enzo was signed as an amateur free agent by the Houston Astros in 1967. The teenager started his professional career with Cocoa in the Florida State League and immediately gave an indication of what his future would be like by hitting .187. At the end of the season he was traded to the Baltimore Orioles and spent three years in the team's farm system, playing for Greensboro, Oklahoma City, Miami, Dallas–Fort Worth, and Rochester. Enzo moved steadily through the minor league ranks, from Class A to Class AAA, despite his weakness at the plate. A typical "good field-no hit" shortstop, he advanced on the strength of his defense. Before the start of the 1971 season he was traded to the San Diego Padres. In his rookie season he finished last among qualifiers in all of the Triple Crown categories, with a .222 BA, 0 HR, and 12 RBIs. Twelve RBIs in 549 at-bats represents one of the least productive seasons in major league history. With a league-leading 33 errors in the field, he almost became the first player ever to have three times as many errors as RBIs. Bill James wrote that San Diego's 1974 double-play combination of Derrel Thomas and Enzo was one of the worst of all time.[23] Yet Hernandez managed to be the Padres' regular shortstop for six years. During spring training in 1978 he was released by San Diego and signed with Los Angeles. He played most of the season with the Dodgers' farm team in Albuquerque. He retired at the end of the season. He has disappeared from America's sports pages, except for stories about the worst hitters of all-time and articles about the long line of Venezuelan shortstops in the major leagues. The Estadio de Beisbol Enzo Hernandez in Anzoategui state, Venezuela, has been named in his honor.

Ranking: Faber System eleventh; *Total Baseball* ninth.

Sonny Jackson

Born: Roland Thomas Jackson, July 9, 1944, Washington, DC
Debut: September 27, 1963; age 19
Last Game: July 9, 1974; age 30
Clubs: Houston NL; Atlanta NL

Jackson got the nickname "Sonny" as a boy and carried it with him into the major leagues, probably because of his slight stature and youthful appearance. He was signed out of Silver Spring's Montgomery Blair High School at age 18 by Billy Jurges, a scout for the Houston Colt .45's. He worked his way up the Houston farm system rapidly—Class A Modesto in 1963, Class AA San Antonio in 1964, and Class AAA Oklahoma City in 1965. In the latter year he hit .330 and led the Pacific Coast League with 193 hits. During each of those minor league seasons, Sonny joined the big club for a few games at the end of the year. He was still considered a rookie in 1966 when he became a full-time big leaguer. He led the league in singles and sacrifice hits, and was second in stolen bases, earning him the runner-up spot for Rookie of the Year honors. After two years in Houston, Jackson was traded to the Atlanta Braves. Hampered by injuries, he never hit well again after that good start, and his fielding left something to be desired. In 1971 the Braves moved him from shortstop to the outfield. He played his last major league game on his thirtieth birthday, and finished the 1974 season at Class AAA Richmond. He played two more seasons in the minors, with the Hawaiian Islanders in 1975 and the Iowa Oaks in 1976. After he retired as a player, Jackson continued in baseball in various capacities, mostly in the Atlanta Braves' farm system. He coached their minor league teams in Kingsport, Savannah, and Richmond, managed the Anderson Braves in 1980–81, served as a roving minor league instructor, and was on the big league staff in 1982–83. After 19 years in the employ of the Braves, he has worked for the San Francisco Giants and the Chicago Cubs.

Ranking: Faber System twelfth; *Total Baseball* eleventh.

Buddy Kerr

Born: John Joseph Kerr, November 6, 1922, Astoria, NY
Debut: September 8, 1943; age 20
Last Game: September 30, 1951; age 28
Clubs: New York NL; Boston NL

Growing up in Queens, Buddy idolized the New York Giants and was thrilled to sign a contract with the club in 1941 at the age of 18. The Giants sent the youngster to their farm club at Fort Smith. During the next two seasons he played for the Jersey City Giants until he was called up to the majors late in 1943. In his first big league at-bat, he hit a home run. Kerr was granted a draft deferment to support his family and played throughout World War II. A weak hitter, Kerr excelled in the field. He led NL shortstops in putouts, assists, double plays, and total chances in 1945, and in fielding percentage in 1946. He set a major league record (since broken) by playing 68 consecutive errorless games at shortstop. According to the Faber System, Buddy was the best all-around shortstop in the NL in 1945[24] and the loop's top fielder in 1946.[25] For his career he ranks sixth among shortstops in fielding points per season.[26] He was named to the NL All-Star team in 1948. Kerr's boyhood hero, Mel Ott, was fired as manager of the Giants in 1948. Buddy and the new manager, Leo Durocher, did not get along, and Kerr was traded to the Boston Braves following the 1949 season. After two years with Boston, he went back to the minor leagues, playing Class AAA ball for Baltimore, Milwaukee, Toledo, and Toronto. In 1956 he became a manager in the Giants' farm system, moving from Cocoa to Selma, Michigan City, Fresno, Quincy, and Springfield. From 1975 through 2000 he worked for the Mets as a special assignment scout. After a short illness, Kerr died in a New York City hospital on November 7, 2006, the day after his 84th birthday.

Ranking: Faber System second; *Total Baseball* seventh.

Tony Kubek

Born: Anthony Christopher Kubek, October 12, 1935, Milwaukee, WI
Debut: April 20, 1957; age 21
Last Game: October 3, 1965; age 29
Club: New York AL

Tony first attracted attention in the sports pages at the age of 14 or 15 (the year of his birth is disputed) when he played for Milwaukee against Waukesha in the annual Stars of Tomorrow game in 1950. Two years later he played in the Hearst All-Star game at the Polo Grounds. The lad's accomplishments were not limited to baseball. In 1952 he made third-string end on Wisconsin's all-state football team. That winter he was the star guard on Bay View High School's basketball squad. He signed with the New York Yankees in 1954 and was assigned to Owensboro of the Kitty League, moving up to Quincy of the Three-I League, and Denver in the American Association. His batting average for the three minor league seasons was .335, earning him advancement to the majors in 1957. He was the AL Rookie of the Year and remained with the Yankees for his entire career, missing only part of the 1962 season when he was in the military. He did not hit as well in the majors as he had in the minors, but his fielding put him on the AL All-Star team four times. During his nine seasons with the Bronx Bombers, Kubek played in the World Series six times. He is most remembered for an incident that happened in Game 7 of the 1960 classic. With the Yankees leading, 7–4, in the eighth inning, Pittsburgh's Bill Virdon hit a grounder that took a bad hop, hitting Tony in the throat and seriously injuring him. Kubek's error contributed to a Pittsburgh rally, setting the stage for Bill Mazeroski's dramatic walk-off homer in the bottom of the ninth. Kubek recovered to play several more years, but a neck and back condition forced him to retire at the age of 29. Tony then became an analyst on NBC's *Game of the Week* telecasts for 24 years and also worked post-season and All-Star games. In addition, he broadcast Toronto Blue Jays games from 1977 to 1989 and Yankees games from 1990 to 1994. He earned respect for the honesty and intelligence of his analyses. In 2008 he earned the Ford Frick Award, which is given annually to a broadcaster by the Baseball Hall of Fame. Kubek returned to Wisconsin, where he lives in Appleton and is a certified teacher of English as a second language. His students are mostly but not exclusively Hmong immigrants from Asia.

Tony Kubek is ranked third by the Faber System, fourth by *Total Baseball*, and second by James.

Manny Lee

Born: Manuel Lora Lee, June 17, 1965, San Pedro de Macoris, Dominican Republic
Debut: April 10, 1985; age 19
Final Game: April 26, 1995; age 29
Clubs: Toronto AL; Texas AL; St. Louis NL

The New York Mets signed the 16-year-old Dominican in 1982 and assigned him to Kingsport of the Appalachian League. In 1983 he played for the Mets' Gulf Coast League team and Little Falls of the New York–Penn League. Despite Lee's poor batting averages with his first three teams, the Mets promoted him to Columbia in the South Atlantic League, where he hit higher than .300 for the only time in his career. At the end of the season the Mets traded Lee to Houston. He never played a game for the Astros, as they did not protect him in the 1984 Rule 5 draft and watched Toronto select him. Still a teenager, Manny made his major league debut with the Blue Jays and spent his entire rookie season with them, although he hit only .200 and had no home runs or RBIs in 64 games. The next year he played 35 games for the Jays but spent most of the season in the minors at Knoxville and Syracuse. In 1987 he again split the season between Toronto and Syracuse. In 1988 Manny had his best year, hitting his major league-high at .291 while playing mostly second base. For the next four years he was a regular in the Jays' lineup at either second base or shortstop. At the end of the 1992 season Manny was granted free agency and signed with Texas, where he was to be the Rangers' starting shortstop. However, injuries limited his playing time. He was playing well in 1994 when the season ended early because of the strike. In October he was made a free agent. In April 1995, Lee signed with St. Louis but was injured during his first game with the Cardinals. He was sent to Louisville on a rehab assignment. After 12 games with the AA club, the Cardinals released him, and Manny announced his retirement.

Ranking: Faber System seventh; *Total Baseball* twelfth.

Kevin Stocker

Born: Kevin Douglas Stocker, February 13, 1970, Spokane, WA
Debut: July 7, 1993: age 23
Last Game: September 29, 2000; age 30
Clubs: Philadelphia NL; Tampa Bay AL; Anaheim AL

Kevin played baseball at Central Valley High School in suburban Spokane and at the University of Washington. He was drafted by the Philadelphia Phillies in the second round of the 1991 amateur draft. The Phillies sent him to Spartanburg in the South Atlantic League and promoted him in 1992 to Clearwater in the Florida League and then Reading in the Eastern League. He started the 1993 season with Scranton/Wilkes-Barre. Although he was hitting only .233 for the International League club, the Phillies called him up in midseason because they needed his glove at shortstop. To the Phils' pleasant surprise, after the promotion Stocker hit .324 in 70 games, the only time in his career he topped the .300 mark. For the next four years, Kevin was a Phillie, with occasional trips back down to Scranton. In November 1997 he was traded to Tampa Bay for Bobby Abreu, surely one of the most lopsided trades in history. Hampered by injuries, he did not fare well in St. Petersburg. In the spring of 2000 the Rays released him, and he signed with Anaheim but hit only .197 for the Angels. In 2001 he played one game for Las Vegas in the Pacific Coast League before his playing career was over. Stocker returned to the Spokane area. At last report he was living in Liberty Lake and was the owner of an Emerald City Smoothie franchise. He has been described as a switch-hitter who could not hit from either side of the plate, but his fielding was good enough to keep him in the majors for seven years.

Ranking: Faber System eighth; *Total Baseball* fifth.

Buck Weaver

Born: George Daniel Weaver, August 18, 1890, Pottstown, PA
Debut: April 11, 1912; age 21
Last Game: September 27, 1920; age 30
Club: Chicago AL

Buck Weaver is remembered primarily as the third baseman on the infamous Chicago Black Sox of 1919. Ty Cobb named him the third baseman on his all-time all-star team. Actually, he played nearly twice as many games at shortstop as at the hot corner. As a teenager he was given the nickname "Buck" because of his passionate style of play and his upbeat, positive attitude. He was playing semi-pro ball in Northampton, Massachusetts, in 1909 when Charley Dooin, manager of the Philadelphia Phillies, signed him to play for the York White Roses in the Tri-State League for $175 a month. In the fall of 1910 the Chicago White Sox bought his contract and assigned him to San Francisco of the Pacific Coast League. After a good year with the Seals, he was called up to the Sox in the spring of 1912. He soon earned another nickname when a *Chicago Tribune* reporter wrote, "Weaver plugged the hole at shortstop by going into the game with a left hand done in bandages. In spite of

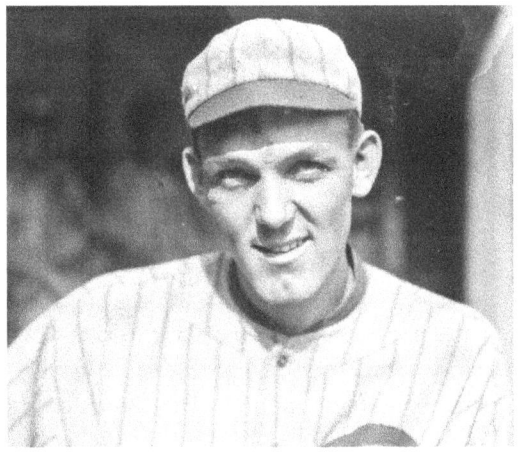

Buck Weaver is remembered mainly as the third baseman on the Chicago Black Sox, but he played more games at shortstop than at third. Although he claimed that he did not participate in fixing the 1919 World Series, he was present in meetings where the fix was discussed. He was banned for failing to report his awareness of the shenanigans (Library of Congress).

that handicap the 'ginger kid' played a splendid game."[27] Buck claimed his proudest accomplishment came when he participated in John McGraw's famous world tour in the winter of 1913-14. Weaver and pitcher Red Faber were the only Sox players to make the trip. In 1914 Buck became field captain of the Pale Hose. He led the AL in sacrifice hits in both 1915 and 1916. In 1917 he switched from shortstop to third base. In the World Series that fall, he and Faber were involved in an embarrassing incident. With Weaver on first base, Faber hit safely to right field and took second on the throw to third, which the Ginger Kid reached safely. With the next batter at the plate, the Giant pitcher took a full windup. Faber took off for third and slid in safely to find Weaver still on the bag. Buck hit .333 in that classic and batted .300 the next season. After the 1918 season ended early because of World War I, Weaver took a job as a mechanic in the Fairbanks-Morse plant in Beloit, Wisconsin, and played for the firm's semi-pro baseball team. In 1919 he hit .296 and led all AL third sackers in Faber System points for hitting and fielding combined.[28]

Weaver attended at least two meetings related to fixing the 1919 World Series. He wanted no part of the fix, accepted no money, and played his best in the Series. He hit .324, made no errors, and impressed sportswriters with his fighting spirit. In 1920 he had his best year at the plate, hit a career-high .331, with an OBP of .365, and scored 102 runs. As is well known, the jury returned a verdict of not guilty on all the accused players. Nevertheless, Commissioner Landis banned the eight from baseball for life, saying, "Regardless of the verdict of juries, no player who ... sits in conference with a bunch of crooked players and gamblers where the ways and means of throwing games are discussed and does not promptly tell the club about it will ever play professional baseball." Weaver was banned, not for fixing a game or taking a bribe, but for refusing to inform on his teammates. His defenders point out that the working-class code is "you don't rat on your buddies." Buck believed it would have been less honorable to turn them in than to keep quiet. Over the years Weaver appealed to Landis for reinstatement, sometimes supported by thousands of petitions, but the judge was adamant. Buck remained in Chicago, barnstorming with other players, playing semi-pro ball, and continually hoping for reinstatement. In the 1930s he was in the drugstore business. In the 1940s he managed a girls' softball team and worked for a florist before taking his final job as a pari-mutuel clerk at a Chicago racetrack. On January 31, 1956, he died at the age of 65 while walking down a Chicago sidewalk on the way to see his tax consultant.

Even after his death, efforts have continued to get Buck reinstated. His career has been amply documented. He was featured in the book by Eliot

Asinof, *Eight Men Out*.[29] John Cusack portrayed Weaver in the movie based on the book. A sympathetic view is presented in Irving Stein's *The Ginger Kid: The Buck Weaver Story*.[30] He is profiled in *Deadball Stars of the American League*. Ranking: Faber System fourth; *Total Baseball* third; James third.

THIRD BASEMEN

	G	R	H	HR	RBI	BA	OBP	Faber System Hit	Field	Total
Doug Baird	617	230	492	6	191	.234	.291	32	246	278
Les Bell	896	404	938	66	509	.290	.346	213	-43	170
Dave Brain	679	254	641	27	303	.252	.292	146	123	269
Andy Carey	938	371	741	64	350	.260	.327	128	240	368
John Castino	666	293	646	41	249	.278	.329	193	331	524
Bill Coughlin	1049	481	972	15	380	.252	.299	217	404	621
Charlie Deal	851	295	752	11	318	.257	.293	56	351	407
Bob Horner	1020	560	1047	218	685	.277	.340	683	265	948
Roy Howell	1112	422	991	80	454	.261	.321	257	105	362
Freddie Lindstrom	1438	895	1747	103	779	.311	.351	606	402	1008
Jim Presley	959	413	875	135	495	.247	.290	230	143	373
Ken Reitz	1344	366	1243	68	548	.260	.290	157	629	786
Red Smith	1117	477	1087	27	514	.278	.353	508	296	804
Jim Tabor	1005	473	1021	104	598	.270	.322	312	202	514
Hank Thompson	933	492	801	129	482	.267	.372	345	168	513
Johnny Vergez	672	258	593	52	292	.255	.311	5	174	179

Doug Baird

Born: Howard Douglas Baird, September 27, 1891, St. Charles, MO
Debut: April 18, 1915; age 23
Last Game: October 2, 1920; age 29
Clubs: Pittsburgh NL; St. Louis NL; Philadelphia NL; Brooklyn NL; New York NL

Douglas Baird grew up in St. Charles, a suburb of St. Louis, and attended Westminster College in Fulton, Missouri. In 1912 he played baseball for Westminster and later became the first alumnus of the college to reach the major leagues. After the college season of 1912 concluded, Doug made his professional debut with Springfield of the Three-I League. In 1915 he was acquired by the Pittsburgh Pirates and played for five different clubs during a six-year big league career. In his rookie season he led the National League in strikeouts and never hit for a high average. He was very fast on the base paths, however, and ranked third in stolen bases and sixth in triples during his initial season. His fielding was good enough to keep him in the Show for a half-dozen years.

After his major league career ended, he played for another seven years in the minors. From 1921 to 1925 he was in the American Association, with Indianapolis and Columbus. In 1926 and 1927 he played for Birmingham and Little Rock in the Southern Association. He hit better in the minors than he ever did in the majors, topping the .300 mark four times. In 1921, while playing for Indianapolis, the speedster broke the AA record with 72 stolen bases. Following his retirement from baseball, he worked for a time as a salesman in the oil business in Winnetka, Illinois. Baird died at the age of 75 on June 13, 1967, in Thomasville, Georgia.

Ranking: Faber System thirteenth; *Total Baseball* ninth.

Les Bell

Born: Lester Rowland Bell, December 14, 1901, Harrisburg, PA
Debut: September 8, 1923; age 21
Last Game: September 27, 1931; age 29
Clubs: St. Louis NL; Boston NL; Chicago NL

Les was a railway clerk playing semi-pro baseball in Columbia, Pennsylvania, when he was "discovered" by Jimmy Sheckard. The young man got his professional career off to a good start, hitting .329 for Lansing in the Central League in 1922, which earned him a step up to the Syracuse Stars of the International League. During the spring of 1923 Les failed both in hitting and in fielding his position and was released in midseason. He was immediately picked up by the Houston Buffaloes, the Texas League farm club of the St. Louis Cardinals. He hit higher than .300 for the Buffs and fielded well at the shortstop position. In 1924 he had a spectacular year at the plate, making 230 hits for a .365 batting average and scoring 145 runs. He got into a few late-season games for the Cards in both 1923 and 1924 and became their regular third baseman in 1925. He had his best major league season in 1926, with a .325 batting average, 17 home runs, and 100 RBIs. He helped the Cardinals win their first World Series title with a dramatic victory over the New York Yankees that October. Bell had one homer and six ribbies in the classic. His productivity declined slightly the next season and he was traded to the Boston Braves. He hit only ten home runs in 1928, but three of the ten came in the same game. He is one of only twelve players to hit both an inside-the-park grand slam and a pinch-hit grand slam during a big league career. After two years in Beantown, he was selected off waivers by the Chicago Cubs. In 1931 he was replaced as the Cubs' third baseman by rookie Billy Jurges, who was a vastly superior fielder. Les played a few games for Louisville in 1932. In the 1940s he emerged as a successful minor league manager with his hometown

Harrisburg Senators in the Inter-State League, where he won the 1941 pennant his first year as skipper. Because of World War II the club suspended operations from 1943 to 1945, but Bell came back as manager from 1946 through 1951, posting four more winning seasons. Les died of cancer at the age of 84 on December 26, 1985, in Hershey, Pennsylvania.

During his career Bell was an adequate major league hitter, but his defensive work at the hot corner pulled his ratings down.

Ranking: Faber System sixteenth of sixteen; *Total Baseball* eighth.

Dave Brain

Born: David Leonard Brain, January 24, 1879, Hereford, England
Debut: April 24, 1901; age 22
Last Game: October 7, 1908; age 29
Clubs: Chicago AL; St. Louis NL; Pittsburgh NL; Boston NL; Cincinnati NL; New York NL

According to his biographer, not much is known about David's early life, but he appeared to have started playing baseball at the age of 19.[31] Available census records show he came to the United States in 1883 and never became a naturalized citizen. His professional baseball career began with Des Moines of the Western League in 1900. Playing third base he hit a robust .305, with 52 extra-base hits, including 13 triples, and stole 27 bases before moving up to the Chicago White Stockings of the American League, which still had minor league status that year. When the AL achieved major league rank in 1901, Brain became a big leaguer for five days until his substandard fielding led to his demotion to St. Paul of the Western League, where he paced the loop with 13 home runs. In 1902 Dave patrolled the hot corner for Buffalo in the Eastern League and posted the best hitting statistics of his professional career. He led the league with 127 runs scored and hit a robust .331 with 44 extra-base hits and 247 total bases, very good numbers for the Deadball Era. He had 37 steals that year.

This productivity earned him another shot at the majors and he made good by playing for five different National League clubs in the next six seasons, mostly at third base but occasionally at other positions. He never hit for a high average in the majors, but he was known as a power hitter. In 1907 he led the league in home runs with ten. Twice he finished among the circuit's ten best in each of the following categories: doubles, triples, total bases, and slugging percentage. His combination of speed and power allowed him to set several records for three-base hits. He is the only player in major league history to have three triples in a game twice in a season. He also holds or shares the record for most triples in a game since 1900, most consecutive triples in a nine-inning game, and most times in a career with three triples in a game. His fielding prowess was a matter of dispute. He covered a lot of ground but committed many errors. For example, in 1906 he led the NL in both putouts and errors by a third sacker. On June 11 of that year he made five errors, the most miscues by a third baseman in a game since 1900. In 1907 he led in total chances per game.

His skills declined rapidly, and he was sold to Columbus of the American Association in 1909 but refused to report because of a salary dispute. He went to Buffalo of the Eastern League and led the league in his specialty — triples — but hit only .234 with two homers. He was out of baseball after 1910. Brain relocated to Los Angeles and worked for the National Biscuit Company for a while, then for the Standard Oil Company from 1918 until 1938, first as a salesman, later as a credit manager. On May 25, 1959, he died in Los Angeles at the age of 80.

Dave Brain is profiled in SABR's *Biography Project*. Ranking: Faber System fourteenth; *Total Baseball* fifth.

Andy Carey

Born: Andrew Arthur Hexem, October 18, 1931, Oakland, CA
Debut: May 2, 1952; age 20
Last Game: October 2, 1962; age 30
Clubs: New York AL; Kansas City AL; Chicago AL; Los Angeles NL

Andy was well schooled for baseball success. He attended Alameda High School, which has sent eleven graduates to the major leagues. In 1949–50 he played for St. Mary's College, which has had 60 alumni in the majors, probably more than any other college of its size in America. After his freshman year at St. Mary's he was signed by the New York Yankees for $60,000, a large amount for those times, earning him notoriety as a "bonus baby." The Yankees assigned him to Kansas City in the American Association, and he spent most of the next three years with the Blues, although he received brief tastes of the major leagues in 1952 and 1953. Carey became the Yankees' regular third baseman in 1954 and hit .302 that season, his best year in the Show. In 1955 Andy led the league in triples. A good fielder, he led AL third sackers in total chances per game and in Faber System fielding points in 1954.[32] In 1955 he again led the league in chances per game as well as in putouts, assists, and double plays. Over the years his playing time decreased as the Yankees were well stocked with infielders.

In 1959 he was stricken with mononucleosis and lost his third-base job. He was unable to win it back the next year and was traded to the Kansas City

Athletics. A year later he was traded to the Chicago White Sox. He had little success with the Sox and was traded to Philadelphia in the spring of 1962. By this time Carey had established a brokerage business in Southern California and his wife, the former movie actress Lucy Marlow, refused to leave their home in Corona del Mar. Rather than play in the East, Andy announced his retirement. In order to accommodate the infielder, the Sox renegotiated their trade with the Phillies and dealt Carey to Los Angeles. Andy did not perform well for the Dodgers. He retired for good at the end of the 1962 season and returned to his brokerage business. In 1963 he was selected as the second baseman on the baseball team for St. Mary's Athletes of the Century.

Ranking: Faber System eleventh; *Total Baseball* seventh.

John Castino

Born: John Anthony Castino, October 23, 1954, Evanston, IL
Debut: April 17, 1979; age 24
Last Game: May 7, 1984; age 29
Club: Minnesota AL

A graduate of Winnetka's New Trier High School, John starred in baseball for the Rollins College Tars, where he was named the Florida College Player of the Year in 1976. He is considered the most prominent Tar to play professional baseball. He was selected by the Minnesota Twins in the third round of the amateur draft. It took him three years to reach the majors, working his way through the system, from Wisconsin Rapids to Visalia to Orlando. Castino had a fine first year with the Twins, hitting .285, leading the league in double plays, and tying Alfredo Griffin for 1979 AL Rookie of the Year honors. In his sophomore season he hit .302, the only time he topped the .300 mark. He continued to field well, leading AL third basemen in assists that year and in putouts the next. Despite John's excellent play at the hot corner, he had to yield the position in 1982 to Gary Gaetti, one of the best fielding third basemen of all time. Castino moved to second base and performed well at the keystone in 1982 and 1983 before he developed a back problem. After the 1982 season he had spinal fusion surgery. In 1984 he again suffered back pain and was placed in a body cast. Although he was unable to play, the Twins kept him on the roster throughout the 1984 and 1985 seasons, finally releasing him in October 1985. Castino returned to Rollins, completed his undergraduate degree, and earned an MBA from St. Thomas University. In 1987 he became an investment advisor. In 2009 he was senior vice president at Wealth Enhancement Group in Wayzata, Minnesota.

Ranking: Sixth in both Faber System and *Total Baseball*.

Bill Coughlin

Born: William Paul Coughlin, July 12, 1878, Scranton, PA
Debut: August 9, 1899; age 21
Last Game: September 23, 1908; age 30
Clubs: Washington NL; Washington AL; Detroit AL

From the age of 17 to his death at the age of 64, Scranton Bill Coughlin devoted his entire life to baseball. The teenager made his professional debut with Pawtucket of the New England League in 1896. In 1898 he moved up to the Eastern League, playing for Providence and Wilkes-Barre. In 1899 he played for Wilkes-Barre and the Kansas City Blues of the Western League before making his major league debut with Washington in the National League near the end of the season. The following year found him back with Kansas City. The first of eight consecutive years as a full-time major leaguer came in 1901. In his rookie year he led the AL in putouts, which he did again in 1906. In his second season he hit .301, the highest average he posted in the majors. He was an excellent fielder and an adequate hitter by the standards of the Dead Ball Era. In 1907 he was the best third baseman in the league, according to the Faber System.[33]

In 1905 he was traded to Detroit and was captain of the Tigers in their pennant-winning seasons of 1907 and 1908. A good base runner, he stole second, third, and home in the same game against his former Washington teammates in 1906. Rowdy Bill was master of the hidden ball trick. Although no definitive list exists, he may have executed the ploy more than any other player in major league history. He pulled it off seven times, including the only time in World Series history, when he victimized Jimmy Slagle in the 1907 Series.

From 1909 to 1917 Coughlin was a player and/or manager in his native Pennsylvania, playing for Williamsport (1909–10), Reading (1911), and Allentown (1912–13) in the Tri-State League. At both Williamsport and Allentown he was a player-manager. From 1914 to 1917 he managed the Scranton Miners but played only the first year in his hometown. In 1919 Coughlin operated a school for umpires in occupied Coblenz, Germany. From 1920 to the end of his life Bill was the head baseball coach at Lafayette College, where he had only one losing season in 23 years and compiled a .675 winning percentage. Coughlin died in Scranton on May 7, 1943, at the age of 64. He was inducted into the Helms Foundation College Baseball Hall of Fame in 1944 and the Lafayette College Hall of Fame in 1977.

Ranking: Faber System fifth; *Total Baseball* fourteenth.

Charlie Deal

Born: Charles Albert Deal, October 30, 1891, Wilkinsburg, PA
Debut: July 19, 1912; age 20
Last Game: October 2, 1921; age 29
Clubs: Detroit AL; Boston NL; St. Louis FL; St. Louis AL; Chicago NL

Young Charlie Deal went straight from the semi-pros to the major leagues without benefit of minor league experience. After he had played a few games for the Detroit Tigers in 1912 and 1913, it appeared he was not quite ready for prime time. He spent most of 1913 with Providence in the International League, where his .312 batting average persuaded the Boston Braves to select him in the Rule 5 draft. During most of 1914 he was a benchwarmer for the Braves until their regular third baseman, Red Smith, broke his leg in the last game of the regular season, clearing the way for Deal to play full-time as the Miracle Braves swept Philadelphia in the World Series. Charlie hit only .125 in the Series but thought he deserved a salary increase for the next year. When the raise was not forthcoming, Deal jumped to the St. Louis Terriers of the new Federal League. Early in 1916 in a transaction between two St. Louis clubs, the Browns purchased Charlie. In turn, they sold him to the Chicago Cubs in midseason. In response to Secretary Baker's work-or-fight order, Charlie worked for the Breckenridge Allegheny Steel Company between the 1918 and 1919 seasons. For the next five years Deal was the regular third baseman for the Cubs, where he emerged as one of the best fielding third sackers in the league, leading the loop in Faber System fielding points three consecutive years, from 1919 through 1921.[34] At the plate he did not show much power but earned a reputation for being hard to strike out. He struck out only 121 times in 851 major league games. Some present-day big leaguers can match that total in half a season. In May 1921 Charlie suffered a broken nose when struck by a batted ball, causing him to miss several days. At the end of the season the Cubs dealt Deal to Los Angeles of the Pacific Coast League, where he played two years, moving to Vernon in 1924, to Portland in 1925, and concluding his career with New Orleans in the Southern Association in 1927. Charlie established his residence in California, living first in Los Angeles and later in Pasadena. In the 1930 census he was listed as retired, although he was only 38 years old. Deal died in a rest home in Covina on September 16, 1979, at the age of 87.

Ranking: Faber System ninth; *Total Baseball* tenth.

Bob Horner

Born: James Robert Horner, August 6, 1957, Junction City, KS
Debut: June 16, 1978; age 20

Last Game: June 18, 1988; age 30
Clubs: Atlanta NL; St. Louis NL

See the entry on Horner in Part One of this book.
Ranking: Faber System second; *Total Baseball* fourth; James third.

Roy Howell

Born: Roy Lee Howell, December 18, 1953, Lompoc, CA
Debut: September 9, 1974; age 20
Last Game: September 29, 1984; age 30
Clubs: Texas AL; Toronto AL; Milwaukee AL

The young redhead was a dominant star at Lompoc High School. In 1972 he was selected in the first round (fourth overall pick) of the 1972 amateur draft by the Texas Rangers. They sent the teenager to their Pittsfield club of the Eastern League for two years, and promoted him to Spokane of the Pacific Coast League in 1974. He hit .281, with 22 home runs and 101 runs scored for Spokane, earning him a promotion to the big leagues late in the season. In early May 1977 he was traded to the Toronto Blue Jays, where he hit .316 for the remainder of the season. He had his greatest day at the plate on September 10—five-for-six, two home runs, four runs scored, and an amazing nine runs batted in. All came off the deliveries of Catfish Hunter and relief pitchers of the AL champion New York Yankees. The following year Howell made the AL All-Star squad. He had three more good seasons in Canada before he became a free agent. He signed with Milwaukee and played for the Brewers for four years but never reached the level of productivity he had displayed earlier. Milwaukee released him in the fall of 1984 and he signed with San Francisco but was released by the Giants before he played a game for them.

In 1985 he played a partial season with Portland. Howell retired from the game and opened an insurance business, but he did not get baseball out of his system. He played a bit with a senior team and managed a team in San Luis Obispo for a year. In 2000 Roy joined the San Diego organization and served as a hitting instructor in Mobile and later in Portland. From 2003 to 2005 Howell managed the Eugene Emeralds, a San Diego farm club. More recently he has been president/manager of the San Luis Obispo Rattlers in the California Collegiate League and has conducted youth baseball clinics in the area. In 2009 he lived with his family in nearby Shell Beach, California.

Ranking: Faber System twelfth; *Total Baseball* thirteenth.

Freddie Lindstrom

Born: Frederick Charles Lindstrom, November 21, 1905, Chicago, IL
Debut: April 15, 1924; age 18
Last Game: May 15, 1936; age 30
Clubs: New York NL; Pittsburgh NL; Chicago NL; Brooklyn NL

See the entry on him in Part One of this book.

Lindstrom is a member of the National Baseball Hall of Fame. Ranking: Faber System and Bill James both have him first; *Total Baseball* places him third.

Jim Presley

Born: James Arthur Presley, October 23, 1961, Pensacola, FL
Debut: June 24, 1984; age 22
Last Game: June 7, 1991; age 29
Clubs: Seattle AL; Atlanta NL; San Diego NL

Jim Presley, nicknamed "Hound Dog" for obvious reasons, was an early bloomer as a baseball star. In 1974 the 12 year old led his team to the Dixie Youth World Series. He was drafted out of Escambia High School by Seattle in the fourth round of the 1979 amateur draft and spent the next eleven years in the Mariners organization, working his way up from Bellingham through Wausau, Lynn, Chattanooga, and Salt Lake before reaching the majors. His best years in Seattle were 1985 through 1987, when he hit more than 20 home runs each season and had 107 RBIs in 1986. Presley was named to the AL All-Star team that summer. He was traded to Atlanta in 1990 but was granted free agency at the end of the year and signed with San Diego. The Padres released him in midseason, and he signed with the Texas Rangers, who assigned him to their Oklahoma City farm club.

In 1997 Jim became a hitting instructor. He started with Lethbridge in the Pioneer League and went to the South Bend Silver Hawks in 1998. Later he joined the Arizona Diamondbacks' organization for five years, usually serving as a hitting coach but managing the Missoula Osprey, the Diamondbacks' Rookie League affiliate, in 2004. Since 2006 he has been a hitting instructor for the Florida Marlins. Somewhere along the line he found time to earn two degrees from the University of West Florida — a bachelor's in health, leisure and sports and a master's in educational leadership. In 2009 he and his family were living in Cantonment, Florida.

Ranking: Faber System tenth: *Total Baseball* fifteenth.

Ken Reitz

Born: Kenneth John Reitz, June 24, 1951, San Francisco, CA
Debut: September 5, 1972; age 21
Last Game: June 3, 1982; age 30
Clubs: St. Louis NL; San Francisco NL; Chicago NL; Pittsburgh NL

Ken was drafted out of Daly City's Jefferson High School by the St. Louis Cardinals in the 31st round of the 1969 amateur draft. As the 730th overall selection, his chances of reaching the major leagues did not appear to be very good, yet he managed to have an eleven-year career in the Show, all but two of them with the Redbirds. He started with the Gulf Coast Cardinals and moved up the farm system, through Cedar Rapids, St. Petersburg, Arkansas, and Tulsa in four years. Never a strong hitter by major league standards, Reitz succeeded with his excellent glove work. He led the NL in fielding percentage five times, tying Heinie Groh's record. Ken won a Gold Glove in 1978 and led third sackers in Faber System fielding in 1978 and 1981.[35] His .970 lifetime fielding average is the highest of any NL third baseman in the league's 133-year history. His ability to suck ground balls off the turf earned him the nickname "Human Zamboni Machine." Reitz played in the 1980 All-Star game. After his major league years were over, Ken played a few games in the minors for Louisville and Tulsa and wound up his playing career with the San Jose Bees in 1987. He was enshrined in the Missouri Sports Hall of Fame in 2009. Currently he is a motivational speaker with the All-American Speakers organization.

Ranking: Faber System fourth; *Total Baseball* sixteenth.

Red Smith

Born: James Carlisle Smith, April 6, 1890, Greenville, SC
Debut: September 5, 1911; age 21
Last Game: September 25, 1919; age 29
Clubs: Brooklyn NL; Boston NL

Red Smith played baseball and football at Alabama Polytechnic Institute (now Auburn University) in 1908–09. After his entry into professional baseball, he returned to Auburn and graduated in 1912. He got his major league start with Brooklyn in 1911. Boston acquired him in the midst of the Miracle Braves' dramatic climb from last place to the pennant in 1914, and he was an important contributor, hitting .314 down the stretch with an OBP of .401. Unfortunately, Smith broke his leg on an awkward slide into a base during the last game of the regular season. Unable to compete in the World Series, he was temporarily replaced at the hot corner by Charlie Deal. Red was a

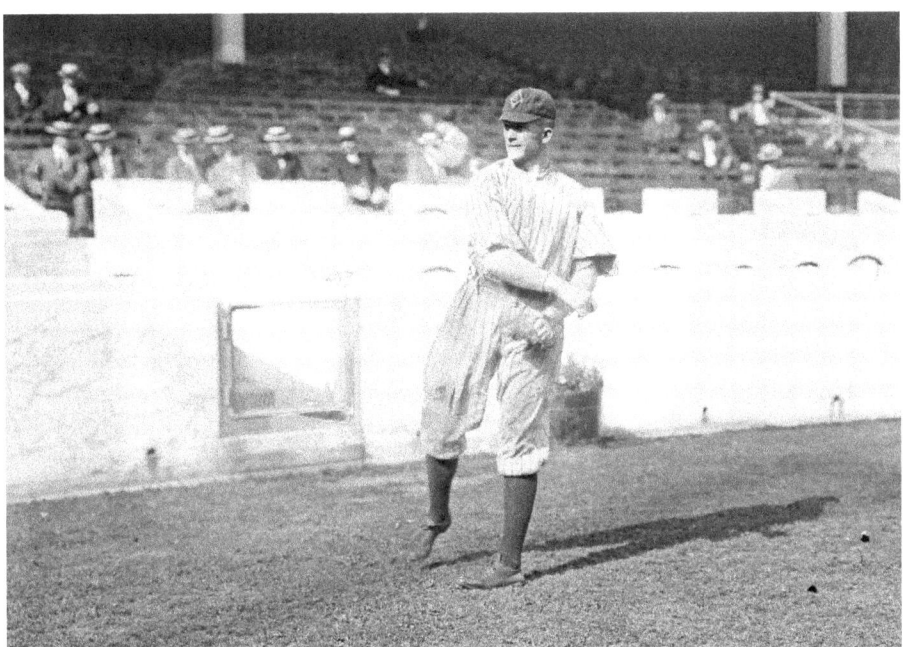

James Carlisle "Red" Smith was a good, solid major league hitter, frequently finishing among the league leaders in every hitting category. In the field he had both positive and negative accomplishments, leading the league in assists four times and in putouts and errors three times. *Total Baseball* ranks him at the top of the list among third basemen who played their final major league game at the age of 30 or younger (Library of Congress).

good, solid hitter throughout his major league career. He led the NL in doubles in 1913 and was in the top five in that statistic four other times. He finished in the top ten in RBIs five times, and ranked among the ten best at least once in batting average, OBP, slugging, hits, total bases, home runs, and bases on balls. In 1915 he slugged the first grand slam ever hit at Braves Field. Because of a low fielding percentage, Red was sometimes considered to be a poor fielder. He led the league in errors three times, but he also led in putouts three times, in assists four times, and in total chances per game once. In 1914 the Faber System rated him as the league's best-hitting third baseman and the best third sacker overall, considering both hitting and fielding.[36] After his major league career was over, Smith managed for a while in the minors. He skippered the Jacksonville Tars of the Southeastern League and the Springfield Senators of the Three-I League for short stretches. Smith died at the age of 76 in Atlanta on October 11, 1966.

Ranking: Faber System third; *Total Baseball* first; James second.

Jim Tabor

Born: James Reubin Tabor, November 5, 1916, New Hope, AL
Debut: August 2, 1938; age 21
Last Game: September 17, 1947; age 30
Clubs: Boston AL; Philadelphia NL

Jim was signed by the Boston Red Sox off the University of Alabama campus, where he played baseball in 1935–36. The youngster, who was sometimes called "Rawhide," moved quickly through the farm system, playing at Little Rock in 1937 and Minneapolis in 1938. His .330 batting average for the Millers earned him a call-up to the majors near the end of the season. He played for the Sox through the 1944 season and missed all of 1945 while serving in the military. After his discharge he was traded to Philadelphia but released after playing only two years with the Phillies. He was a good hitter, with considerable power and some speed on the bases. His major league highs were .289 batting average, 21 home runs, 101 runs batted in, and 17 stolen bases. On July 4, 1939, Tabor became the second man in major league history to hit two grand slams in the same game. Jim was an unreliable third baseman who occasionally made a spectacular play but led the league in errors five times. *Who's Who in Baseball* touted him in 1939 as an ideal hot corner workman, tall and rangy, with a whipcord arm. Tabor's main problem was excessive drinking. In 1941 he was suspended briefly for drinking and missing a game. His teammate Doc Cramer told writer Peter Golenbock, "Tabor would get drunk and be half drunk when he came to the park. The Sox hired two private investigators to shadow him. Tabor locked them in the bathroom and went on to the next bar."[37] After the Phillies released him, Rawhide played from 1948 to 1952 in the Pacific Coast League for Sacramento, Los Angeles, San Diego, and Portland, twice hitting higher than .300. On August 22, 1953, he died of a heart attack in Sacramento at the age of 36.

A biography of Jim Tabor is included in the book *Lefty, Double-X, and the Kid: The 1939 Red Sox, a Team in Transition*, published by Rounder Books in 2009. Ranking: Faber System seventh; *Total Baseball* eleventh; James fourth.

Hank Thompson

Born: Henry Curtis Thompson, December 8, 1925, Oklahoma City, OK
Debut: July 17, 1947; age 21
Last Game: September 30, 1956; age 30
Clubs: St. Louis AL; New York NL

Hank began his professional baseball career as a 17-year-old right fielder with the Kansas City Monarchs in the Negro American League in 1943. In

1944–45 he served in the military with the 1695th Combat Engineers and fought at the Battle of the Bulge. After his return to civilian life he played mainly at second base but occasionally appeared at shortstop or in the outfield for the Monarchs. Following the 1946 season he was a member of a Negro All-Star team that played against major league stars in a barnstorming tour organized by Bob Feller. Feller's praise of Thompson's play created interest on the part of major league owners after Jackie Robinson broke the color barrier. In July 1947 the St. Louis Browns made conditional purchases of Thompson and Willard Brown for $2500 each and agreed to pay an additional $5000 for each player kept longer than a month. The players endured less than desirable conditions while with the Browns and were returned to Kansas City in August. In 1948 Hank was purchased by the New York Giants and assigned to their Jersey City farm club in the International League. He was promoted to the majors in 1949 and played mostly at third base during eight seasons with the Giants. In 1950 Hank hit .289 with 20 home runs and 91 RBIs. During the Giants' thrilling come-from-behind chase for the 1951 pennant, Thompson hit eight home runs in the final stretch. In the World Series against Cleveland in 1954 he set a record by walking seven times and tied another mark by getting a hit in every game of the Series. He was considered adequate in the field.

After his major league career was over, Hank played for the Minneapolis Millers but quit before the end of the 1957 season. For a time he was a cab driver in New York City. In 1963 he was convicted in Texas of armed robbery, sentenced to ten years in prison, and was paroled in 1967. In 1968 he became a playground director for the Fresno Recreation Department. He died in a Fresno hospital on September 30, 1969, after suffering a seizure the night before and never regaining consciousness. He was 43 years old.

Ranking: Faber System eighth; *Total Baseball* second; James fourth.

Johnny Vergez

Born: Jean Louis Verges, July 9, 1906, Oakland, CA
Debut: April 14, 1931; age 24
Last Game: June 13, 1936; age 29
Clubs: New York NL; Philadelphia NL; St. Louis NL

Johnny played baseball at Alameda High School, and earned this tribute in the school's 1925 yearbook: "Around the hot corner was Frenchy Vergez, who fielded well and led the boys with the willows."[38] A year later Vergez made his professional debut with Terrell of the Texas Association. After a season in the Lone Star State, Johnny moved to Ogden of the Utah-Idaho League.

Midway through the 1928 season he returned to the city of his birth to play for the Oaks in the Pacific Coast League. He hit higher than .300 in both 1929 and 1930 for the Oaks, earning advancement to the major leagues with the New York Giants. In the majors Johnny was never able to attain a high batting average. In 1933 he was having perhaps his best year at the plate, hitting .271 with 16 home runs and 72 RBIs in 123 games, when stricken with appendicitis. Although he had helped the Giants win the pennant, he was unable to play in the World Series. In an unusual move in November 1934, Vergez was traded for his former Alameda High School teammate, Dick Bartell, in a package deal between the Giants and the Phillies. He played in Philadelphia only one year before being sold to the Cardinals. He concluded his major league career after playing only a few games in St. Louis in 1936. Vergez was a better fielder than he was a batsman. He led the NL in assists in 1933 and topped the circuit in 1935 in putouts, double plays, and fielding percentage. The Faber System rated him as the loop's best fielder at the hot corner in 1935.[39]

After his major league career ended he returned to the Pacific Coast League, where he played for Sacramento from 1936 to 1938 and for Oakland from 1939 to 1943, until the PCL temporarily suspended operations due to World War II. During his time with the Oaks Johnny served at least one year as manager. Later he marked as a scout for the Giants. He died of kidney failure at the University of California–Davis Medical Center on July 15, 1991, at the age of 85.

Ranking: Faber System fifteenth; *Total Baseball* twelfth.

CATCHERS

Player	G	R	H	HR	RBI	BA	OBP	Faber System Bat	Field	+	Total
Fred Carroll	754	546	820	27	366	.284	.370	408	80	31	519
Dave Nilsson	837	389	789	105	470	.284	.356	351	53	0	404
Mickey O'Neil	672	177	475	4	179	.238	.292	-302	307	8	13
Ellie Rodriguez	775	220	533	16	203	.245	.356	164	274	0	438
Earl Williams	889	361	756	138	457	.247	.318	313	105	70	488

+ refers to bonus points for handling pitchers

Fred Carroll

Born: Frederick Herbert Carroll, July 2, 1864, Sacramento, CA
Debut: May 1, 1884; age 19

Last Game: August 18, 1891; age 27
Clubs: Columbus AA; Pittsburgh AA; Pittsburgh NL; Pittsburgh PL

After playing baseball for one year at St. Mary's College, Fred joined his teammate Ed "Cannonball" Morris on a journey into professional baseball. The two men remained batterymates for eight years, starting with the minor league Reading Actives in 1883 and continuing into the majors, first in Columbus and then for six seasons in Pittsburgh. Fred hit the ground running. Without specifying his criteria, Bill James named Carroll as the second-best young catcher in baseball, behind only Johnny Bench.[40] During his brief major league career, Carroll finished in the top ten in every important hitting statistic at least once. His best year was 1889, when he hit .330 and led the league in OBP at .486, and in on-base plus slugging percentage with a remarkable .970. Fred was not particularly adept at fielding his position and sometimes moved to first base or the outfield, but his ability to handle pitchers kept him behind the plate most of the time. He participated on the All-American team that accompanied the Chicago White Stockings in their world tour in 1888–89. During most major league offseasons, Carroll, Morris, and others played winter ball in the California League.

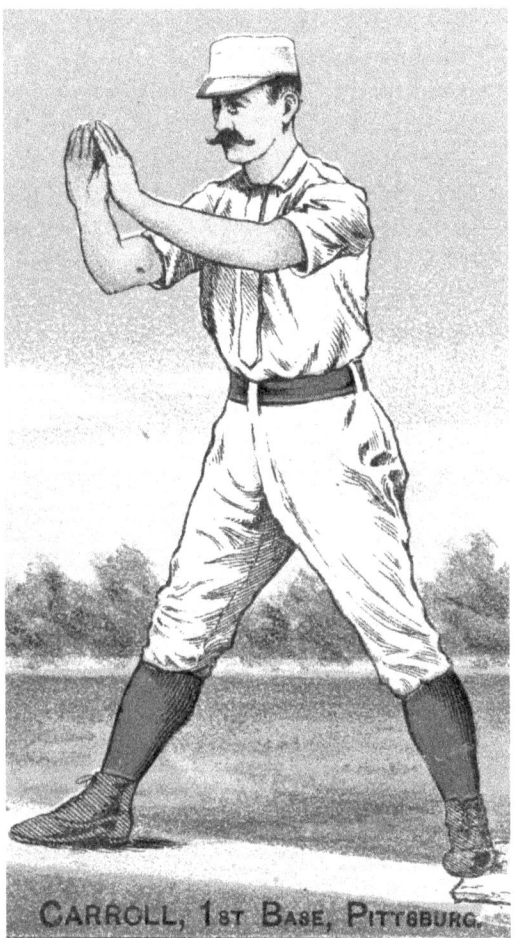

Fred Carroll was named by Bill James as the second-best young catcher in baseball, behind only Johnny Bench. During his brief major league career, Carroll finished in the top ten in every batting category at least once. He was not particularly adept at fielding his position and was sometimes moved to first base or the outfield. His ability to handle pitchers kept him behind the plate most of the time (Library of Congress).

Fred never liked living in the East and returned to the West Coast when the Pirates released him late in the 1891 season. He immediately joined the Oakland club in the California League. In 1892 Carroll led the league in both batting average and home runs but left the Colonels after clashing with the club owner. In 1893 he played for San Francisco. During his two and a fraction years in the California League, Carroll played mainly in the outfield and hit better than .300 each year. In 1894 Fred played exclusively in the outfield for Grand Rapids in the Western League and hit .389. Included among his 223 hits that year were 51 doubles, 13 triples, and 22 home runs. He still had speed as well as power, as demonstrated by his 71 stolen bases. In 1895 he divided the season between Grand Rapids and Kansas City and closed out his professional career by hitting an amazing .414. Carroll remained in California and prospered in the freight business. He died in San Rafael on November 7, 1904, at the age of 40.

Fred Carroll is profiled in *Baseball's First Stars*. Ranking: number one by all three sources.

Dave Nilsson

Born: David Wayne Nilsson, December 14, 1969, Brisbane, Australia
Debut: May 18, 1992; age 22
Last Game: October 3, 1999; age 29
Club: Milwaukee AL

Dave first attracted international attention as a 15 year old when he won the Helms Award as the MVP in the Claxton Shield Series, an annual event to determine the baseball championship of Australia. Shortly after his 17th birthday he was signed by the Milwaukee Brewers. He made his professional debut in American ball later that year and hit .394 for the Helena Brewers of the Pioneer League. Despite this stellar beginning he progressed slowly through the Brewer system, playing for Beloit, Stockton, El Paso, and Denver before being called up for a few games with the big club in 1992. Due to injury problems he had several rehab assignments in the minors, starting in 1993 and continuing throughout most of his career. In 1995 he missed the first two months of the major league season because of Ross River fever, contracted while playing winter ball. He had three rehab stints that year and hit higher than .400 in each of them. When he was healthy he was a very good hitter. His best year was 1996, when he hit .331 with a .407 OBP, 17 home runs, and 84 RBIs. Before the 2000 season he was granted free agency so he could represent his country in the Olympics. After the games concluded, he was offered a conditional contract by the Boston Red Sox, but the offer was withdrawn when Nilsson failed a medical exam on his left knee. In 2003 the Sox again reached an agreement with Dave but he decided not to play, having lost the desire to play in the States.

As the baseball seasons in North America and Australia come during different times of the year, Nilsson was able to play Down Under during his major league career. He made the Australian Baseball League (ABL) all-star team multiple times and holds the league record for batting average and slugging percentage. Dave managed in the ABL four years. In 1999 he captained the team that won Australia's first-ever International Cup. He was named Player of the Tournament and to the All-World team. He captained the Australian Olympic team in 2000 and represented his country again in the 2004 Olympics and in the 2006 World Baseball Classic. Nilsson owned the now-defunct International Baseball League of Australia. In addition, he has played in Japan and Italy. He was inducted into the Baseball Australia Hall of Fame in 2005 and the Sport Australia Hall of Fame in 2008. In 2009 Nilsson was head coach of the Australian MLB Academy.

Ranking: Faber System fourth; *Total Baseball* third.

Mickey O'Neil

Born: George Michael O'Neil, April 12, 1900, St. Louis, MO
Debut: September 12, 1919; age 19
Last Game: June 19, 1927; age 27
Clubs: Boston NL; Brooklyn NL; Washington AL; New York NL

Mickey broke into organized ball as a 17 year old with Alton in the Three-I League in 1917 and spent most of the rest of his life in the game. He caught for teams in Nashville, Toronto, and Rochester before making it to the Boston Braves near the end of the 1919 season. He was a very weak hitter, with a career batting average of .238. He never came close to leading the league in any offensive category. Frustrated at his inability to hit, he once dropped his bat and swung futilely at the ball with his bare hand, missing, of course. Behind the plate was a different matter, however. He was an excellent fielder, twice leading the league in assists. His greatest boast was that he caught more than 2000 games in the majors and minors and never broke a finger. O'Neil had the misfortune of playing most of his major league career for weak teams in Boston and Brooklyn. Perhaps to compensate he developed a great sense of humor and became something of a comedian on the field, protesting umpire's calls vigorously but never with ill humor, whether he was at the plate or behind it. Perhaps association with the Daffiness Boys in Brooklyn brought out this side of his personality. At any rate he became a well-liked and entertaining performer.

After his major league career ended Mickey played 15 years in the minors for one or two years each in Toledo, Louisville, New Orleans, Shreveport, Tyler, and Trois Rivieres, and for five years in Memphis and seven years in Jackson, Mississippi. That adds up to more than 15 years, but several times he played for two teams in the same season. He was a playing manager at Jackson in the Kitty League from 1940 to 1942 and managed the club again in 1952 and 1953. At other times he managed in the Ohio State, Carolina, Georgia-Florida, and Northern leagues, scouted for the Pittsburgh Pirates, and coached one year for the Cleveland Indians. The man got around, reportedly making friends wherever he went. O'Neil wound up his career as president, general manager, and field manager of the Hot Springs Bathers of the Cotton States League in 1954. He died at his home in St. Louis on April 8, 1964, just four days before his 64th birthday.

Ranking: Faber System and *Total Baseball* fifth in both.

Ellie Rodriguez

Born: Eliseo Rodriguez Delgado, May 24, 1946, Fajardo, PR
Debut: May 26, 1968; age 22
Last Game: October 3, 1976; age 30
Clubs: New York AL; Kansas City AL; Milwaukee AL; California AL; Los Angeles NL

Although he was born in Puerto Rico, Ellie grew up in the Bronx idolizing Yogi Berra. In 1964 he was signed by the Kansas City Athletics as an amateur free agent. The teenager spent the season with farm clubs in Wytheville and Daytona Beach. At the end of the year he was selected by the New York Yankees in the first-year player draft. The Yanks started him at Greensboro and moved him up the system to Columbus, Binghamton and Syracuse. He reached the Show in 1968 and made his major league debut for the Yankees on May 26, two days after his 22nd birthday. What a birthday present it must have been for him to don the catcher's gear for the team of his boyhood dreams! However, he played in only nine games for the Bronx Bombers before they sent him back to Syracuse. In October he was chosen by the Kansas City Royals as the 13th pick in the expansion draft. Although he hit only .236 his rookie season, he was selected for the All-Star game. After two years in Kansas City, he was traded to Milwaukee. He had his best year at the plate in 1972, hitting .285 with a .382 OBP. He made the AL All-Star squad again that year. In 1974 Ellie was traded to the California Angels and led the AL in Faber System fielding and total points that season.[41] He led the league in putouts, assists, and total chances per game. He also tied the AL record for putouts in a nine-inning game and set a mark for putouts in an extra-inning game. Both of these records were due largely to the efforts of Nolan Ryan, who struck out 19 in each game. Only two of Ellie's putouts were not from Ryan's punchouts. In 1976 Rodriguez was traded to the Dodgers and spent one season in Los Angeles before being released the next spring. A traveling man, Ellie played for eleven different clubs in thirteen years. More recently, Rodriguez has been a player development consultant for the Atlantic League of Professional Baseball and is in charge of scouting Latin America for the circuit.

Ranking: Faber System third; *Total Baseball* second.

Earl Williams

Born: Earl Craig Williams, Jr., July 14, 1948, Newark, NJ
Debut: September 13, 1970; age 22
Last Game: September 25, 1977; age 29
Clubs: Atlanta NL; Baltimore AL; Montreal NL; Oakland AL

As a youngster Earl played Little League baseball and starred in baseball, basketball, and football at Montclair High School. He earned a basketball scholarship to Ithaca College but gave it up when he was taken by Atlanta in the first round of the 1965 draft of American Legion players. However, the Braves paid the tuition for the first three years so Earl could attend Ithaca during the offseason. He was only 17 when he started his professional career as a pitcher with the Braves in the Gulf Rookie League. The Braves converted him to a first baseman/outfielder and promoted him to West Palm Beach and Greenwood. Attending college necessitated his reporting late to spring training before Williams gave it up after 1968. He had his best minor league season with Greenwood in 1969, hitting .340 and clubbing 33 home runs, earning him advancement to Shreveport and Richmond in 1970, and a call-up to the Show that September.

Atlanta general manager Paul Richards decided to make Earl a catcher and sent him to Puerto Rico to learn that trade. Without any minor league experience at the position, Williams became Atlanta's catcher in 1971 and won NL Rookie of the Year honors, largely because of his outstanding hitting — 33 home runs and 87 RBIs. Despite Earl's ambivalent attitude toward catching, his work behind the plate drew praise from his teammates, not only for his fielding but also for his work with the pitchers. Earl was only the second catcher to win Rookie of the Year honors. Johnny Bench, the first, was awash in endorsements; Earl received none. This bothered him, as he thought it might be because of his race. A sportswriter described Williams as militant.

In 1972 Earl reported to camp overweight, was hospitalized briefly with migraine headaches, and fell into disfavor with some of his teammates, who considered him "brash and cocky."[42] In 1972 he was traded to Baltimore. He suffered an ankle sprain that was slow to heal, and got into some name-calling incidents with teammates. By August Oriole fans had begun riding him, and Earl shouted back at them, using intemperate language. Williams became unpopular with fans, fellow players, and management. He felt, perhaps correctly, that much of the criticism was racially motivated. His productivity fell off, and at the age of 24 his career started a downward slide. He was traded back to Atlanta for two years, then to Montreal for one, and ended his stay in the majors after one year in Oakland.

Earl went to the Mexican League for two years. In 1979 he hit .343 with 20 homers and a league-leading 112 RBIs. In 1980 he played for Campeche, but his numbers fell off drastically. In 1981 he reported to the Pittsburgh Pirates' spring training camp and signed a contract with their Portland farm club but never played for the Beavers. After 1980 he never played another game of professional baseball, blaming racism and his own unsavory reputation, immaturity, and willingness to speak out. In recent years he has been associated with the Earl Warren Training Program, a project started by the Legal Defense Fund of the NAACP for the purpose of increasing the number of black attorneys in the United States. He has received favorable notice in the press for working with public school students in New Jersey's inner cities.

Ranking: Faber System second; *Total Baseball* fourth.

RIGHT FIELDERS

Player	G	R	H	HR	RBI	BA	OBP	Faber System Hit	Field	Total
John Cassidy	634	353	650	5	191	.246	.271	271	125	396
Tony Conigliaro	876	464	849	166	516	.264	.327	496	187	683
Mike Davis	963	419	778	91	371	.259	.313	231	173	404
Jake Evans	472	215	435	1	168	.238	.264	-20	377	357
Steve Evans	978	478	963	32	466	.287	.374	537	151	688
Doc Gessler	880	370	831	14	363	.280	.370	446	125	571
Danny Green	923	552	1021	29	423	.293	.359	517	241	758
Ken Harrelson	900	374	703	131	421	.239	.325	384	239	613
Butch Huskey	642	259	555	86	336	.267	.318	105	76	181
Harry Lumley	730	300	728	38	305	.274	.328	331	120	451
Jack McGeachy	608	345	604	9	276	.245	.265	-120	256	376
Alex Ochoa	807	320	597	46	261	.279	.344	108	156	264
Hosken Powell	594	241	470	17	160	.259	.314	72	145	217

								Faber System		
Player	G	R	H	HR	RBI	BA	OBP	Hit	Field	Total
Bobby Roth	811	427	804	30	422	.284	.367	364	133	497
Ron Swoboda	928	285	624	73	344	.242	.324	55	182	337
Chicken Wolf	1198	779	1440	18	593	.290	.327	654	605	1259
Ross Youngs	1211	812	1491	42	592	.322	.399	895	252	1147

John Cassidy

Born: John P. Cassidy, about 1856, Brooklyn, NY
Debut: April 24, 1875; age 18 or 19
Last Game: August 12, 1885; age 29
Clubs: Brooklyn NA; New Haven NA; Hartford NL; Chicago NL; Troy NL; Providence NL; Brooklyn AA

Very little is known about the early days of John Cassidy. Sources dispute the year of his birth; some say 1857, others suggest 1855. The year 1856 seems more likely. His age was reported as 24 in the census taken in June 1880. It is known that he was an Irish-American lad playing on the sandlots of Brooklyn when he made his professional debut with the Atlantics of Brooklyn in 1875. When the National League was formed, John joined the Hartford club. He was one of the first ten left-handed players in the league. In 1877 he had by far his best season in the majors, hitting .378. He was runner-up for the batting crown that year. He finished third in slugging percentage, fourth in on-base percentage, and fifth in total bases, winning honors as the Faber System right fielder of the year.[43] He never came close to having another season like that, as his batting average plummeted. In 1879, due to injury or illness, he played only nine games for Troy. Nevertheless, when the reserve clause was introduced in November, he was one of the five Trojans protected for the 1880 season. In the nineteenth century, active players were sometimes used as umpires. Cassidy umpired a few games in three different leagues — the NA in 1875, the NL in 1882, and the AA in 1884. He lived less than six years after retiring from baseball, dying from dropsy (now called edema) in Brooklyn on July 2, 1891, probably at the age of 35.

Ranking: Faber System eleventh; *Total Baseball* sixteenth.

Tony Conigliaro

Born: Anthony Richard Conigliaro, January 7, 1945, Revere, MA
Debut: April 16, 1964; age 19
Last Game: June 12, 1975; age 30
Clubs: Boston AL; California AL

Tony could have been one of the greatest stars in the history of baseball if not for an unbelievable string of bad luck that extended even after his career was over. A three-sport star at St. Mary's High School in suburban Lynn, Tony excelled in football, basketball, and baseball and was considered one of the finest all-around athletes in the state. A pitcher and a power hitter in prep school, he was scouted by a majority of the major league baseball teams and signed with the Boston Red Sox in 1962 for a $22,000 bonus. He played basketball at Oswego College in the winter of 1962-63. During spring training in 1963 the Red Sox converted him into an outfielder, and he was regarded as one of the most outstanding players in camp. The Sox assigned him to their Wellsville farm club in the New York–Pennsylvania League, where he swatted 24 home runs. Unfortunately, he missed the first three weeks of the season because of a broken thumb, the first in a string of injuries that haunted him. He recovered in time to hit .363 in 83 games, earning a promotion to the big leagues in 1964. The young man got off to a great start, having already clouted 24 home runs by July 26, when he was hit by a pitch that broke his forearm. He was out of action for five weeks, which probably cost him Rookie of the Year honors, which went to Tony Oliva. Conigliaro usually crowded the plate and was hit again in 1965, when a pitch broke his wrist. Despite losing more than three weeks because of the injury, he still hit 32 homers, becoming the first 20 year old to lead the league in four-baggers. By the midsixties Tony was the most popular player in New England. He had tremendous talent, charisma, and an engaging personality. He had a good singing voice, signed a recording contract, cut a few records, and was a frequent guest on TV shows. His roommate, Rico Petrocelli, said Tony had matinee idol good looks and was a chick magnet, dating actresses and Playboy bunnies, but avoiding fancy nightclubs.[44]

During spring training in 1967 Conigliaro was hit by a pitch that broke his shoulder blade but he recovered quickly. At 22 he became the youngest AL player ever to reach 100 career home runs. On the night of August 18, a pitch thrown by Jack Hamilton crashed into the side of Tony's face, just below the eye socket. He was knocked unconscious, blood streaming down his face. He was carried from the field on a stretcher and taken by ambulance to a hospital. His left eye was swollen completely shut, his cheekbone was fractured, and his jaw dislocated. Whether his retina was permanently damaged would not be determined for some time. He did not play again for 18 months until suddenly his vision improved. In 1969 he was back on the field and earned the AL Comeback Player of the Year award. In 1970 he hit 36 homers and knocked in 116 runs, but his vision began to deteriorate late in the season. The Red Sox traded him to the Angels in 1971, but he could barely see out of his left eye and retired in midseason. After three years out of the game, Tony tried to make a comeback with the Red Sox — both in Boston and in Pawtucket — in 1975 but soon retired for good. He moved to San Francisco and became a sportscaster for a Bay Area TV station.

In January 1982 Conigliaro flew to Boston to interview for a job as a baseball analyst for Red Sox games on cable television. After the interview his brother Billy was driving him to Logan Airport for the flight back to California when Tony slumped over, the victim of a heart attack. By the time Billy could get him to the nearest hospital, Tony was in a coma. He never fully recovered and spent the rest of his life in a vegetable state, mostly in a nursing home in Salem and sometimes at his parents' house. He died in Salem on February 24, 1990, at the age of 45. Petrocelli said that was about the time Tony should have been preparing to enter the Baseball Hall of Fame.

Conigliaro is profiled in a book by Petrocelli and Chaz Scoggins.[45] Ranking: Faber System fifth; *Total Baseball* ninth; James second.

Mike Davis

Born: Michael Dwayne Davis, June 11, 1959, San Diego, CA
Debut: April 10, 1980; age 20
Last Game: October 1, 1989; age 30
Clubs: Oakland AL; Los Angeles NL

Mike was signed as a teenager by the Oakland Athletics after being selected in the third round of the 1977 amateur draft. Assigned to Medicine Hat in the Pioneer League, he hit .315 and moved up to Modesto of the California League the following year and batted .335. In 1979 he split the season between Modesto and Waterbury. He started the 1980 season at Oakland but did not hit well and was sent down to Ogden in the Pacific Coast League. He spent most of the next two seasons in the PCL with Tacoma, although he did have a few games in Oakland each year. After six years he finally became a big league regular in 1983. His best year in the majors came in 1985, when he hit .287 with 24 home runs. He stole 24 bases that season, scored 92 runs, and batted in 82. In July 1987 he kicked a dugout door in anger, injuring his knee, and fell into a long slump. At the end of the season, the A's released him and he signed as a free agent with the Dodgers. He did not hit well in Los Angeles but gained some notoriety in the 1988 World Series. In Game 1 he drew a walk from Dennis Eckersley, stole second, and scored on Kirk Gibson's dramatic game-winning homer. In Game 5 Mike's two-run homer was the winning margin as the Dodgers clinched the championship. Despite these heroics, his major league career ended that October. In 1990 he played for the San Jose Giants in the California League and concluded his baseball career with Indianapolis of the American Association in 1991.

Ranking: Faber System tenth; *Total Baseball* tied for eleventh.

Jake Evans

Born: Uriah L. P. Evans, September 22, 1856, Baltimore, MD
Debut: May 1, 1879; age 22
Last Game: May 19, 1885; age 28
Clubs: Troy NL; Worcester NL; Cleveland NL; Baltimore AA

Exactly when and why young Evans acquired the nickname "Bloody Jake" is not known for certain. Obviously, it was a baseball appellation. In census returns he was invariably reported as "Uriah." Jake started his professional career in 1877 at the age of 20 with the Rhode Island club of the New England League. In 1878 he played for New Bedford of the International Association. He made his major league debut with Troy in 1879 and was placed on the protected list by the Trojans the first year the reserve clause was in effect. Jake was a weak hitter, seldom batting over .250, and hit only one home run in his entire big league career. In the field, he excelled. At various times he led his circuit in double plays, assists, and fielding percentage. In 1882 he set the all-time record for Faber System fielding points by a right fielder.[46] Despite a mediocre performance at the plate, Bloody Jake was the outstanding player at his position in 1882.[47] Over his short career Evans amassed the most Faber System fielding points per season of any right fielder in history.[48] He died in Baltimore on January 16, 1907, at the age of 50.

Ranking: Faber System thirteenth; *Total Baseball* eighth. How could he have been such a great fielder, yet rank so low? The answer is he was a really poor hitter.

Steve Evans

Born: Louis Richard Evans, February 17, 1885, Cleveland, OH
Debut: April 16, 1908; age 23
Last Game: October 3, 1915; age 30
Clubs: New York NL; St. Louis NL; Brooklyn FL; Baltimore FL

How he came to be known as Steve is a mystery. After learning baseball on the sandlots of his native Cleveland, Evans signed his first professional contract with the Dayton Veterans of the Central League in 1907, thus becoming a Veteran and a rookie at the same time. In midseason the Veterans sold him to Fairmont of the Western Pennsylvania League, where he was spotted by a scout for the New York Giants, Hall of Famer Dan Brouthers. Steve opened the 1908 season with the Giants but was sent to Monteal of the Eastern League, where he played first base for the remainder of the season. The St. Louis Cardinals purchased him and switched him to the outfield. He was the regular right fielder for the Cards for the next five years. Evans led the league in being hit by a pitch three years in a row, once getting plunked three times in a single game. In 1910 he was hit 31 times, the most ever by a left-handed batter in the NL. In 1914 Steve jumped to Brooklyn in the new Federal League. He hit .348 for the Tip-Tops, with a .416 OBP, 93 runs scored and 96 runs batted in. He led the league in slugging with a .556 average and in triples with 15. In 1915 he split the season between Brooklyn and Baltimore, again putting up outstanding numbers, including a league-leading 34 doubles. When the Federal League folded, Evans signed with Toledo of the American Association, where he hit .298, with 33 doubles, 16 triples, 10 home runs, and 101 runs scored. He had another good year for the Mud Hens in 1917, then retired from baseball.

Although Steve was a very good ballplayer, he was perhaps better known as a prankster and comedian. He had a lighthearted, cheerful personality and enjoyed life very much. Among his pranks were presenting a fan with a gift box containing a pocket watch that exploded when the man opened it and taking the field on a hot summer day in St. Louis with a Japanese paper parasol over his shoulder. He accompanied the Chicago White Sox on their world tour with the Giants in the winter of 1913-14. On the way to the port of embarkation, he walked through the train informing players that a free breakfast was being served in the dining car. Only when presented with the bill did the players realize they had been taken. In Egypt he stood on one side of the Sphinx and caught a baseball thrown over it by Ivy Wingo. He and Buck Weaver demonstrated the tango for patrons at a fancy Egyptian hotel. Evans was one of the best singers and dancers on the tour and loved demonstrating his talent. A few years later he almost went too far with one prank. On a postseason hunting trip with Elmer Knetzer and Jack Lewis, the ballplayers went to an all-night restaurant in Prairie du Chein for an early-morning breakfast. When the waitress asked what they were doing up so early, Evans said they were there to rob the bank, but not to tell anyone. The frightened girl promised not to tell, but after the players got back to their hotel, the town bell rang and the sheriff and an armed posse confronted the players. Steve had some tall explaining to do in order to get out of trouble that time.

Following his retirement from baseball, Evans worked as a supervisor for the State of Ohio. After a long illness he died at his home in Cleveland on December 28, 1943, at the age of 58.

Steve Evans is profiled in *Deadball Stars of the National League* and in the SABR *Biography Project*. Ranking: Faber System fourth; *Total Baseball* tied for fourth; James fourth.

Doc Gessler

Born: Henry Homer Gessler, December 23, 1880, Greensburg, PA
Debut: April 23, 1903; age 22
Last Game: October 7, 1911; age 30
Clubs: Detroit AL; Brooklyn NL; Chicago NL; Boston AL; Washington AL

According to one account Gessler attended Ohio University, Washington and Jefferson College, and became a physician, graduating from Johns Hopkins Medical School before his baseball career began. This seems unlikely, as he was playing in the major leagues at the age of 22. His biography in the *New York Times* stated that before entering baseball, Harry distinguished himself on the football field for Washington and Jefferson and Johns Hopkins. Web sites for Ohio and Hopkins do not mention him, but Washington and Jefferson lists him on their baseball squad in 1900 and 1901. At any rate he was already called "Doc" when he started his big league career in 1903. For some time he apparently played ball during the summer, practiced medicine during the offseason, and continued his studies at Hopkins.

While playing for the Chicago Cubs in 1906, Doc participated in one of the freakiest double plays of all time. In a game against Boston, Gessler was playing center field. With one out and Boston's Sam Brown on second base, Allie Strobel hit a fly ball. Doc caught the fly and, thinking it was the third out, put the ball in his pocket and headed for the dugout. Seeing this, Brown rounded third and headed for home. Gessler finally realized what was happening and fired the ball to the catcher, who tagged Brown to complete the double play. In 1907 Doc was demoted to the minor leagues, where he hit .326 at Columbus, earning another shot at the majors. Back in the big time, he had his best season in 1908 as he hit .308, led the league with a .394 OBP, and ranked third in slugging percentage. Over the years Gessler appeared among his league's top ten performers in every leading batting category at least once. In the field he was not quite up to par.

By 1909 he had established a medical practice in Indiana, Pennsylvania, and had invested in an oil business in Oklahoma. Following two good years with the Boston Red Sox, Doc was traded to Washington. In 1912 he was sold to Kansas City but refused to report to the Blues. He returned to Johns Hopkins and played baseball under an assumed name until he was exposed. In 1913 he appeared in 35 games for Kansas City before retiring as an active player. When the Federal League was formed in 1914, Gessler was named as manager of the Pittsburgh Rebels. After only a few games at the helm, he was deposed as skipper and remained with the organization for a while as a scout. When he registered for the draft in 1917, Gessler was a physician, residing in Tulsa. According to both the *New York Times* and the *Washington Post*, Dr. Harry H. Gessler, 45, died at his home in Indiana, Pennsylvania, on Christmas Day 1924, after a long illness. Other sources report the place of his death variously as Greensburg and Pittsburgh.

Ranking: Faber System seventh; *Total Baseball* tied for fourth.

Danny Green

Born: Edward Green, November 6, 1876, Burlington, NJ
Debut: August 17, 1898; age 21
Last Game: October 8, 1905; age 28
Clubs: Chicago NL; Chicago AL

Danny got his start in professional baseball at the age of 19 with Carlisle of the Cumberland Valley League in 1896. He played with the Springfield Ponies in the Eastern League in 1897 and 1898, hitting over .300 both years. He reached the National League with the Chicago Cubs in 1898. In 1901 he played center field for the Cubs and led the NL in putouts and total chances per game. He also had a good year at the plate that season, hitting .313 and stealing 31 bases. After four years in the NL, he jumped to the White Sox of the AL in 1902. He was an excellent hitter and base runner, finishing in the top ten in his league in on-base percentage and stolen bases four consecutive years. During one game when he was with the White Sox, Green called umpire Jack Sheridan an abusive name. Sheridan punched Green, one of the few times in major league history when an umpire struck a player. The combatants were separated and Sheridan was arrested but did not lose his position as an umpire.

In 1905 Green suffered an injury to his throwing arm, and he was released to Milwaukee of the American Association. While playing for the Brewers, Danny was struck in the head by a pitch, causing an injury from which he never fully recovered. He was sold to Sioux City of the Western League, but he hit only .226 for the Packers in 1909. In 1910 he went down to the lowest minor league classification, Class D, and played a few games for the Burlington Pathfinders in the Central Association. His health did not permit him to play longer. He returned to New Jersey and died three days after his 38th birthday on November 9, 1914, at an institution outside Camden known as the Blackwood Insane Asylum. His mental health problems were said to be linked to a brain injury he had received when hit by a pitch in Milwaukee several years earlier.

Ranking: The Faber System, *Total Baseball*, and Bill James are unanimous in ranking Danny Green third among early leaving right fielders.

Ken Harrelson

Born: Kenneth Smith Harrelson, September 4, 1941, Woodruff, SC
Debut: June 9, 1963; age 21
Last Game: June 20, 1971; age 29
Clubs: Kansas City AL; Washington AL; Boston AL; Cleveland AL

As a boy Ken attended Benedictine Military School in Savannah, where he played baseball, basketball, football, and golf. He hoped to get a basketball scholarship from the University of Kentucky, but when that did not materialize he turned to baseball. The Kansas City Athletics drafted the 17 year old as an amateur free agent in 1959, and he worked his way up the farm system, one rung at a time. He started at Olean of the New York–Pennsylvania League, then to Sanford (Florida League), Visalia (California League), Binghamton (Eastern League), and Portland (Pacific Coast League), playing one year at each level until he reached the big leagues in 1963. The following year he was sent back to the PCL, this time to Dallas, which had replaced Portland as the A's farm club. In 1965 he returned to the majors for the rest of his career. During the 1966 season he was traded to the Washington Senators, but the A's acquired him again a year later. He had been with Kansas City only a few weeks when he denounced owner Charlie Finley as a menace to baseball. The A's immediately released him, whereupon the Boston Red Sox signed him to replace the injured Tony Conigliaro. In 1968 "Hawk," as he was called because of his distinctive nose, had his best year in baseball. He made the all-star team, led the league in runs batted in, and was among the AL's top ten in batting average, on-base percentage, slugging average, runs scored, total bases, home runs, and bases on balls. He also had his best season in the field, leading the league with a perfect 1.000 average, and topping AL right fielders in Faber System fielding points and total points (fielding plus hitting).[49] That was his last good season. In the remainder of his career he compiled a cumulative batting average of .220. In 1969 Harrelson broke his leg sliding into second base in an exhibition game and missed most of the season. In 1971 Hawk retired to pursue a professional golf career.

After a few years of minimal success in golf, Hawk turned to broadcasting and found his niche in life. He started announcing Red Sox games over a Boston TV station in 1975 but was fired after the 1981 season for publicly criticizing decisions of Red Sox owner Haywood Sullivan. From 1982 to 1985 Hawk announced White Sox games, but left the broadcasting booth during the 1986 season to become the White Sox general manager. This did not work out, as he fired field manager Tony La Russa and assistant GM Dave Dombrowski, two very competent baseball men. During 1987–88 Hawk did play-by-play for Yankee games on the Baseball Network. Since 1990 he has been the main announcer for White Sox games. He is an obvious "homer," openly rooting for the Sox, whom he calls "the Good Guys." He has certain catch phrases he uses over and over again, the most notable being his call after a White Sox home run: "You can put it on the booooard. Yes!" His mannerisms rub some people the wrong way, but he is quite popular with many White Sox fans and has been nominated several times for broadcasting awards. During the season he lives in Granger, Indiana, and in Orlando during the offseason.

Ranking: Faber System sixth; *Total Baseball* tenth.

Butch Huskey

Born: Robert Leon Huskey, November 10, 1971, Anadarko, OK
Debut: September 8, 1993; age 21
Last Game: October 1, 2000; age 28
Clubs: New York NL; Seattle AL; Boston AL; Minnesota AL; Colorado NL

A 17-year-old third baseman out of Eisenhower High School in Lawton, Oklahoma, Butch was selected by the New York Mets in the seventh round of the 1989 amateur draft. With the exception of a few games with the big club in the fall of 1993, Huskey spent four years in the Mets' minor league system. He won the Doubleday Award, given annually to the MVP of each of the Mets' farm clubs, while playing for Sarasota in the Gulf Coast League in 1989. He won it again at Columbia in 1991, as he led the Sally League in home runs and RBIs. He took the award for the third time in 1993, playing for Binghamton in the Eastern League. Moving up the system, Butch played for Norfolk in the International League in 1994. He won his fourth and final Doubleday Award in 1995 as he hit .284 with 28 homers and 87 RBIs for Norfolk. In 1996 Huskey had his first full season in the majors. At 6'3" and 244 pounds, Huskey was husky, and sports reporters commented on the appropriateness of the name. He had his best major league season in 1997 when he hit .287 with 24 home runs and 81 ribbies. In the field he had problems. He could not handle the hot corner and was tried at first base before being moved to right field. The Mets traded him to Seattle after the 1998 season, but he did not fare well with the Mariners. He played briefly with four different clubs in the next two years and retired at the age of 29.

Ranking: Faber System seventeenth; *Total Baseball* sixteenth. His statistics suffered from the fact that he was frequently used as a pinch-hitter, reducing his times at bat and chances in the field. Further, his movement from position to position negatively impacted his rating as a fielder. Only once in his entire major league career did he play as many as 100 games in a year at the same position.

Harry Lumley

Born: Harry Garfield Lumley, September 29, 1880, Forest City, PA
Debut: April 14, 1904; age 23
Last Game: May 19, 1910; age 29
Club: Brooklyn NL

Although he was born in Pennsylvania, Harry moved with his parents to Lestershire (now called Johnson City), New York, as a child. He played semi-pro ball with the Endicott-Johnson Shoe Company club. In 1901 the youngster made his professional debut with the Rome club in the New York State League, hitting a robust .350. In 1902 he played for St. Paul in the American Association and hit a league-leading 18 home runs. He started the next season with Colorado Springs but spent most of 1903 with Seattle, where he led the PCL with a .387 average. He was selected by Brooklyn in the 1903 Rule 5 draft and spent his entire major league career with the Superbas. He was named by both the editors of the *Baseball Encyclopedia* and a SABR committee as the ex-post-facto Rookie of the Year for 1904. Harry certainly deserved the award as he led the league in home runs and triples, finished second in RBIs and total bases, and was sixth in hits and slugging average. He hit even better the next two seasons, raising his average each year. In 1906 he hit .326, third-best in the league, and led the circuit in slugging. Despite rheumatism and a split finger that cause him to miss 20 games, Harry placed in the top ten in OBP, hits, total bases, doubles, triples, home runs, and stolen bases. After that stellar season, injuries and a tendency to gain weight caused his productivity to decline. In 1907 he broke an ankle while sliding; in 1909 he had a shoulder injury. Bill James called him a "flameout of the 1900s."[50] In 1909 Lumley served as Brooklyn's manager. In the spring of 1910 Harry's wife died and he asked for a leave of absence. He never returned to Brooklyn. In 1911 and 1912 he was playing manager of the Binghamton Bingos and led the New York State League in batting in the latter season. The 1920 census showed him as working for an insurance company. Afterwards he operated the Terminal Café in Binghamton until failing health caused him to give it up in 1937. He died in that city on May 22, 1938, at the age of 57.

Lumley, who was nicknamed "Judge," is profiled in *Deadball Stars of the National League* and in SABR's *Biography Project*.

Ranking: Faber System ninth; *Total Baseball* sixth.

Jack McGeachey

Born: John Charles McGeachey, May 13, 1864, Clinton, MA
Debut: June 17, 1886; age 22
Last Game: August 24, 1891; age 27
Clubs: Detroit NL; St. Louis NL; Indianapolis NL; Brooklyn PL; Philadelphia AA; Boston AA

The son of Scottish immigrants, John dropped out of school by the age of 16 and was following his father's trade as a dyer in a textile mill. He made his start in professional baseball at Holyoke in 1884. He played for Waterbury the next year. In 1886 he played for four different clubs — Long Island and Providence in the Eastern League and Detroit and St. Louis in the National League. The only stability in his career came from 1887 to 1889, when he spent three years with the same club, the Indianapolis Hoosiers. In 1890 he joined the Brooklyn club in the short-lived Players League. Jack split his final major league season in 1891 between the Philadelphia and Boston clubs in the American Association. His last season in professional baseball came with the Augusta Kennebecs of the New England League in 1895. McGeavey was a weak hitter, never batting higher than .269 or driving in more than 65 runs in a big league season. He showed speed on the base paths, however, with a high of 49 stolen bases in 1888. What kept him in the majors for six seasons was his fielding, which was above average for right fielders of his era. McGeachy spent his final years in Cambridge. The 1910 census showed him as a clerk for a drug company. In 1920 he was a bartender. He died in Cambridge on April 5, 1930, at the age of 65.

Ranking: Faber System twelfth; *Total Baseball* seventeenth among seventeen.

Alex Ochoa

Born: Alex Ochoa, March 29, 1972, Miami Lakes, FL
Debut: September 18, 1995; age 23
Last Game: September 29, 2002; age 30
Clubs: New York NL; Minnesota AL; Milwaukee NL; Cincinnati NL; Colorado NL; Anaheim AL

Alex was selected by the Baltimore Orioles in the third round of the 1991 amateur draft. He went on to play for 15 different professional clubs, but the Orioles were not among them. The young man started with the Orioles' farm club in the Gulf Coast League in 1991 and worked his way up the ladder — Kane County, Frederick, Bowie, and Rochester. In 1995 Baltimore traded its promising young farmhand to the New York Mets, who assigned him to their Norfolk affiliate. The Mets gave him a taste of big league life in September, sent him back to Norfolk for part of 1996, then called him up again. He had a big day for the Mets on July 3, when he hit for the cycle with five hits, three RBIs, and three runs scored. During the next six years Alex played for six different major league clubs. His best season was 2000, when he hit .316 with 13 home runs for Cincinnati. After the 2002 season Ochoa was granted free agency and went to Japan, where he played for the Chunichi Dragons for four years, the longest time he spent with one club in his entire career. In 2007 he signed as a free agent with the Boston Red Sox, who sent him to their Pawtucket farm. Unable to make the grade with the PawSox, Alex returned to Japan and wound up his 17-year playing career with the Hiroshima Carp. In 2009 he became an assistant coach with the Red Sox.

Alex Ochoa was never a star but he was a good journeyman who could play all three outfield positions and hit well enough to merit a long career in professional baseball.

Ranking: Faber System fifteenth; *Total Baseball* tied for eleventh.

Hosken Powell

Born: Hosken Powell, May 14, 1955, Selma, AL
Debut: April 5, 1978; Age 22
Last Game: July 1, 1983; Age 28
Clubs: Minnesota AL; Toronto AL

Hosken was selected from Florida's Chipola Junior College in the nineteenth round of the 1975 amateur draft, but the young outfielder did not sign with the Pirates. The Minnesota Twins chose him as the third pick in the first round of the supplemental draft held that spring. Powell advanced quickly through the Twins' system, starting with Elizabethton in the Appalachian League in 1975, where he hit .329 and led the Rookie league in RBIs. At Reno in 1976 he hit .345 and led the Class A California League with 118 runs scored. In 1977 he leaped all the way to Tacoma of the Class AAA PCL, where he hit .326 and scored 107 times. In his first three years in the minors, Powell never hit less than .316, earning rapid advancement to the big leagues. He was unable to duplicate that success at the major league level. His best season came in his second year with the Twins, when he hit a solid .293. After the 1981 season Hosken was traded to Toronto. During his second year with the Blue Jays he slumped, and he was released in July 1983. Still a young man,

Powell signed with the Milwaukee organization and played briefly for the Vancouver Canadians but never fulfilled the promise that he had shown a few years earlier. Not yet thirty, he ended his career by hitting .213 in 57 games for Vancouver in 1984. At last report he was living in Pensacola.

Ranking: Faber System sixteenth; *Total Baseball* fifteenth.

Bobby Roth

Born: Robert Frank Roth, August 28, 1892, Burlington, WI
Debut: September 1, 1914; age 22
Last Game: October 1, 1921; age 29
Clubs: Chicago AL; Cleveland AL; Philadelphia AL; Boston AL; Washington AL; New York AL

At the age of 17 Bobby began his professional baseball career with Green Bay of the Wisconsin-Illinois League in 1910. After a poor start, he was released and caught on with Red Wing in the Minnesota-Wisconsin League. In 1911 he played third base for Racine, where he hit .255 and made 44 errors in 114 games. In 1912 and 1913 he moved from team to team, making enough moves to earn him the nickname "Globetrotter." His play improved to the point where he was pur-

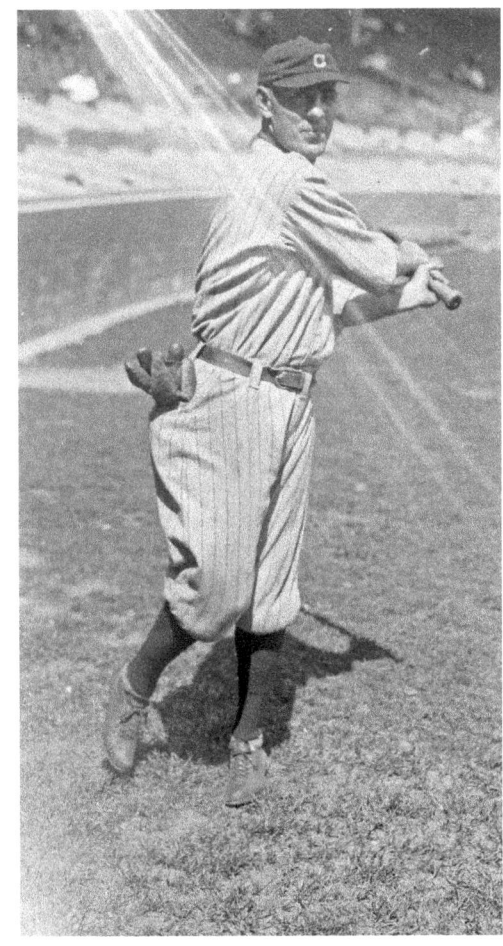

Bobby "Braggo" Roth was an entertaining talker who boasted so much about his accomplishments that he acquired the nickname "Braggo." Although perhaps not as great as he claimed, Roth was a very good hitter. Several times from 1915 to 1918 he was among the league leaders in doubles, triples, home runs, and stolen bases. Hampered by injuries and unpopular with his teammates, his major league career ended at the age of 29 (Library of Congress).

chased by Kansas City. Bobby had a good year for the Class AA Blues in 1914, batting .293 with eight home runs and 91 runs scored. His manager at KC, Bill Armour, switched him from third base to the outfield. Roth was an entertaining talker who boasted so much about his accomplishments that he acquired the nickname "Braggo." The new appellation stuck. Toward the end of the 1914 season Braggo was purchased by the Chicago White Sox and performed well, hitting .294 with six triples in 34 games. In 1915 Roth slumped at the plate and played inconsistent defense, leading to a trade to Cleveland. With the Indians Braggo's productivity increased. His seven home runs were enough to lead the AL in this deadball year. Several times from 1915 to 1918 he was among the league leaders in doubles, triples, home runs, slugging average, and stolen bases. In 1916 an unruly crowd at Sportsman's Park in St. Louis began throwing objects onto the field. A bottle hit Roth, and he hurled the missile back into the crowd. A ruckus ensued and Roth was ejected from the game for his own safety. In 1918 he suffered a back injury that shelved him for three weeks and plagued him throughout the season. Needing pitching, the Indians traded Roth to Philadelphia in 1919. Bobby's personality did not go over well with A's manager Connie Mack, and soon the Globetrotter was traveling again to Boston, Washington, and New York. Hampered by injuries, Roth did not play well and was released by the Yankees after the 1921 season.

At the age of 29 he had played for five different clubs in the last three years, and none of them wanted him any longer. Bobby went back to Wisconsin and played semi-pro ball for a year. In 1923 he returned to Kansas City. Although he was hitting .339 at the time, the Blues released him on August 3 for indifferent play. He was charged with not running out ground balls and poor play in the outfield. His teammates were not sorry to see him go. A Kansas City newspaper reported the Blues considered holding a celebration when he was dropped.[51] The St. Paul Saints picked him up immediately. Roth finished the 1923 season with a combined average of .324 for the two Class AA clubs, with 32 doubles, eight triples, 12 home runs, 110 runs scored, 97 RBIs, and 19 stolen bases — quite a season for someone accused of dogging it. Nevertheless, the Saints did not invite him back for another year. He had worn out his welcome again. As one newspaper reported it, Roth "was the exasperating grain of dust in the eye of whatever ball team he became associated with."[52] After playing semi-pro ball in the Chicago area for several years, Roth had one more fling at the professional game in 1928. He hit .283 in 67 games for the Hollywood Stars in the PCL, but hit only one home run and stole only one base.

On September 11, 1936, in Chicago, Roth was a passenger in a car driven by a friend when their vehicle was struck by an oncoming newspaper delivery truck. The friend was killed instantly; Roth died later in the day in a Chicago hospital from severe head injuries. He was 44 years old.

Bobby "Braggo" Roth is profiled in *Deadball Stars of the American League* and in SABR's *Biography Project*. Rank: Faber System eighth; *Total Baseball* seventh.

Ron Swoboda

Born: Ronald Alan Swoboda, June 30, 1944, Baltimore, MD
Debut: April 12, 1965; age 20
Last Game: September 30, 1973; age 29
Clubs: New York NL; Montreal NL; New York AL

The Mets signed Swoboda out of the University of Maryland in September 1963. The youngster spent only one season in the minors—at Williamsport and Buffalo—before being called up to the majors. Despite inconsistent hitting and erratic fielding, he quickly became a favorite of Met fans, partly because of his vivacious personality and engaging sense of humor. The Mets of 1965 were woefully weak, as shown by their 112 losses. Ron's 19 home runs provided one of the highlights of that dismal season and gave the fans hope for better things in the future. That brighter future arrived in 1969 when the Miracle Mets not only won the NL pennant, but also knocked off the heavily favored Baltimore Orioles in the World Series. Although he hit only .235 that season, Ron played a key role in the drive to the pennant, batting in 26 runs in the final five weeks of the campaign. Normally considered a poor fielder, Swoboda made a spectacular diving catch of a line drive by Brooks Robinson to snuff out a Baltimore rally in the ninth inning of Game 4 at Shea Stadium. Ron never mastered the art of hitting the curveball and was traded to Montreal in 1971. The Expos quickly traded him to the Yankees, who sent him to their farm club in Syracuse for a while, and then released him following the 1973 season. He signed as a free agent with Atlanta, but the Braves released him during spring training in 1974. Swoboda unsuccessfully attempted a comeback with the Mets during spring training in 1976.

After his retirement as a player, Ron has worked as a television sportscaster in New York and more recently in New Orleans. In 2009 he was a color commentator for telecasts of New Orleans Zephyrs games. He was a 2009 recipient of the Thurman Munson Award, given annually to a sports figure for excellence in community philanthropic work. Among other contributions Swoboda helped Habitat for Humanity in rebuilding homes destroyed by Hurricane Katrina in the Ninth Ward.

Ranking: Faber System fourteenth; *Total Baseball* thirteenth.

Chicken Wolf

Born: William Van Winkle Wolf, May 12, 1862, Louisville, KY
Debut: May 2, 1882; age 19
Last Game: August 21, 1892; age 30
Clubs: Louisville AA; St. Louis NL

See the entry on Wolf in Part One of this book.
Chicken Wolf is profiled in *Baseball's First Stars* and in SABRs *Biography Project*. Ranking: Faber System first; *Total Baseball* second. He is not ranked by James.

Ross Youngs

Born: Royce Middlebrook Youngs, April 10, 1897, Shiner, TX
Debut: September 25, 1917; age 20
Last Game: August 10, 1926; age 29
Club: New York NL

See the entry on Ross Youngs in Part One of this book.
Ranking: Faber System second; *Total Baseball* and Bill James both rank him first.

CENTER FIELDERS

Player	G	R	H	HR	RBI	BA	OBP	Faber System Bat	Field	Total
Rich Becker	789	345	570	45	243	.256	.358	90	293	383
Joe Birmingham	771	284	667	7	265	.263	.294	46	466	512
Charlie Dexter	771	424	749	16	346	.261	.318	97	65	162
John Dobbs	582	305	585	7	207	.263	.325	158	245	403
Happy Felsch	749	383	829	38	446	.293	.347	431	442	873
Dick Johnston	746	453	751	33	386	.251	.285	146	324	470
Benny Kauff	859	521	961	49	454	.311	.389	683	332	1014
Bill Lange	813	691	1056	39	579	.330	.400	714	484	1220
Rudy Law	749	379	656	18	199	.271	.325	196	214	410
Jim McTamany	813	693	794	19	334	.256	.373	550	304	854
Rowland Office	899	259	626	32	242	.259	.315	5	213	218
Homer Smoot	680	308	763	15	269	.290	.336	296	273	569
Fred Snodgrass	923	453	852	11	351	.275	.367	394	407	801
Farmer Weaver	753	423	856	9	344	.278	.330	111	281	392
Jimmy Welsh	715	387	778	35	288	.290	.340	131	360	491
Whitey Witt	1139	632	1195	18	302	.287	.362	295	240	635
Marvel Wynne	940	300	664	40	244	.247	.297	81	250	331

Rich Becker

Born: Richard Godhard Becker, February 1, 1972, Aurora, IL
Debut: September 10, 1993; age 21
Last Game: October 1, 2000; age 28
Clubs: Minnesota AL; New York NL; Baltimore AL; Milwaukee NL; Oakland AL; Detroit AL

Rich was a baseball star at Aurora West High School, making the Upstate Eight All-Conference team in 1990. The Minnesota Twins selected him in the third round (85th pick overall) of the 1990 amateur draft, and sent him to their Elizabethton club in the Appalachian League. He moved up the chain quickly, to Kenosha in 1991, Visalia in 1992, and Nashville in 1993. He made the big league club that September and split the 1994 and 1995 seasons between the Twins and their Salt Lake farm club in the PCL. His best year in the bigs came in 1996, when he hit .291 and scored 92 runs. In 1998 he was traded to the New York Mets for Alex Ochoa and never recovered his hitting stroke, bouncing between five clubs in three years until he was out of the majors after the 2000 season. Although he was a good fielder, his glove work was not enough to keep him in the majors as his batting productivity declined. In 2001 he played Class AAA ball with Calgary in the PCL and Toledo in the American Association. In 2003 he played for Fargo-Moorhead in the independent Northern League and hit a respectable .289. In October Joliet claimed him off waivers, but he never played for the Jackhammers.

Ranking: Faber System fourteenth; *Total Baseball* seventh.

Joe Birmingham

Born: Joseph Leo Birmingham, August 6, 1884, Elmira, NY
Debut: September 12, 1906; age 22
Last Game: June 25, 1914; age 29
Club: Cleveland AL

Joe's first baseball was played in his hometown for a semi-pro team sponsored by the Fishing Tackle Manufacturers of America. Later he played both college football and baseball at Notre Dame and then at Cornell in 1904–05. He made his professional debut with the Amsterdam-Gloversville-Johnstown club of the New York State League. He spent less than a full season in the minors, as his contract was purchased by the Cleveland Naps in August for $1500. "Dode," as he was sometimes called, hit higher than .300 only once in the majors, as he posted a .304 mark in 1911. However, he was an outstanding fielder, with one of the strongest throwing arms in baseball. He led the AL in Faber System fielding points three times (1908, 1910, and 1911).[53] Bill

James placed him on his Gold Glove team of the 1900s.[54] At the age of 28, Joe was named manager of the Naps in 1912. His tenure as manager was an unhappy one. He feuded with second baseman Nap Lajoie when he benched the future Hall of Famer during a batting slump in 1913. In 1915 he blamed owner Charlie Somers' interference for an injury to Joe Jackson when the owner insisted that Jackson be moved to first base. Somers immediately fired Birmingham.

Dode was out of baseball for the rest of 1915 but came back as playing manager of Toronto of the International League in 1916. That job lasted only one year. In 1917 Joe played for Reading in the New York State League. In 1918 he played only three games for Toledo. In 1919–20 he was a playing manager again, this time with Pittsfield in the Eastern League. Under his leadership the Hillies won the pennant. He concluded his professional baseball career as a non-playing manager with Albany of that circuit in 1921. Unfortunately for Joe's managerial reputation, the Senators finished in the basement while Pittsfield won another flag. However, Joe kept his interest in baseball. He appeared at old-timers games and scouted for the New York Giants. During World War II he worked in a Brooklyn shipyard. Later he became an umpire in the Mexican League. He died in a Tampico hotel room from a heart attack on April 24, 1946, at the age of 61.

Ranking: Faber System eighth; *Total Baseball* thirteenth.

Charlie Dexter

Born: Charles Dana Dexter, June 15, 1875, Evansville, IN
Debut: April 17, 1896; age 20
Last Game: September 27, 1903; age 28
Clubs: Louisville NL; Chicago NL; Boston NL

Although it is reported that Charlie attended Sewanee College (now the University of the South), there is no evidence that he played baseball there. He first appears in the sports pages as a catcher and outfielder with Louisville in 1896 at the age of 20. His best year in the majors came in 1898, when he hit .314, stole 44 bases, and scored 76 runs for the Colonels. After four years with Louisville, Dexter played another four seasons in the majors, with Chicago and Boston, but he never hit well in either place. In 1901 and 1902 he played every position on the field except pitcher. After his major league career ended, he played and managed a few years in the minors. Charlie played first base and second base for Louisville, now in the American Association, in 1904 and 1905, managing the club during part of the latter season. In 1906 he played first base for Des Moines in the Western League and hit a career-best

.333. His average fell precipitously the next two years as he played first base and outfield for the Champions and managed them to a last-place finish in the league in 1908. Following his retirement from baseball he remained in Iowa, managing a music store in Des Moines in 1917 and working as a buyer for a clothing store in the capital city in 1920. In Cedar Rapids on June 8, 1934, he committed suicide by shooting himself. He was 58.

Charlie Dexter is a member of the Evansville Sports Hall of Fame. Ranking: Faber System seventeenth of seventeen; *Total Baseball* fourteenth.

John Dobbs

Born: John Gordon Dobbs, June 3, 1875, Chattanooga, TN
Debut: April 30, 1901; age 25
Last Game: September 20, 1905; age 30
Clubs: Cincinnati NL; Chicago NL; Brooklyn NL

John got his start in professional baseball at the age of 20 with his hometown Chattanooga Warriors in 1895. From there he went to Mobile, Terre Haute, Springfield, Wheeling, and Utica before making his big league debut with the Cincinnati Reds in 1901. His best year in the majors came in 1902 when he hit .299 and led the NL in Faber System fielding points as a left fielder.[55] John never came close to hitting that well again, but he continued to be an excellent fielder, usually playing in the center garden. After his major league career was over, he remained active in baseball the rest of his life. He played five years in Nashville, Chattanooga, and Montgomery and managed for a quarter of a century, 23 years in the Southern Association and one year each in the Sally and Piedmont leagues. As a manager he won 1,918 games while losing 1,487 for a winning percentage of .563. His teams won five pennants in the Southern Association; the Chattanooga Lookouts in 1909, the New Orleans Pelicans in 1915, the Memphis Chicks in 1924, and the Birmingham Barons in 1928 and 1929 were all league champions. In 1933 Dobbs became co-owner as well as manager of the Charlotte Hornets in the Piedmont League. The Hornets won the first half of a split season in 1934. Two days before the playoffs for the title were scheduled to begin, John Dobbs died of a heart attack in Charlotte on September 9 at the age of 59.

Ranking: Faber System and *Total Baseball* both rank him twelfth.

Happy Felsch

Born: Oscar Emil Felsch, August 22, 1891, Milwaukee, WI
Debut: April 14, 1915; age 23

Last Game: September 26, 1920; age 29
Club: Chicago AL

See the entry on Happy Felsch in Part One of this book. Felsch is profiled in *Deadball Stars of the American League* and in the *SABR Biography Project.* Ranking: Faber System third; *Total Baseball* fourth; James second.

Dick Johnston

Born: Richard Frederick Johnston, April 6, 1863, Kingston, NY
Debut: August 12, 1884; age 21
Last Game: August 16, 1891; age 28
Clubs: Richmond AA; Boston NL; Boston PL; New York PL; Cincinnati AA

Dick started his professional baseball career with the Richmond Virginias of the Eastern League on May 1, 1884. On August 4 Richmond left to join the American Association, and the 21-year-old Johnston was now a major leaguer. The next year he became a National Leaguer and played five years for the Boston Red Caps. His best season came in 1888, when he hit .296, led the league in triples with 18, and was second in total bases and third in runs scored, hits, doubles, and home runs. He finished the season in the circuit's top ten in slugging, runs batted in, and batting average. That was to be his only year as a batting star. He was an excellent fielder, topping the NL in putouts and total chances per nine innings in 1886 and 1887, and was named the best fielding center gardener by the Faber System both years.[56] Dick jumped to the Players League in 1890 and wound up his major league career with Cincinnati in the American Association in 1891. In 1892 he was back in the Eastern League with New Haven and Elmira. In 1894 he returned to his hometown of Kingston and closed out his professional playing career in the New York State League. Later Johnston followed a variety of occupations. He was a printer in Kingston in 1900, a haberdashery clerk in Newburgh in 1920, and a guard in a corrections facility in Detroit in 1930. He died in Detroit on April 4, 1934, two days before his 71st birthday.
Ranking: Faber System tenth; *Total Baseball* eleventh.

Benny Kauff

Born: Benjamin Michael Kauff, January 5, 1890, Pomeroy, OH
Debut: April 20, 1912; age 22
Last Game: July 2, 1920; age 30
Clubs: New York AL; Indianapolis FL; Brooklyn FL; New York NL

See the entry on Kauff in Part One of this book.

Benny Kauff is profiled in *Deadball Stars of the National League* and in SABR's *Biography Project*. Ranking: Faber System second; *Total Baseball* first; James third.

Bill Lange

Born: William Alexander Lange, June 6, 1871, San Francisco, CA
Debut: April 27, 1893; age 21
Last Game: October 15, 1899; age 28
Club: Chicago NL

See the entry on Lange in Part One of this book.

Bill Lange is profiled in *Nineteenth Century Stars*. Ranking: Faber System and James both rank him first; *Total Baseball* places him second.

Rudy Law

Born: Rudy Karl Law, October 7, 1956, Waco, TX
Debut: September 12, 1978; age 21
Last Game: October 4, 1986; age 29
Clubs: Los Angeles NL; Chicago AL; Kansas City AL

Although he was born in Texas, Rudy grew up in California and attended Ravenswood High School in East Palo Alto. He was signed as an amateur free agent by the Los Angeles Dodgers in 1975 and assigned to their Bellingham farm club in the Northwest League. His .335 batting average earned him a promotion to Lodi in 1976, where he excelled by hitting .386. After batting .312 and stealing 79 bases at Albuquerque in the PCL in 1978, he got a late-season call-up to the Dodgers. He moved back and forth between Albuquerque and Los Angeles the next three years. With blazing speed on the base paths, he was one of the fastest players in baseball. Rudy did not have great base running instincts, but his incredible speed enabled him to set a Dodger record for steals by a rookie. Four times he ranked among the top ten base stealers in the AL. He had little power at the plate but frequently was able to beat out ground balls for hits. In the outfield he did not always get a good jump on fly balls, but his outstanding speed enabled him to make up for mistakes. In 1983 he led the AL in fielding percentage. Law had a weak throwing arm, and runners often took an extra base on hits to center field. Bill James wrote that Law had the worst outfield arm of the 1980s.[57] The Dodgers traded Rudy to the White Sox in the spring of 1982, and the speedster had his best major league seasons in Comiskey. He hit .318 in 1982 and pilfered 77 sacks in 1983.

The Sox released him in 1986 and he played his final major league season for Kansas City. Law played a few games for San Bernardino of the California League before hanging up his spikes in 1987.

Rudy has continued his interest in baseball, acting as an unofficial ambassador for major league baseball in general and the Los Angeles Dodgers in particular. He has been active in a movement to encourage black inner-city youths to take up the game. Recently he has worked with the Urban Youth Academy in Compton and the Eastside Little League in Baldwin Park, among other sites.

Ranking: Faber System eleventh; *Total Baseball* tenth.

Jim McTamany

Born: James Edward McTamany, July 1, 1863, Philadelphia, PA
Debut: August 15, 1885; age 22
Last Game: October 5, 1891; age 28
Clubs: Brooklyn AA; Kansas City AA; Columbus AA; Philadelphia AA

Jim started his professional baseball career with the Lancaster Ironsides of the Eastern League in 1884. The next year he played for Lancaster and Baltimore before making his major league debut with Brooklyn late in the season. Jim established himself as a good outfielder, leading the league in total chances per nine innings in 1886 and in assists and double plays in 1887. After four years with Brooklyn he went to Kansas City for the 1888 season. In 1889 the Columbus Solons purchased him from the Cowboys for $1000. McTamany had two outstanding years with Columbus, drawing more than 100 walks and scoring more than 100 runs each year, with an OBP of over .400. In 1890 Jim led the AA in both bases on balls and runs scored, and ranked seventh in doubles and ninth in OBP. So adept was he at drawing bases on balls that he led the league in five of his six full seasons in the AA. His ability to draw walks helped him attain a career OBP of .373 while batting only .256. The difference between his BA and OBP is one of the largest in major league history. According to the Faber System, in 1889 and again in 1890 McTamany was the best center fielder in the AA when both hitting and fielding are considered.[58]

After his great year in 1890, Jim slumped and played only one more campaign in the majors. In 1892 he hit only .220 for Rochester of the Eastern League and fell to York of the Pennsylvania State League in 1893 and Indianapolis in the Western League in 1894. Out of the majors at 28, his professional career was over at age 31. Two mysteries remain about McTamany. Why did his productivity decline so rapidly after 1890? And why do modern baseball researchers virtually ignore him? Bill James wrote that McTamany had one of the best final seasons of any center fielder,[59] yet no biographical sketches of him exist. Jim died in Lenni, a suburb of Philadelphia, on April 16, 1916, at the age of 52.

Ranking: Faber System fourth; *Total Baseball* third.

Rowland Office

Born: Rowland Johnie Office, October 25, 1952, Sacramento, CA
Debut: August 5, 1972; age 19
Last Game: April 20, 1982; age 30
Clubs: Atlanta NL; Montreal NL; New York AL

Rowland played baseball at C. K. McClatchy High School in Sacramento. It has been reported that he also played for Sacramento City College, but his name does not appear on the college's list of alumni who played in the majors. He was selected by the Atlanta Braves in the fourth round (93rd overall pick) of the 1970 amateur draft. The youngster started his professional career with Greenwood in the Western Carolinas League in 1971, moved up to Savannah of the Southern League in 1972, and when he joined the Braves that August, he was the youngest player in the major leagues. Rowland was sent down to Richmond of the International League in 1973 but made the Braves' starting lineup in 1974. He was not quite a star for the Braves, but he played well enough to be a regular in seven of his eleven big league seasons. One of the highlights of his career was his leap over the seven-foot-high center field fence to rob Mike Ivie of a homer in 1975. It has been called the greatest defensive play ever made in Atlanta–Fulton County Stadium. In the middle of the 1976 he had a hot streak when he hit in 29 consecutive games. The Braves granted him free agency after the 1979 season, and he signed with Montreal. The Expos released him in the spring of 1982 and he signed with the Phillies, who sent him to their Oklahoma City farm club. He hit only .183 in 26 games for the '89ers, earning another release. The Yankees picked him up, played him in two games and sent him to Columbus in the International League, where he closed out his professional career by hitting a respectable .297.

Ranking: Faber System sixteenth; *Total Baseball* seventeenth out of seventeen.

Homer Smoot

Born: Homer Vernon Smoot, March 23, 1878, Galestown, MD
Debut: April 17, 1902; age 24
Last Game: October 7, 1906; age 28
Clubs: St. Louis NL; Cincinnati NL

Homer played baseball and football at Washington College in Chestertown, Maryland, in the late 1890s. During those same years he played semipro ball at Cambridge and Salisbury and across the state line in Delaware at Purcell and Laurel. He started his professional career in 1900 with the Allentown Peanuts in the Atlantic League. When that circuit folded, he moved to the Eastern League, where he played for Worcester and Providence the remainder of the season. With Worcester in 1901 he led the league with a .356 batting average. In 1902 Smoot joined the St. Louis Cardinals in the National League and immediately became the team's regular center fielder. He started a string of batting more than 500 times that season, becoming the only player in major league history to play five or more years and have at least 500 at-bats every season he played. Smoot, sometimes called "Doc," was a good hitter for the Deadball Era, ranking in the NL's top ten in almost every offensive category at least once — batting average, slugging, hits, singles, doubles, triples, home runs, RBIs, extra-base hits, and sacrifices. He was also a fine fielder, leading the league in putouts his rookie year. After four excellent seasons his level of play declined in 1906, probably because of rheumatism. Homer was traded to the Chicago Cubs, who sold him to Toledo of the American Association at the end of the season. He hit better than .300 in each of three seasons with the Mud Hens. From Toledo he went to Louisville and Kansas City in the AA, then to Wilkes-Barre of the New York State League, where he ended his playing career in 1912.

Doc suffered from rheumatism for several years.[60] The affliction became more severe over time, probably accounting for his early departure from the major leagues and certainly leading to his retirement in 1912. Homer coached for one season at his alma mater and managed the Salisbury Indians of the Eastern Shore League in 1925. However, he spent most of his final years farming, raising chickens, and operating a feed store in Salisbury. On March 28, 1928, he died of spinal meningitis in Salisbury two days after his fiftieth birthday.

Homer Smoot is profiled in SABR's *Biography Project*. Ranking: Faber System seventh; *Total Baseball* sixth.

Fred Snodgrass

Born: Frederick Carlisle Snodgrass, October 19, 1897, Ventura, CA
Debut: June 4, 1908; age 20
Last Game: October 5, 1916; age 28
Clubs: New York NL; Boston NL

In 1907 Fred was a catcher for St. Vincent's College when the collegians played an exhibition game against the New York Giants. The youngster made quite an impression on New York manager John McGraw. When McGraw came to Los Angeles to attend horse races the next February, he inquired about Snodgrass. Learning that Fred was catching for a semi-pro team called the Hoegee Flags, McGraw left a message for the young man to come see him at his hotel. When Snodgrass arrived the manager offered him a contract and Fred's professional career began. At the age of 20, with no minor league experience, Snodgrass was a Giant. He sat on the bench for most of the 1908 and 1909 seasons, unable to get much playing time behind Roger Bresnahan or Chief Meyers. In 1910 the Giants switched Fred to the outfield, and he was their regular center fielder for the next six years. He hit .321 in 1910 with an OBP of .440. Although he did not have much power, he posted some good numbers, with career highs of 91 runs scored, 77 RBIs, and 51 stolen bases. Wearing a baggy uniform and crowding the plate, he became expert at getting hit by pitches. The Giants of 1911 to 1913 were a rough and tough bunch and a very good ball club. Snodgrass fit right in, and he helped them win three straight pennants.

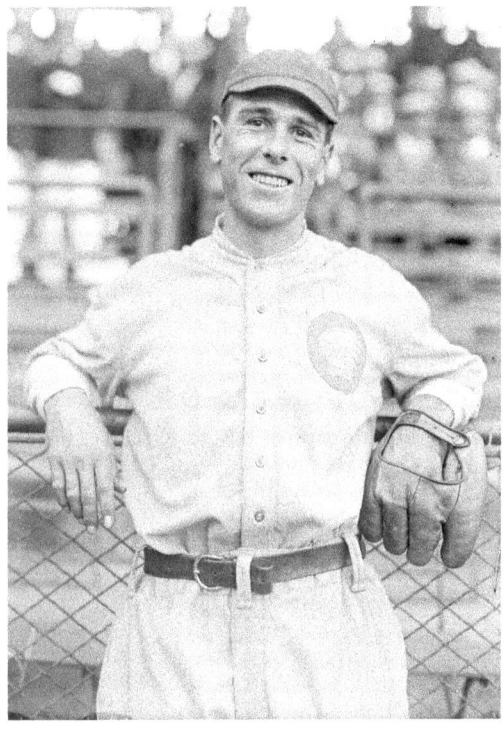

Fred Snodgrass is remembered as the goat of the 1912 World Series, when he dropped an easy fly ball that contributed to the Giants losing the Series to the Red Sox. That one miscue should not tarnish the reputation of this fine ballplayer. He was among the better center fielders of his era (Library of Congress).

He did not fare so well in the World Series, however. At the start of the 1911 Fall Classic against the Philadelphia A's, the Giants sharpened their spikes with files in full view of their opponents in an effort to intimidate A's fielders. Twice Fred slid hard into third baseman Frank Baker, ripping the fielder's pants both times and inflicting a wound the second time that took several minutes to heal. Snodgrass was, perhaps unfairly, charged with being the dirtiest player in baseball, and unfounded reports circulated that he had been shot by an irate fan. In the 1912 Series against the Red Sox, Snodgrass committed the famous muff that dogged him the rest of his life. In the twelfth inning of a tie game he dropped an easy fly ball that allowed what proved to be the winning run to get on base. He carried the stigma of that error to his grave. Even his obituary in the *New York Times* was headlined: "Fred Snodgrass, 86, Dead; Ball Player Muffed 1912 Fly."[61] The over-reaction to his miscue was unfair; dropping a fly ball is not an unusual occurrence in our national pastime. Neither his teammates nor his manager blamed him for losing the Series, but the newspapers did. Actually, Snodgrass was an excellent fielder. The Faber System rated him as the league's best all-round center fielder in 1910 and the best fielder at the position in 1911.[62]

The Giants released him in 1915, and he played parts of two seasons with the Boston Braves before returning to California. He played one year in the Pacific Coast League, then retired to go into the appliance business. He became a successful businessman and banker in Oxnard, served three terms on the city council, and was appointed mayor in 1937. After 11 months he resigned and moved to Ventura, where he bought a ranch and grew walnuts and lemons. On April 5, 1974, he died in Ventura at the age of 86, leading to that unfortunate headline in the *Times*.

Fred Snodgrass in profiled in *Deadball Stars of the National League* and in SABR's *Biography Project*. Ranking: Faber System and *Total Baseball* fifth; James fourth.

Farmer Weaver

Born: William B. Weaver, March 23, 1865, Parkersburg, WV
Debut: September 16, 1888; age 23
Last Game: September 29, 1894; age 29
Clubs: Louisville AA; Louisville NL; Pittsburgh NL

Weaver probably acquired his nickname due to his rural background. Very little is known about his life outside the major leagues. He started his big league career with Louisville in the American Association and remained with the Colonels when they moved to the National League. Except for thirty games with Pittsburgh in 1894, Weaver spent his entire time in the Show with Louisville. Farmer was not a very powerful hitter, although he topped the .290 mark twice. His speed helped him, as he stole 45 bases in 1890 and scored 101 runs. He had one memorable day at the plate. On August 12, 1890, he hit for the cycle while making six hits in the game. No other major leaguer duplicated that feat until Ian Kinsler did it on Jackie Robinson Day in 2009. Farmer was an excellent fielder. In 1891 he led league in putouts, assists, and percentage — the Triple Crown for fielders. He led the AA in Faber System fielding points that season.[63] Although he was primarily an outfielder, Weaver also caught a few games and played all four infield positions. After he retired from baseball, he worked for the Goodyear Tire and Rubber Company in Akron. He died in Akron on January 23, 1934, at the age of 68.

Ranking: Faber System thirteenth; *Total Baseball* ninth.

Jimmy Welsh

Born: James Daniel Welsh, October 9, 1902, Denver, CO
Debut: April 14, 1925; age 22
Last Game: September 28, 1930; age 27
Clubs: Boston NL; New York NL

Although Jimmy was born in Denver, he grew up in Oakland and started his professional baseball career with the Oaks in the Pacific Coast League. From there he went to Seattle, where he hit .350 in 1924. The Boston Braves purchased his services for a hefty $50,000 and installed him as their regular right fielder. As a rookie he hit .312 in 1925, which was his career high. During his major league career, he averaged .290. Welsh was an excellent fielder, leading NL right fielders in assists in 1925 and 1926. The Faber System rated him as the league's top right fielder in 1925.[64] In 1927 the Braves moved him to center field, where he continued his fielding brilliance, leading the loop in total chances per nine innings in 1930. Bill James wrote that Welsh should have won a Gold Glove that year.[65] In 1928 the Braves traded Jimmy and Shanty Hogan to the New York Giants for Rogers Hornsby, but reacquired him the next year. After the 1930 season the Braves traded Jimmy to the Cubs, who sent him to their farm club in Los Angeles. Unable to agree on a contract with their new acquisition, the Angels sent Jimmy to the Mission club in San Antonio. Jimmy suffered a finger injury in 1931, and the Missions released him in the spring of 1932. He was then signed by Seattle and spent two years there, before winding up his PCL career with Oakland in 1935. He played some semi-pro ball in Alameda County before hanging up his spikes. Welsh died in Oakland on October 30, 1970, at the age of 68.

Ranking: Faber System ninth; *Total Baseball* eighth.

Whitey Witt

Born: Ladislaw Waldemar Wittkowski, September 28, 1895, Orange, MA
Debut: April 12, 1916; age 20
Last Game: August 18, 1896; age 30
Clubs: Philadelphia AL; New York AL; Brooklyn NL

The son of Polish parents, Whitey anglicized his name to Lawton Walter Witt. The nickname "Whitey" was bestowed in recognition of his blond hair. It is said that Witt attended Bowdoin College, but there is no record of his having played baseball for the Polar Bears. The Philadelphia A's signed him out of high school for $300 a month and installed him immediately as their regular shortstop. He missed the entire 1918 season because of World War I. After his return he played mainly in center field. In 1923 Witt led AL center fielders in fielding percentage. He did not have much power at the plate, but he was a good bunter and could beat out infield hits. After an unimpressive beginning, he improved his hitting and batted higher than .300 three times and scored 100 runs or more twice between 1920 and 1923. The A's traded him to New York in 1922, and he led the AL in bases on balls that season.

On September 16 he was involved in an incident that brought him more notoriety than anything else in his career. The Yankees and the St. Louis Browns were involved in a tense pennant race that season. As the Browns batted in the last half of the ninth inning, trailing 2–1, Witt set out in pursuit of a fly ball, only to be hit in the forehead by a pop bottle hurled from the stands by an irate fan. Whitey was carried from the field on a litter but came back to play the next day with his head swathed in bandages. AL president Ban Johnson offered a $1000 reward for the arrest of the offending fan. No one claimed the reward, and Johnson launched his own investigation. In what Tom Meany called "the biggest farce in baseball jurisprudence," Johnson announced after the investigation that no fan had thrown the bottle after all. He concluded that the bottle had been lying in the center field grass and when Whitey inadvertently stepped on it, the bottle flew up and hit him in the head.[66] Witt's good friend and fellow outfielder Babe Ruth said, "It's a wonder they didn't accuse Whitey of trying to commit suicide."[67] In one reference book it is stated that this incident occurred on the day the Yankees clinched the pennant.[68] Actually, the Yankees sewed up the flag the following Monday when, with his head still bandaged, Witt hit a two-run ninth-inning single to win the game for the New Yorkers, 3–2.

After the 1925 season the Yankees released Witt, and he played his final major league season for Brooklyn in 1926. In 1927 Whitey played 19 games for Kansas City in the American Association. He hit .377 and had an OBP of .472 — not a bad way to close out a baseball career. After his retirement, Witt purchased a farm in Alloway Township, New Jersey, and opened Whitey's Irish Bar in nearby Salem, which became a popular gathering place for fans and players. He died from a heart attack at his home on July 14, 1988. He was 92.

Ranking: Faber System sixth; *Total Baseball* fifteenth. Regardless of his stats, he is best remembered for being felled by that pop bottle.

Marvell Wynne

Born: Marvell Wynne, December 17, 1959, Chicago, IL
Debut: June 15, 1983; age 23
Last Game: October 3, 1990; age 30
Clubs: Pittsburgh NL; San Diego NL; Chicago NL

Only a few major league teams hold tryout camps each year. Among those that do, most do not require pitching prospects to run. Teenaged Marvell Wynne was fortunate to attend a camp that was an exception to the rule. As a pitcher, he would not have made the grade at the Kansas City camp in 1978. However, as Art Stewart, director of scouting for the Royals, said, "He ran for us and flew like the wind. If he hadn't run we would never have known."[69] The Royals signed him as an amateur free agent and made him an outfielder. It took nearly five years in the minors for Marvell to be ready for prime time. He started in the Gulf Coast League in 1979 and played for Charleston in the Sally League in 1980. Kansas City traded him to the Mets organization in 1981. Marvell played for the Jackson Mets in the Texas League in 1981, and moved up to the top minor league rung with Tidewater of the International League in 1982. During the 1983 season he was traded to Pittsburgh and made his major league debut with the Pirates in June. His speed made him a good fit for the expansive outfield at Three Rivers Stadium. In 1986 he was traded to San Diego, where Jack Murphy Stadium had an even deeper center field. However, he did not hit well and was traded again, this time to the Chicago Cubs, where he became a part-time player. In October 1990 he was purchased by the Hanshin Tigers and played one year in Japan. Wynne was never a good hitter and relied primarily on his speed and defense to keep him in baseball. In 1984 he batted 653 times without hitting a home run. No one has had more at-bats in a homerless season since then. However, he is in the record books for two home run feats. On April 13, 1986, he hit a pinch-hit home run for the Padres, stayed in the game, and hit another homer in the same contest. Exactly one year later, on April 13, 1987, he led off the game with a home run. Second up, Tony Gwynn followed with a dinger. Third man up, John Kruk, hit a four-bagger. For the first time in major league history, the first three men to bat in a game hit consecutive home runs. Since retiring as a player, Marvell has been replaced in the sports limelight by his son, Marvell Wynne II, who in 2009 was playing major league soccer with Toronto FC.

Ranking: Faber System fifteenth; *Total Baseball* sixteenth.

LEFT FIELDERS

Player	G	R	H	HR	RBI	BA	OBP	Bat	Faber System Field	Total
Shad Barry	1100	516	1073	10	391	.267	.321	265	321	419
Beals Becker	875	367	763	45	292	.276	.335	285	162	447
Curt Blefary	974	394	649	112	382	.237	.342	355	167	522
Lee Magee	1015	467	1031	12	277	.276	.325	323	347	670
Carlos May	1165	545	1127	90	536	.274	.357	659	223	882
Kevin Mench	702	309	629	89	330	.269	.326	126	193	319
Mike Menosky	810	363	685	18	252	.278	.369	279	252	531
Darby O'Brien	709	577	805	20	394	.282	.344	320	214	534
Spike Shannon	694	383	677	3	183	.259	.337	342	288	630
Gary Thomasson	900	315	591	61	294	.249	.330	115	66	181

Shad Barry

Born: John C. Barry, October 27, 1878, Newburgh, NY
Debut: May 30, 1899; age 20
Last Game: October 7, 1908; age 29
Clubs: Washington NL; Boston NL; Philadelphia NL; Chicago NL; Cincinnati NL; St. Louis NL; New York NL

Shad played baseball at Niagara University from 1896 to 1899 and went straight from the campus to the big leagues, with no detour into the minors. The nickname "Shad" was a compliment, probably given in recognition of his style or sense of fashion. After only one season with Washington, Barry was purchased by Boston for $7500, a good price for a ballplayer in those days. During his ten years in the majors, Shad played for seven different teams, all of them in the National League. His best season came in 1905, when he hit .304 and scored 100 runs. Playing in the Deadball Era, he did not put up power numbers; his three home runs in 1902 ranked fifth in the league. He never led the league in any statistical category, but his versatility made him a valuable utility man. In addition to the outfield, he played all four infield spots, ranging from 42 games at shortstop to 295 at first base. He had a really poor year at the bat in 1908, and his big league career ended at the age of 29. During World War I Shad Barry was in charge of all baseball operations of the American Expeditionary Forces in Europe. He died November 27, 1936, in Los Angeles, California. His baseball career overlapped that of another John "Jack" Barry, the famous shortstop of the Philadelphia Athletics. This similarity in names caused some confusion in newspaper accounts of Shad's death.
Ranking: Faber System eighth; *Total Baseball* tenth.

Beals Becker

Born: David Beals Becker, July 5, 1886, El Dorado, KS
Debut: April 19, 1908; age 21
Last Game: October 6, 1915; age 29
Clubs: Pittsburgh NL; Boston NL; New York NL; Cincinnati NL; Philadelphia NL

As a schoolboy Beals was a three-sport star at Wentworth Military Academy in Lexington, Missouri. He played left end on the football eleven, was the center on the basketball squad, and pitched and played outfield on the baseball team. The recipient of Wentworth's Champion Athlete Award in 1905, he is the only graduate of the academy to play major league baseball. He pitched for a club in Oklahoma that summer. In 1906 he joined the Wichita Jobbers and won the Western Association batting championship the following year, the first of four minor league batting titles he was to win. In 1908 Beals received his first taste of major league ball with the Pittsburgh Pirates. The Corsairs sent him down to Little Rock in July, but Boston purchased him and brought him back to the Show in August. For eight seasons he toiled in the big leagues, playing with five different clubs. An inability to hit left-handed pitching consistently kept him from becoming a major star. Even with this weakness, he hit .316 in 1913 and .325 the next year. He led the NL in home runs four times, in slugging thrice, in batting twice, and in triples and total bases once each. He never pitched in the NL, playing mostly in the outfield with an occasional game at first base.

One source wrote, "After his major league career ended, Becker bounced around the minor leagues for a number of years."[70] Actually, he played for Kansas City of the American Association for six years and Seattle of the Pacific Coast League for two years—hardly bouncing around. At Kansas City he won the batting championship in 1916 and led the AA in home runs the same year. Somehow he had learned how to hit southpaws. In 1917 he repeated, again winning both those titles as well as leading the loop in hits. In 1919 he hit .332 but won no crowns. In 1920 Becker retired from baseball to own and operate a billiards and pool establishment in Lemoore, California. The Blues tried to entice him back to Kansas City and succeeded in 1922. His first year back in baseball, Beals won another batting title, hitting a hefty .367 with 26 home runs. He hit .301 the following year. In July 1924 Becker was released by Kansas City and immediately joined the Seattle club in the PCL, where he hit .310 for the remainder of the year. He played one more year for Seattle and retired in 1925. Becker was a friendly and witty conversationalist and reportedly very popular with fellow players and fans alike. He owned a farm in Kansas and had several business interests in California. He died on August 16, 1943, at the home of his sister in Huntington Park at the age of 57. Ranking: Faber System seventh; *Total Baseball* fourth.

Curt Blefary

Born: Curtis Le Roy Blefary, July 5, 1943, Brooklyn, NY
Debut: April 14, 1965; age 21
Last Game: October 4, 1972; age 29
Clubs: Baltimore AL; Houston NL; New York AL; Oakland AL; San Diego NL

Curt was a star athlete at New Jersey's Mahwah High School. He was an all-state halfback in football. He played third base and caught for the baseball team and was named to the "Best of the Century Team" by the Bergen *Record*.[71] He was good, and he knew it, leading to a reputation for cockiness. In the fall of 1961 he starred for the Wagner College football team. Before the 1962 baseball season began, the New York Yankees signed him as an amateur free agent for $18,000 and sent him to Greensboro of the Carolina League to learn to play the outfield. The young left-handed hitter showed flashes of potential and signs of an ill temper. He also suffered a minor leg injury. The Yankees did not protect him from becoming a first-round waiver pick by Baltimore. The Orioles kept him at Greensboro for part of the 1963 season, then sent him to Elmira in the Eastern League, where Curt played first base and caught. In the fall of 1963 Baltimore sent him to the Florida Instructional League and counseled him on controlling his temper. He was promoted to Rochester of the International League in 1964 and had a good season, hitting 31 home runs and leading the loop in walks.

In 1965 Blefary made his big league debut, playing in the Baltimore outfield and winning AL Rookie of the Year honors. Although he never attained a high batting average, he hit with power and showed good discipline at the plate. He ranked in the top ten in bases on balls four times in his first five years. In both 1965 and 1966 he was in the top ten in both OBP and slugging percentage. In 1967 he ranked eighth in home runs and seventh in RBIs. In the outfield he demonstrated limited range, with a strong but inaccurate throwing arm. At various times he tried other positions, usually first base. After the 1968 season Curt asked for a trade and was sent to Houston. Blefary blasted his ex-manager in the press. Blefary was a misfit in Houston and again asked for a trade, complaining that his manager had not handled him correctly. The Astros traded him to the Yankees. Again he was unhappy with his manager and once more asked to be traded. It was becoming a refrain. He played 21 games for the Yankees, 58 for Oakland, and 74 for San Diego. After he was released by the Padres in 1972, he signed as a free agent with Atlanta but never played a game for the Braves. They released him during spring training in 1973. No one else wanted him. He did not understand it, saying perhaps he had been too outspoken.

Out of baseball, Blefary tried a variety of other jobs. He sold insurance and automobiles; he worked in bars and fast food restaurants; he drove a truck. He found no joy in any of these endeavors. Eventually, he bought a nightclub, Curt's Coo Coo Lounge, in Dania, Florida. In the 1980s he acknowledged that he had a drinking problem. He tried Alcoholic Anonymous for 11 years but that did not help. In 1994 he completed Sam McDowell's alcohol rehabilitation program. But it was too late. He developed chronic pancreatitis, caused by years of alcohol abuse. The disease took his life. He died at his home in Pompano Beach on January 28, 2001, at the age of 57. His biographer wrote that Curt "had three productive seasons before his intertwined personal demons, alcohol and anger, overcame his terrific natural ability."[72]

Curt Blefary is profiled in SABR's *Biography Project*. Ranking: Faber System sixth; *Total Baseball* and Bill James both ranked him first at his position, although James assigned him to right field.

Lee Magee

Born: Leopold Christopher Hoernschemeyer, June 4, 1889, Cincinnati, OH
Debut: July 4, 1911; age 22
Last Game: September 28, 1919; age 30
Clubs: St. Louis NL; Brooklyn FL; New York AL; St. Louis AL; Cincinnati NL; Brooklyn NL; Chicago NL

The young son of German immigrants started his profes-

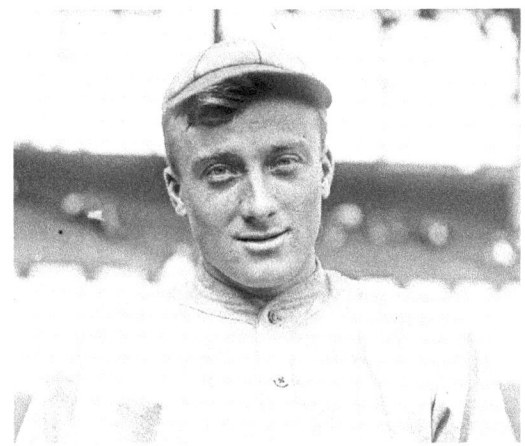

Lee Magee was a good outfielder and second baseman. He fielded adequately at either position and hit as well as the average major leaguer. However, he made a mistake that cost him his baseball career. In 1918 Magee and a teammate were bribed by a gambler to throw a game. Upon confessing, Lee was banned from the sport for life (Library of Congress).

sional baseball career as a 16 year old under the name of Magee in Meridian of the Cotton States League in 1906. As Lee Magee he advanced through the minor league system to Springfield of the Three I League, Burlington and Waterloo of the Iowa State League, Seattle of the Northwestern League, and Louisville of the American Association in 1910. However, in the federal census that year he was still listed as Leopold C. Hoernschemeyer. In 1917 he registered for the draft as Leo C. Magee. By then he was an established major leaguer, having come up as an infielder at St. Louis in 1911. From 1912 on he played mostly in the outfield, although he continued to play second base and other infield positions. In 1913 he led the NL in Faber System fielding points as a left fielder.[73] He stayed with the Cardinals until 1915, when he jumped to the Federal League. Lee hit .323 for the Tip-Tops that season, his only year in the Show when he topped the .300 mark. He ranked in the top ten among the Feds in batting average, slugging percentage, runs scored, and total bases. He played second base that year and led FL second sackers in errors and in total chances per nine innings. After the Federal League collapsed, Magee played for five different clubs in the next four years. In 1918 he had a good year at the plate for the Cincinnati Reds, ranking in the NL's top ten in slugging, total bases, doubles, and triples. He was at the keystone sack for the Reds that year and led the loop in errors and double plays. In 1919 he split the season between the Brooklyn Robins and the Chicago Cubs. It was to be his last year in organized baseball.

In 1918 Magee and teammate Hal Chase agreed to throw a game against the Boston Braves. Each player gave the gambler a check for $500 in return for a promise of one-third of the winnings. Unfortunately for the conspirators, the Reds won the game despite Magee's two errors. Lee stopped payment on the check. When the Reds came to Boston in 1919, the gambler had Lee served with papers for non-payment of debt. During a subsequent investigation, Magee confessed to the deal, although he insisted he had intended to bet for the Reds, not against them. Magee, Chase, and Heinie Zimmerman, who was also implicated, were banned from baseball for life.

After his expulsion from baseball, Magee moved to Columbus, Ohio. In 1930 he was a representative of a finance company. Later he owned the Commerce Coal Company. He died on March 14, 1966, in Columbus at the age of 76.

Ranking: Faber System second; *Total Baseball* fifth.

Carlos May

Born: Carlos May, May 17, 1958, Birmingham, AL
Debut: September 6, 1968; age 20

Last Game: October 2, 1977; age 29
Clubs: Chicago AL; New York AL; California AL

See the entry on him in Part One of this book.
Ranking: Faber System first; *Total Baseball* third; James second.

Kevin Mench

Born: Kevin Ford Mench, January 7, 1978, Wilmington, DE
Debut: June 16, 1999; age 21
Last Game: September 28, 2008; age 30
Clubs: Texas AL; Milwaukee NL; Toronto AL

Kevin was an outstanding baseball star in high school, college, and the minors, but he was unable to perform consistently at a high level in the majors. He played at St. Mark's High School in Wilmington and four years at the University of Delaware, where he immediately became one of the nation's top stars. As a freshman he hit 15 homers, and more than doubled that output with 33 dingers in his sophomore season. He earned National Player of the Year honors from *Collegiate Baseball* and was a consensus All-American. He led the Blue Hens to the NCAA Tournament in both 1998 and 1999. In the 1999 amateur draft Mench was selected by the Texas Rangers in the fourth round with the 118th overall pick. He hit .362 for Pulaski in the Appalachian League and .304 for Savannah in the Sally League. In 2000 he hit .334 with 27 homers and 121 RBIs for Charlotte. The next year he hit 26 homers for Tulsa, earning himself a promotion to the majors in 2002. He did not stick with the Rangers, although he hit .260 with 15 home runs and garnered some votes for AL Rookie of the Year. From 2002 through 2004, Kevin was shuttled between Texas and their farms in the Pacific Coast and Texas leagues. His best year in the majors was 2004, when he hit .279 with 26 homers in 125 games. During 2006 he was traded to Milwaukee, where he did not play well. He became a free agent after the 2007 season and returned to Texas, which promptly traded him to Toronto. He split the 2008 season between the Blue Jays and their AAA affiliate in Syracuse. In 2009 he played for the Hanshin Tigers in Japan.

The highlight of Kevin's major league career was his streak in 2006, when he hit home runs in six consecutive games. He was very popular in Texas, less so in Milwaukee and Toronto. His Texas teammates joked about Kevin's outsized head and feet. He wore a size 8 hat and size 12½ shoes. In 2005 the Rangers nominated him for the Roberto Clemente Award, given annually to the MLB player who combines baseball skills with outstanding community service. In 2005 Mench was inducted into the University of Delaware Athletics Hall of Fame.

Ranking: Faber System ninth; *Total Baseball* sixth.

Mike Menosky

Born: Michael William Menosky, October 16, 1894, Glen Campbell, PA
Debut: April 18, 1914; age 19
Last Game: October 7, 1923; age 28
Clubs: Pittsburgh FL; Washington AL; Boston AL

The son of Hungarian immigrants, Mike was working as a coal miner at the age of 15. Fortunately, he was able to get out of the mines in a few years. In 1913 he played baseball at Indiana Normal School (now called Indiana University of Pennsylvania) and got in a few games with Allentown in the Tri-State League. The next year he was in the major leagues for part of the season with Pittsburgh of the Federal League. Menosky spent most of 1915 and 1916 back in the minors at New Haven and Minneapolis. In 1917 he was in the majors again with Washington and played the rest of his major league career in the AL, three years with the Nats and four with the Boston Red Sox. He missed the entire 1918 season while serving in the military during World War I. Called "Leaping Mike" for his acrobatic outfield catches, he was better than average both as a hitter and as a fielder. His best year at the bat was 1921 when he hit .300 for the Sox and scored 80 runs. The Vernon club of the PCL purchased him from Boston in 1924, and he hit .328 on the Coast. In 1925 he hit .297 for Rochester in the International League. After that his skills declined rapidly. He fell all the way to Uniontown in the Mid-Atlantic League in 1926. The next year he tried out with Nashville in the Southern Association but was released before playing a game for the Vols. He made one last comeback attempt with Binghamton of the New York–Pennsylvania League in 1929 and hit a respectable .281, but gave it up after one year. In 1930 he was a marine mechanic in Cleveland. For many years from the 1930s to the 1950s he served as a probation officer in Detroit. Leaping Mike died in Detroit on April 11, 1983, at the age of 88.

Ranking: Faber System fifth; *Total Baseball* seventh.

Darby O'Brien

Born: William D. O'Brien, September 1, 1863, Peoria, IL
Debut: April 16, 1887; age 23
Last Game: October 15, 1892; age 29
Clubs: New York AA; Brooklyn AA; Brooklyn NL

William was the son of Irish immigrants, and "Darby" was a nickname frequently given to men of Irish descent in the nineteenth century. For a time there were two Darby O'Briens playing simultaneously in the big leagues. Left fielder O'Brien played for some clubs with colorful nicknames: Winona Clippers; Omaha Omahogs; Keokuk Hawkeyes; Denver Mountain Lions and Mountaineers; New York Metropolitans; and Brooklyn Bridegrooms (sometimes called the Trolley Dodgers).

Darby made his professional debut with Winona of the Northwestern League in 1884, played for Denver in the Colorado State League and Omaha and Keokuk of the Western League in 1885, and Denver in the same circuit in 1886. He broke into the big leagues with the Metropolitans in 1887 and hit .301 as a rookie, one of three seasons in which he topped the .300 mark. Darby was an outstanding hitter, finishing among the top ten in his league at least once in batting average, slugging, runs scored, hits, total bases, doubles, home runs, and extra-base hits. In 1889 he scored 146 runs and had 80 RBIs. He was a whiz on the base paths, stealing 91 bases in 1889 and averaging 54 stolen bases per year over his career. O'Brien was also an excellent fielder, leading left fielders in fielding percentage in 1890 and in Faber System fielding points in 1887 and again in 1891.[74] Consumption brought his stellar career to a halt after only six years in the majors. He died of the disease at his Peoria home on June 15, 1893, at the age of 29, exactly eight months after playing his last game. He is a member of the Greater Peoria Sports Hall of Fame.

Ranking: Faber System fourth; *Total Baseball* second.

Spike Shannon

Born: William Porter Shannon, February 7, 1878, Pittsburgh, PA
Debut: April 15, 1904; age 26
Last Game: September 30, 1908; age 30
Club: St. Louis NL

Shannon attended Grove City College, but the institution keeps no data on its baseball players of that era. The first record of his playing professional baseball was with Indianapolis of the Western Association in 1901. In 1902 he hit .344 for St. Paul. In 1903 Shannon led the American Association in runs scored with 132, while batting .308 and stealing 41 bases. It has been said his cunning on the base paths was the likely origin of his nickname "Spike." At season's end the St. Louis Cardinals drafted him from St. Paul under the Rule 5 draft. According to the Faber System he was the league's best left fielder in his rookie year.[75] He led the loop in fielding percentage that season and the next. Spike led the league in singles in 1906, and in runs scored and times on base in 1907. He ranked in the top ten in stolen bases, runs scored, and singles three times each. Twice he was among the leaders in hits, bases on balls, times on base, and sacrifices.

Never a big star, Spike was a good major league player for five years, then returned to the minors with the Kansas City Blues in the American Association from 1909 through 1911. Out of baseball for a while, he was associated with lead and zinc mining in Quapaw, Oklahoma, in 1920. By 1930 he was back in baseball as an umpire in the Southern Association. He earned considerable notoriety for his actions in a game between Memphis and New Orleans. With the score 4–3 in favor of Memphis and New Orleans at-bat in the last of the ninth, darkness began to descend. With no lights on the field in those days, fans demanded the game be called because of darkness. If the game had been called, the score would have reverted to the last complete inning and the two runs the Chicks scored in the top of the ninth would have been wiped out, giving the Pelicans a 3–2 win. New Orleans started stalling, waiting for the coming dark that would end the game. Shannon warned them to stop killing time, but the Pelicans kept finding ways to delay. At last, the umpire forfeited the game to Memphis. Fans vented their outrage by throwing pop bottles on the field. Shannon received a knot on his head but proved his courage in the face of hostility. Spike had married a Minnesota girl and usually considered the Twin Cities his home. He died in Minneapolis on May 16, 1940, at the age of 62.

Ranking: Faber System third; *Total Baseball* eighth.

Gary Thomasson

Born: Gary Leah Thomasson, July 29, 1951, San Diego, CA
Debut: September 5, 1972; age 21
Last Game: October 6, 1980; age 29
Clubs: San Francisco NL; Oakland AL; New York AL; Los Angeles NL

After playing baseball at Oceanside High School, Gary was taken by the San Francisco Giants in the seventh round of the 1969 amateur draft, the 160th pick overall. He started his professional career with Great Falls in the Pioneer League and hit .359. He moved up rapidly: Decatur of the Midwest League in 1970; Amarillo in the Texas League in 1971; Phoenix of the PCL in 1972, with a promotion to the big club in September. In 1973 he made the Topps All-Rookie team. He spent six years in San Francisco, mainly as the fourth outfielder or back-up first baseman. He never developed into a star. In the spring of 1978 he was traded to Oakland, which sent him to the New York three months later. In 1979 the Yankees traded him to Los Angeles. After two seasons the Dodgers sold him to the Yomiuri Giants. It is said that he was given the biggest contract ever awarded a player in the Nippon League. If so, he must have proved a great disappointment to the Japanese club. Although he homered 20 times, he hit only .249 and came close to setting a league strikeout record. In 1980 he injured his knee, ending his baseball career.

Ranking: Faber System tenth and last; *Total Baseball* ninth.

PART FOUR

All Pitchers

All 90 pitchers who logged at least 15 decisions in each of five or more major league seasons and appeared in their final big league contest at the age of thirty or younger are profiled in alphabetical order in Part Four. Each entry starts with summary data presented in a standard format similar to that utilized in Part Three. A "Record" line has been added, presenting the following data based solely on major league performance, from left to right as follows: wins; losses; winning percentage; earned run average; weighted average; and Faber System points. Information about minor league achievements and other life experiences may be presented in the text.

Biographical sketches by other writers are noted if they appear in any of these five sources: *Baseball's First Stars*; *Deadball Stars of the American League*; *Deadball Stars of the National League*; *Nineteenth Century Stars*; and the SABR Biography Project.

Rankings are provided based upon the Faber System, *Total Baseball*, and Bill James's analyses. The Faber System rates all eligible pitchers, *Total Baseball* rates virtually every pitcher who ever appeared in a major league game, and James ranks only the 100 leading moundsmen. None of the three sources segregates early leavers from other hurlers, but rankings of those with short careers can be derived from the ratings given. The number of players ranked whose careers ended by age 30 is: Faber System, 90; *Total Baseball*, 90; and James, 5. Despite using different methodologies, the Faber System and *Total Baseball* usually provide results that are not considerably different. On those rare occasions when the rankings are far apart, the disparity is usually due to one of two factors. First, Faber System results are based on pitching only, whereas the encyclopedia considers hitting as well. Good hitting pitchers, such as Ben Sanders, tend to do far better in *Total Baseball* rankings. The other major difference lies in the decision about which seasons are included in calculating the ratings. The Faber System counts only those seasons in which the pitcher is involved in fifteen or more decisions. On the other hand, *Total Baseball* counts all seasons equally. For example, the authors of that tome rate Denny McLain as having a below-average career, despite his performing well in almost every pitching category. The reason for this seeming anomaly is that seasons in which he pitched only a few games are given the same weight as those in which he won 20 games or more. Naturally, the Faber System gives McLain a much higher ranking than does *Total Baseball*.

Mark Baldwin

Born: Marcus Elmore Baldwin, October 29, 1863, Pittsburgh, PA
Debut: May 2, 1887; age 23
Last Game: September 30, 1893; age 29
Record: 154–165 .483 3.37 -10,459 227
Clubs: Chicago NL; Columbus AA; Chicago PL; Pittsburgh NL; New York NL

Mark began playing amateur baseball in the Pittsburgh area at the age of 16. In 1892 he played for the Agricultural College of Pennsylvania (now Pennsylvania State University). His professional career began in 1885 with an independent club in Cumberland, Maryland. He then advanced to McKeesport in the Western Pennsylvania League. In 1886 he won 23 games for Duluth in the Northwestern League, attracting the attention of major league teams. Cap Anson of the National League champion Chicago White Stockings signed Baldwin to pitch in the post-season series against the American Association St. Louis Browns. Charles Comiskey, manager of the Browns, refused to let the late signee into the competition, which meant Mark's major league debut was delayed until the following spring. Baldwin had a good fastball, an adequate curve and an acceptable changeup but was plagued with control problems. Pitching for Columbus in 1889, he led the American Association in games pitched, innings, and strikeouts. In the following season he led the Players League in the same three categories, plus wins. The 274 free passes he dealt in 1889 are the second most in walks one season in major league history, and only two fewer than the number issued by Amos Rusie the following season. That negative is more than offset by the 368 strikeouts he amassed in the same season, a number that has since been bettered only by Nolan Ryan and Randy Johnson.

After his major league career ended, Mark pitched briefly for Rochester in the Eastern League before helping found a semi-pro club in Auburn, New York, where he was a co-owner and manager as well as pitcher.

Baldwin had three brushes with the law. In 1891 Chris von der Ahe, president of the St. Louis Browns, caused Baldwin to be arrested and jailed overnight on conspiracy charges for trying to induce former players who had played in the Players League in 1890 to sign with Pittsburgh instead of returning to their original clubs. The charges were dismissed, and Baldwin sued von der Ahe for false imprisonment. After lengthy court action, the Browns executive was forced to pay the pitcher $3000. In 1892 Mark was arrested for aiding Homestead workers in their violent strike against the Carnegie Steel Company but was never brought to trial. While in Auburn he was fined $5 for playing baseball on Sunday in violation of the "Blue Laws."

In 1896 Baldwin quit baseball to pursue his childhood dream of becoming a doctor. He became a successful general practitioner and surgeon, practicing mainly in Pittsburgh and Columbus. Baldwin died in Pittsburgh on November 10, 1929, at the age of 66.

Mark Baldwin is profiled in *Baseball's First Stars* and in the *SABR Biography Project*. Ranking: Faber System 51st; *Total Baseball* 22nd.

Ted Blankenship

Born: Theodore Blankenship, May 10, 1901, Bonham, TX
Debut: July 2, 1922; age 22
Last Game: May 24, 1930; age 29
Record: 77–79   .494   4.29   -299   215
Club: Chicago AL

During his baseball career Ted Blankenship was dogged by bad luck. In 1921 his contract was purchased by the Chicago White Sox from a team in the Texas League, but his major league start was delayed by an automobile accident, causing him to miss the first half of the 1922 season. The Black Sox scandal divested the Chicagoans of eight of their better players, leaving a mediocre team. During his time with the Sox, Blankenship won 77 games. Only Ted Lyons and Red Faber won more for the Pale Hose during those years. Despite weak support, the hard-luck hurler had a fine season in 1925, only to break a finger the following year. It was all downhill after that. In 1929 and 1930 he pitched a few games in the American Association, but he had no more success in Toledo and Indianapolis than he had in the Windy City. The 1925 season was one to remember, however. Among all American League pitchers that year he had the second-lowest WHIP, the third-lowest earned run average, and ranked fourth in shutouts.

F. C. Lane wrote in *Baseball Magazine,* "Ted had a lot of stuff for a pitcher. He could, as the boys say, make the ball whistle."[1] Ted Blankenship died in Atoka, Oklahoma, on January 14, 1945, at the age of 44.

Ranking: Faber System 55th; *Total Baseball* tied for 70th. Could he have been ranked higher had Lady Luck been on his side?

Tommy Bond

Born: Thomas Henry Bond, April 2, 1856, Granard, Ireland
Debut: May 5, 1874; age 18
Last Game: September 11, 1884; age 28
Record: 193–115   .627   2.25   13,582   303
Clubs: Atlantics NA; Hartford NA; Boston NL; Worcester NL; Boston UA; Indianapolis AA

Bond started out as a teenaged fireballer but learned how to throw the curve from his Hartford Blues teammate Candy Cummings and became one of the best curveball pitchers of the 1870s. In his first big league season he won 31 games, which puts him in a tie for ninth in most games won by a rookie. He nearly became the first professional hurler to throw a no-hitter, holding the New York Mutuals hitless until Joe Start hit a double with two out in the ninth inning. Tommy became fed up with the abusive manner of Hartford manager Bob Ferguson, and in a ploy to escape to friendlier confines, he accused the manager of throwing games. The club's board of directors investigated, found Ferguson innocent, and kicked Bond off the team, freeing him to sign with the Boston Red Stockings. During each of his first three years in Boston, he won 40 games, becoming the only National League pitcher to win 40 or more games three years in a row. His 154 wins were the most by any hurler in the 1870s, and his .694 winning percentage was the best of the decade. Bill James wrote that Bond's 1878 season was the best by any pitcher in the 1870s.[2] In 1877 he became the first hurler to win the NL mythical Triple Crown for pitchers, leading in wins, strikeouts, and earned run average. The following season he again led the circuit in those categories, as well as in shutouts and winning percentage. According to the Faber System he was twice the NL Pitcher of the Year.[3] The *Baseball Encyclopedia* names him its ex post facto Cy Young winner three times.[4]

He ranks in the top ten among all pitchers for the lowest career earned run average and the lowest on-base percentage by opponents.

By 1880 Bond had pitched more than 500 innings per season for the past three years and the strain of throwing curveballs had given him a painfully sore arm. After pitching in three games in 1881 he retired at the age of 25. In 1882 he managed the Worcester club for part of the season and pitched a few games. He tried a comeback in the Union Association the next year but soon gave it up. After retiring for good he worked for 35 years in the Boston City Assessor's office and helped coach baseball at Harvard University.

Tommy Bond died January 24, 1941, in Boston at the age of 84.

He is profiled in *Nineteenth Century Stars*. The land of his birth has honored him by presenting the Tommy Bond Best Pitcher Award to the top hurler in the Irish Baseball League each year. His ranking: Faber System 25th; *Total Baseball* 38th; James fifth.

Henry Boyle

Born: Henry J. Boyle, September 20, 1860, Philadelphia, PA
Debut: July 9, 1884; age 23
Last Game: October 2, 1889; age 29
Record: 89–111   .445   3.06   3525   160
Clubs: St. Louis UA; St. Louis NL; Indianapolis NL

Handsome Henry Boyle was one of about two dozen young men who used the upstart Union Association as a springboard to careers in the National League. Boyle got off to a terrific start in the new circuit with 15 wins against only three losses in 1884 while compiling a 1.74 earned run average. His strikeouts-to-walks ratio (8.8 to 1) is the ninth best ever recorded in major league history. He found the National League tougher going, though, never posting a winning record in the senior circuit. However, he led the loop in earned run average with an impressive 1.76 mark in 1886. Perhaps the reason he never posted a winning record in the NL was the mediocre performance of the St. Louis and Indianapolis clubs for which he toiled. Boyle is almost forgotten today, but David Nemec relates an anecdote involving him. In common with other leagues of the time, the Union Association required balls hit into the stands to be returned for continued use. In a game between the Washington Nationals and the St. Louis Maroons, Boyle hit a foul ball out of the park. When the ball was retrieved, Washington argued in vain that the ball was too lopsided to be kept in play and refused to continue the game, whereupon the game was forfeited to St. Louis.[5]

Henry Boyle died May 25, 1932, in Philadelphia at the age of 71. Ranking: Faber System 75th; *Total Baseball* tie for 32nd.

Ralph Branca

Born: Ralph Theodore Joseph Branca, January 6, 1926, Mount Vernon, NY
Debut: June 12, 1944; age 18
Last Game: September 9, 1956; age 30
Record: 88–68   .564   3.79   -710   210
Clubs: Brooklyn NL; Detroit AL; New York AL

Ralph Branca will forever be linked with Bobby Thomson, who hit "the shot heard around the world" off Branca to deprive the Brooklyn Dodgers of the 1951 National League championship. Despite twelve seasons in the big leagues and nearly 100 victories, he is remembered for one pitch. That pitch, of course, came in the ninth inning of the deciding playoff game as the Giants came from behind to win a game Dodger fans thought was in the bag. Instead of celebrating a victory, the crestfallen fans listened to the hysterical screaming of announcer Russ Hodges, "The Giants win the pennant! The Giants win the pennant!" Branca had won 21 games for the 1947 Dodgers as he led them to their first World Series appearance in more than a quarter-century. In 1949 Ralph had a .722 winning percentage as the Dodgers again copped the flag. After 1951 Ralph won only 12 more games in what was left of his career. Perhaps Branca suffered emotionally as a result of that traumatic loss, but a physical injury contributed more to his downfall than any psychological factor. During spring training in 1952 a folding chair gave way. Branca landed hard, his coccyx on a pop bottle. His pelvis was out of whack. A chiropractor realigned it, and Ralph was able to pitch pain-free but with a stiffness in his back that rendered his pitching ineffective. That summer he went on the disabled list but came back and tried to resume his career with little success.

After retirement he became a broadcaster for the New York Mets. In 2009 the 83-year-old ex-pitcher was living at the Westchester Country Club in Rye, New York.

Branca is not considered among baseball's elite, but he did have his time in the limelight. Ranking: Faber System 59th; *Total Baseball* 48th.

Tom Brewer

Born: Thomas Austin Brewer, September 3, 1931, Wadesville, NC
Debut: April 18, 1954; age 22
Last Game: September 27, 1961; age 30
Record: 91–82   .526   4.00   4607   292
Club: Boston AL

Tom Brewer signed with the Boston Red Sox as a 19-year-old amateur free agent off the campus of Elon College in 1951 and spent his entire major league career with the Sox. His best year was 1956, when he won 19 games and lost nine. He ranked second in the American League in shutouts that season and pitched in the All-Star game. He had an excellent curveball but was not always able to get it over the plate, ranking in the top five in the league four times in bases on balls, five times in wild pitches, and three times in hit batsmen. Despite his lack of control, he had a winning record for a Red Sox team that was never a pennant contender during his years with the club. He was the most effective right-handed starter the Bostonians had during the 1950s. He retired after the 1961 season, reportedly citing his disappointment with his teammates as the reason.

For the past several years Brewer has served as a volunteer pitching coach with the Cheraw High School Braves in Cheraw, South Carolina. March 21, 2009, was declared Tom Brewer Day in Cheraw as townspeople honored him for his contributions to the school and the community. As part of the festivities the high school baseball field was named Tom Brewer Field.

Ranking: Faber System tied for 28th; *Total Baseball* tied for 32nd.

Ernie Broglio

Born: Ernest Gilbert Broglio, August 27, 1935, Berkeley, CA
Debut: April 11, 1959; age 23
Last Game: July 2, 1966; age 30
Record: 77–74 .510 3.74 2939 243
Clubs: St. Louis NL; Chicago NL

Just as the name of Ralph Branca will be forever joined with that of Bobby Thomson, so too will the names Ernie Broglio and Lou Brock always be linked. The 1964 trade that sent Broglio from St. Louis for Brock has been called the most lopsided in history. Four other players (Doug Clemens, Bobby Shantz, Jack Spring, and Paul Toth) were also involved in the deal, but Broglio and Brock were the principals. To the chagrin of the Cub fans, Ernie had little success in Chicago, winning only seven games while losing 19 in three seasons with the Cubs. On the other hand, Brock went on to a Hall of Fame career with the Cardinals, leading them to the 1964 World Series and setting a major league stolen base record, since broken by Rickey Henderson. At the time the trade did not seem that uneven. Broglio was considered one of the best pitchers in baseball; Brock was an unproven outfielder.

Ernie signed with the Oakland Oaks of the Pacific Coast League as a teenager. He also pitched for Vancouver of the PCL and Modesto and Stockton of the California League before being called up to the majors. He had his best season for St. Louis in 1960, when he tied Warren Spahn for the National League lead in wins with 21, was second in earned run average, allowed the fewest hits per nine innings, and had the fourth-most strikeouts in the league. He finished third in voting for the Cy Young award and was named the Faber System Pitcher of the Year.[6] He won 18 games in 1963, the year before the infamous trade. Broglio later claimed he was damaged goods at the time of the trade and that the Cardinals knew it. In 1961 he had taken 20 cortisone shots in his shoulder. Ernie's lack of success after the trade led his becoming the target of boo-birds in Wrigley Field. He was exceedingly unpopular with the fans when he was released by the Cubs in midseason 1966. Glad to escape the wrath of Chicago fans, Broglio played for Buffalo of the International

League in 1967 before retiring from baseball to become a full-time representative for a San Jose liquor business in 1968.

Ernie Broglio had one season (1960) when he was arguably the best hurler in the National League. Ranking: Faber System 46th; *Total Baseball* 35th.

Britt Burns

Born: Robert Britt Burns, June 8, 1959, Houston, TX
Debut: August 5, 1978; age 19
Last Game: September 30, 1985; age 26
Record: 70-60 .538 3.66 12,202 292
Club: Chicago AL

After an outstanding high school pitching record (35 wins and only two losses), Burns was selected in the third round by the Chicago White Sox in the 1978 amateur draft. Within a few months he made his first start for the Pale Hose but was sent down to the minors for seasoning. Returning to the majors in 1980, he had six successful big league seasons. Although he never led the league in any major pitching category, he had several top five finishes. In 1980 he had the third-lowest WHIP (walks plus hits per 9 innings). In 1981 he was second in the league in strikeouts. In 1982 his won-lost percentage was third best in the circuit. He ranked second in shutouts in both 1983 and 1985. In 1985 he won 18 games.

After his outstanding year in 1985, Britt was traded to the New York Yankees. A chronic degenerative hip condition, however, prevented him from pitching for the Yankees or ever again in the big leagues. Out of baseball, Burns bought a dude ranch in Colorado that offered guests a wide variety of outdoor activities, such as hunting, fishing, and horseback riding. Hiking in the mountains and hunting elk helped Britt get back in shape, and he tried his hand at pitching again but was unable to make it back to the majors as a pitcher. He did catch on with the Florida Marlins, however, as a pitching coach for one of their minor league affiliates. For eight years he was with the Marlins organization, rising eventually to serve as their minor league pitching coordinator. In 2008 he accepted that same position with the Houston Astros.

Given the fact that a degenerative hip forced him out of the majors at the age of 26, Burns has made a larger mark on the sport than might be expected. Ranking: Faber System tied for 28th; *Total Baseball* tied for 30th.

Kid Carsey

Born: Wilfred Carsey, October 22, 1870, New York, NY
Debut: April 8, 1891; age 20

Last Game: July 20, 1901; age 30
Record: 116–138 .457 4.95 343 277
Clubs: Washington AA; Philadelphia NL; St. Louis NL; Cleveland NL; Washington NL; Brooklyn NL

A feisty little (5'7") pitcher, infielder, outfielder, manager, and promoter, Kid Carsey was a colorful character. As a teenager pitching for the Oakland Colonels of the California League in 1890, Carsey earned a reputation as a "favorite of the ladies." During the season the Kid and his manager, Tip O'Neill, became involved in a dispute over the cost of two tickets the manager sold to his pitcher. The day the season ended the two stripped to the waist and behind locked doors decided to settle the matter in a bare-knuckle boxing match. Both contestants suffered severe bruises before other ballplayers halted the match.

Carsey advanced to the major leagues the following year and lost 37 games. Despite this sad start, he remained in the majors for most of the next decade. In 1897 he took a "vacation" following a dispute with Chris von der Ahe, the owner of the St. Louis Browns. The Kid, while pitching for St. Louis, also had an interest in a semi-pro team called West New York. The latter club had some difficulties and Carsey took a few days off to tend to the matter. Von der Ahe fined Carsey $300, which the hurler refused to pay. As von der Ahe would not allow the Kid to play until the fine was paid, Carsey took his vacation from St. Louis and pitched for his West New York team. The dispute was resolved when von der Ahe sold the Browns and the new owner rescinded the fine.

After 1899 Carsey went back briefly to the minor leagues. One of the clubs for which he pitched was the Anaconda Serpents of the Montana State League. The Serpents released him on September 6, but he wasn't notified until two days later. Meeting club manager Arthur Clarkson on the street after receiving the notice, Carsey hit the manager in the face, breaking two teeth. Clarkson fled across the street with Carsey in hot pursuit. Friends separated the two. It was then discovered that in striking Clarkson, the Kid had severed a tendon in his right hand. While in the hospital receiving treatment for his injured hand, he was arrested on charges of assault.[7]

In 1901 Carsey received one more shot at the major leagues, pitching his final game for Brooklyn on July 30 at the age of 30. For several years he remained active in the sport, mainly as a promoter. In 1911 he secured a franchise for a Washington entry in the proposed United States League, which never got off the ground.

In 1913 four thousand baseball fans crowded Washington's old Union Park to see a widely advertised game, promoted by Carsey, between the

Chicago Bloomer Girls and a men's team. When it was discovered that the Bloomer Girls were actually men wearing wigs, a riot broke out, and three policemen were injured by flying bricks and bottles as they escorted the "girls" to safety. Meanwhile, Carsey had departed with $700, the entire gate receipts, which did not improve the mood of the crowd, many of whom went to the police station demanding that something be done to get their money back.[8]

Carsey is profiled in *Baseball's First Stars*. Surprisingly, none of the above episodes is mentioned in the article, which is confined to a discussion of the Kid's playing career and his pitching style, which was said to include a slow curve but no speedy delivery. The article reports that little is known about Carsey's post-baseball life. Wilfred "Kid" Carsey died in obscurity in Miami on March 29, 1960, at the age of 69.

Ranking: Faber System 34th; *Total Baseball* 89th.

Bob Caruthers

Born: Robert Lee Caruthers, January 5, 1864, Memphis, TN
Debut: September 7, 1884; age 20
Last Game: May 19, 1893; age 29
Record: 218–99   .688   25,182   479
Clubs: St. Louis AA; Brooklyn AA; Brooklyn NL; St. Louis NL

See the entry on Bob Caruthers in Part Two of this book.

A biographical sketch of Caruthers appears in *Nineteenth Century Stars*.

Ranking: Faber System fifth; *Total Baseball* second; James fourth.

Dan Casey

Born: Daniel Maurice Casey, November 20, 1862, Binghamton, NY
Debut: August 18, 1884; age 21
Last Game: October 4, 1890; age 27
Record: 96–90   .516   -3290   168
Clubs: Wilmington UA; Detroit NL; Philadelphia NL; Syracuse AA

Casey made his major league debut in 1884 when the Wilmington Delawareans moved from the Eastern League to the ill-fated Union Association. In the majors he twice had 20-game winning seasons for the Philadelphia Phillies. In his best season, 1887, he led the National League in both earned run average and shutouts, finished third in won-lost percentage, and placed fourth in wins. After he retired from baseball he worked for many years as a trolley car conductor in his native Binghamton before moving to Silver Spring, Maryland. According to *Time* he was almost forgotten by baseball people until one day in 1938 he walked into a Washington newspaper office and introduced himself as the original Casey — the mighty Casey of Ernest Thayer's famous poem "Casey at the Bat." Dan convinced the newspapermen that he was the genuine article. He explained that it was a game against the New York Giants in the old Philadelphia ballpark on August 21, 1887. Tim Keefe and Dan were locked up in a pitcher's duel. With the Giants leading, 4–3, in the bottom of the ninth, two men out, and runners on second and third, Casey came to bat. The septuagenarian said, "A week before I'd busted up a game with a lucky homer and folks thought I could do it again." But, alas, mighty Casey struck out, and there was no joy in Philadelphia.

According to the since-debunked Abner Doubleday myth, baseball's centennial was coming up in 1939. In order to add pizzazz to the celebration, baseball officials decided to honor as many forgotten heroes of the game as they could find. Casey was presented a lifetime pass to all ballparks and featured on a nationally broadcast radio program. At a game between the International League's Baltimore Orioles and the Jersey City Giants, the 76-year-old Casey reenacted the scene from the poem by swinging futilely at a pitch from Rogers Hornsby. The May 30, 1938, issue of *Time* carried a page-length article about Casey, entitled "Mudville Man."

Dan Casey died in Washington on February 8, 1943, at the age of 81. Ranking: Faber System tied for 69th; *Total Baseball* 21st. This is among the greater differences between the two rankings.

Icebox Chamberlain

Born: Elton P. Chamberlain, November 5, 1867, Warsaw, NY
Debut: September 13, 1886; age 18
Last Game: May 13, 1896; age 28
Record: 157–120 .567 3.57 8848 376
Clubs: Louisville AA; St. Louis AA; Columbus AA; Philadelphia AA; Cincinnati NL

At the age of 17 Chamberlain began his professional career in Hamilton, Ontario, in 1885 and led the Canadian League with 189 strikeouts. He started the next year with Macon of the Southern League and moved up to the major leagues with the Louisville Colonels of the American Association before the end of the season. He was pitching in the big leagues at age 18.

According to historian Lee Allen, Elton got his nickname because he was said to possess "austere calm in the face of all hostility by the enemy."[9] He was reputed to have speed, a good curve, and excellent judgment. Some say the new pitching distance that went into effect in 1893 put him out of business. His best season came in 1888. On September 1 that year the St. Louis Browns purchased him from Louisville and he won 11 games in the final month of the season to help the Browns win the AA pennant. His overall record of 25 wins against only 11 losses gave him a .694 winning percentage and won him accolades as the Faber System Pitcher of the Year in the American Association.[10] His 1889 record is in dispute, but he won either 32 or 34 games that season. He had two other years in which he won more than 20 games. In 1890 he led the AA in shutouts. Four times he finished among the top five in his league in earned run average, three times in winning percentage, and once in strikeouts. On September 23, 1893, he had a no-hitter going against Boston when the game was called because of darkness after seven innings.

He is one of three nineteenth century pitchers known to have been ambidextrous. Pitching for the Louisville Colonels against the Kansas City Cowboys on May 9, 1888, the right-handed Chamberlain switched to his left arm in the last two innings of the game. On the negative side Icebox is remembered as the first major league pitcher ever to give up four home runs in one game to the same hitter — Boston's Bobby Lowe on May 3, 1894. He gained considerable notoriety from an off-the-field incident. An outfielder called Jocko Halligan considered himself to be quite a barroom brawler. One night he thrashed one player and then spotted another potential victim, Icebox Chamberlain, who was sitting at the bar. Jocko was unaware that Elton was watching his approach in the large mirror behind the bar. Just as Halligan was about to attack, the pitcher wheeled and flattened him with a bar mallet.[11]

After 1894 Chamberlain never won another big league game. His last appearance in the majors came at the age of 28 in the spring of 1896. During the winter meetings that December he was appointed a National League umpire, but that employment did not last. Reports out of Buffalo in June 1898 said that Chamberlain was thinking about becoming a boxer. He tried a comeback with Buffalo of the Western League in 1899 but failed to win a game for that franchise.

Elton Chamberlain died at 61 in Baltimore. He is profiled in *Nineteenth Century Stars*. Ranking: Faber System 14th; *Total Baseball* 19th.

Dean Chance

Born: Wilmer Dean Chance, June 1, 1941, Plain Township, Wayne County, OH
Debut: September 11, 1961; age 20
Last Game: August 9, 1971; age 30.
Record: 128–115   .527   2.92   10,196   385
Clubs: Los Angeles AL; California AL; Minnesota AL; Cleveland AL; New York NL; Detroit AL

Dean Chance had an almost unbelievable record as a high school pitcher. Hurling for tiny Northwestern High School in West Salem, Ohio, he pitched an incredible 17 no-hitters. As a freshman the farm lad played in overalls because the high school didn't have enough uniforms to go around. He soon earned his uniform, however. As a junior he tossed eight no-hitters, and he threw eight more as a senior when he led the Huskies to the Class A state championship in 1959. He pitched every inning of every game in the postseason tournaments. After graduation he received a $30,000 bonus to sign with the Baltimore Orioles and was assigned to their Bluefield, West Virginia, affiliate in the Appalachian League.

In the 1960 expansion draft Dean was drafted from Baltimore by the Los Angeles Angels. He remained with the Angels until he was traded to the Minnesota Twins after the 1966 season. Chance had a terrific sinking fastball and good control. His best year with the Angels came in 1964, when he won 20 games, led the league with a sensational 1.65 earned run average, and tossed a league-leading 11 shutouts. He won the Cy Young award and *The Sporting News* and Faber System AL Pitcher of the Year awards that season. His first year in Minnesota saw him post another 20-win season, during which he pitched two no-hitters. On August 6, he pitched a rain-shortened, five-inning perfect game against the Boston Red Sox. On August 26 he hurled a 2–1 no-hitter against Cleveland in which the Indians scored one run in the first inning on two walks, an error, and a wild pitch. During his career he won 13 games by a score of 1–0. The only big leaguers to win more games by that score were Walter Johnson, Grover Cleveland Alexander, Christy Mathewson, and Bert Blyleven. His hitting was another matter, however. His career batting average of .066 is the fourth lowest ever posted by a pitcher.

After 1968 his career rapidly declined. His last major league appearance came for the Detroit Tigers in 1971, a couple of months after his 30th birthday. Chance then turned his attention to boxing. He became the manager of several fighters, the best known being Ernie Shavers. In the 1990s he founded the International Boxing Association. In 2009 he was living on a 300-acre farm in his native Wayne County, raising black angus cattle, and running the IBA from the basement of his home.

Ranking: Faber System 13th; *Total Baseball* 11th.

Ken Chase

Born: Kendall Fay Chase, October 6, 1913, Oneonta, NY
Debut: April 23, 1936; age 22
Last Game: October 1, 1943; age 29
Record: 53–84   .387   4.27   -15,281   77
Clubs: Washington AL; Boston AL; New York NL

Ken Chase was a hard-throwing left-hander whose control problems prevented him from achieving the kind of success some had predicted for him. Signed at a tryout camp by the Washington Senators during his senior year in high school, the 17-year-old son of a dairy farmer started his professional career immediately after graduation. His minor league seasoning was at Chattanooga and Panama City. Called up by the Senators in April 1936, he was sent back to Chattanooga after appearing in only one big league game. He opened the 1937 season in Tennessee but got another chance during the season and stayed in the majors through 1943.

Called the "Milkman," Chase pitched some excellent baseball but wildness was his downfall. Twice he ranked fifth in the American League in strikeouts. In 1940 he had the fifth-best earned run average in the circuit, but in that same season he led the league in bases on balls and wild pitches. He was in the top five in walks three times and in wild pitches four times. Surprisingly, he had a great deal of success against Ted Williams, who called the Milkman "the toughest southpaw I ever batted against."[12] It is said that "the Splendid Splinter" instigated the trade that brought Chase to the Red Sox just so he wouldn't have to face his nemesis again.

At the end of the 1943 season Ken retired to his dairy farm and pitched for the Sidney Cardinals, who competed in an extraordinarily tough semi-pro league, centered on the huge Bendix-Scintilla Magneto plant, which drew defense workers from far and wide. After the war Chase retained his interest in the semi-pro league. When an old-timers game was scheduled in 1961, he worked himself back in shape and pitched three scoreless innings for the old-timers as they lost to the Milford Macs. The 47-year-old Chase gave up only one hit, and walked only one — his son, Dick.

Ken Chase lived the rest of his life in the Oneonta area, becoming a realtor after his farming days were over. He died in Oneonta in 1985 at the age of 71. Ranking: Faber System 88th; *Total Baseball* 66th.

Ray Collins

Born: Raymond Williston Collins, February 11, 1887, Colchester, VT
Debut: July 19, 1909; age 22
Last Game: October 7, 1915; age 28
Record: 84–62   .575   2.51   2219   236
Club: Boston AL

Born on a farm in Vermont, Collins attended the University of Vermont where he played varsity basketball, tennis, and baseball while earning a degree in economics. His success on the baseball diamond led to offers from major league clubs as early as his sophomore year. However, he waited until after graduation to sign with the Boston Red Sox, going directly to the big leagues without a minor league trial. For several seasons he was one of the best left-handed pitchers in baseball, possessing excellent control. For five consecutive years he ranked in the top seven in the American League in the fewest walks per nine innings. He finished in the top ten in earned run average three times; in wins twice; in won-lost percentage twice; in shutouts four times; and in strikeouts-to-walks ratio four times. In 1915 he suddenly lost effectiveness. Newspapers at the time made no mention of an injury, and the reason for the downturn remains a mystery. He threw his last major league pitch on October 7 at the age of 28. In December he announced his retirement, saying he was discouraged at his inability to regain his previous form. He returned to his Vermont farm, working the fields, selling maple syrup, and eventually turning the farmhouse into a bed-and-breakfast. He was very active in community affairs and served in the state legislature. He died at his hometown hospital on January 9, 1970, at the age of 82.

Collins is profiled in *Deadball Stars of the American League*. Ranking: Faber System 48th; *Total Baseball* 24th.

Larry Corcoran

Born: Lawrence J. Corcoran, August 10, 1859, Brooklyn, NY
Debut: May 1, 1889; age 20
Last Game: May 20, 1887; age 27
Record: 177–89   .665   2.36   7370   305
Clubs: Chicago NL; New York NL; Washington NL; Indianapolis NL

At the age of 17, Larry was pitching for the Mutual and Chelsea clubs in his native Brooklyn. Before he was out of his teens he had pitched for several minor league clubs, and future stardom was predicted for the young hurler. He pitched his first major league game at the age of 20, and piled up 43 victories for the Chicago NL team in 1880. He followed with 31 wins the next year, for the second-most victories ever by a pitcher in his first two major league seasons, behind only Matt Kilroy's 75 triumphs in 1886–87. The editors of the *Baseball Encyclopedia* named him their ex post facto Cy Young award winner in both 1880 and 1881.[13] Corcoran pitched three no-hitters during his brief major league career, setting a National League record that stood for more than 80 years, from 1884 to 1965, when Sandy Koufax tossed his fourth no-no. He tied for the NL lead in wins in 1881 and was the circuit's strikeout champion in 1880. In 1882 he led the league in won-lost percentage and earned run average. Due to an inflammation on his right index finger, Larry

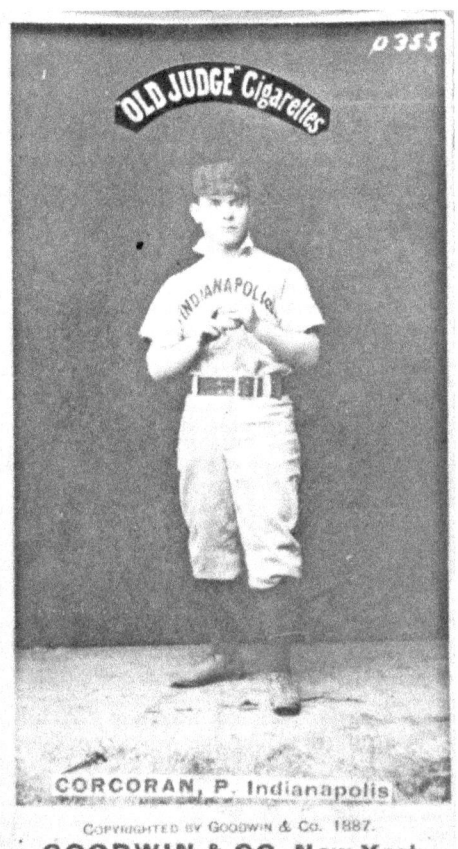

CORCORAN, P. Indianapolis
COPYRIGHTED BY GOODWIN & CO. 1887.
GOODWIN & CO. New York.

At the age of 20 Larry Corcoran made his major league debut in 1880 and won 43 games. The following season he won 31 games. In the entire history of major league baseball only one pitcher has compiled more victories in his first two seasons than did Corcoran. He was the best pitcher in baseball for a time. In his brief career he pitched three no-hitters. Only Sandy Koufax has pitched more no-hit games in the National League. Larry was well on his way to becoming one of the greatest pitchers of all time, having won 170 games in only five years, when he injured his shoulder muscles in 1885. His effectiveness was over at the age of 25 (Library of Congress).

joined the ranks of the ambidextrous on June 16, 1884, pitching four innings from the port side. He is credited with being the first hurler to signal pitches to his catcher. Pitching with a wad of chewing tobacco in his mouth, he would shift the position of the chew to let his catcher know whether a curve or a fastball was coming. During his first five seasons in the majors Corcoran posted 170 victories. If he could have continued that pace for another five years, he would have logged his 300th win well before his 30th birthday. It didn't happen. Early in the 1885 season he strained the muscles in his shoulder so severely that he couldn't throw for several weeks. When he showed no improvement, Chicago released him. He was signed by the New York Giants, then went to Washington and to Indianapolis but never won another major league game after 1885. His effectiveness was over at the age of 25. He ranks in the top ten among all major league pitchers in several categories. His .688 winning percentage is fifth, as is his .264 opponents batting average. His 47 putouts in one season are the sixth most ever made by a pitcher. His 43 wins, 57 complete games, and 268 strikeouts are among the top rookie performances.

After his last major league game he appeared briefly as a minor league player and umpire. By the spring of 1891 he had to give up all such activity because of kidney disease, perhaps brought on by heavy drinking. On October 14, 1891, he died of Bright's disease in Newark at the age of 32.

Larry Corcoran is profiled in *Nineteenth Century Stars*. Injury and illness denied him the place in the Baseball Hall of Fame that could have been expected given his early record. Ranking: Faber System 24th; *Total Baseball* tied for 49th.

Frank Corridon

Born: Frank Joseph Corridon, November 25, 1880, Newport, RI
Debut: April 15, 1904; age 23
Last Game: September 7, 1910; age 29
Record: 70–67 .511 2.80 277 224
Clubs: Chicago NL; Philadelphia NL; St. Louis NL

Corridon was nicknamed "the Fiddler" because he was an enthusiastic violinist. In the major leagues the Fiddler never quite lived up to the reputation he had built by winning 28 games for the Providence Grays of the Eastern League in 1902. He came up with the Chicago Cubs in 1904 but had the misfortune to be traded in midseason to the Philadelphia Phillies. Although he was a better than average major league hurler, it was difficult to gain a lot of recognition pitching for the Phillies of that era. His best season was 1907 when he won 18 games. He pitched three consecutive seasons, from 1907 through 1909, without giving up a home run.

One day in early April 1907 Corridon was pitching for the Phillies against the New York Giants at the Polo Grounds. Frank was breezing along with a one-hitter when the crowd became incensed at several calls that went against the home team. It had snowed the night before the game, so plenty of ammunition was on hand. The fans began pelting the umpires with snowballs. At the end of the eighth inning, several hundred fans rushed the field and the umpires forfeited the game to Philadelphia.

Frank was one of several pitchers who claimed to have invented the spitball. According to his story, he accidentally learned the pitch while hurling for Providence. He discovered that a ball that had landed in a puddle and was wet on one side did unexpected things when he threw it. His claim to have been the inventor of the pitch is not universally accepted, as the origin of the wet one is not known. The extent to which Corridon utilized the pitch is in dispute. He once said he had struck out Honus Wagner with a spitter in an exhibition game but never used it thereafter for fear of hurting his arm. Later he illogically claimed that throwing the wet one shortened his career.

In the big leagues he was known chiefly for his fastball. He also threw a curve and an occasional change-up. Several of his ex-teammates said they never saw him use the spitter.

During the 1909-10 offseason the Phillies traded Corridon to Cincinnati. The Reds in turn traded the pitcher to St. Louis a few days later. The Fiddler never had much success with the Cardinals and left the team late in the 1910 season. After that he continued in the game at a lower level. For example, in 1913 he was pitcher and manager for the Springfield Ponies of the Eastern Association. It was reported that while on the mound he was a constant threat to base runners because he could throw with either hand and potential base stealers never knew which hand held the ball. After the association disbanded, Frank pitched for several years for semi-pro clubs in his hometown.

Corridon died February 21, 1941, in Syracuse, New York, at the age of 60. After his death officials of Newport named a highway after him to honor the only native son of the city to reach the major leagues. Ranking: Faber System 52nd; *Total Baseball* 67th.

Doc Crandall

Born: James Otis Crandall, October 8, 1887, Wadena, IN
Debut: April 24, 1908; age 20
Last Game: August 31, 1918; age 30
Record: 102–62 .622 2.92 10,454 322
Clubs: New York NL; St. Louis NL; St. Louis FL; St. Louis AL; Boston NL

Born on a farm in northwestern Indiana into a family of ballplayers, Otis was pitching semi-pro baseball at the age of 14. In 1906 the teenager made his professional debut with Cedar Rapids of the Three-I League. At the end of the 1907 season he was drafted by the New York Giants. His rookie year was the only season in which he started more than he relieved. From 1909 through 1913 he led the National League in relief appearances each year, becoming baseball's first relief specialist. Damon Runyon pinned the nickname "Doc" on him for his demeanor on the mound. "Crandall is the Giants' ambulance corps," the legendary Runyon wrote. "He is first aid to the injured. He is the physician of the pitching emergency, and they sometimes call him old Doctor Crandall. He is without equal as an extinguisher of batting rallies."[14] Doc was also a good hitter who was used sometimes as a pinch-hitter and plied his trade in both the infield and the outfield.

His best year on the mound came in 1910 when he won 17 games against only four losses. He pitched complete games in 13 of his 18 starts that season and also relieved 24 times. He had another excellent year in 1911, winning 15 of 20 decisions. In the World Series he was the winning pitcher in Game 5. In 1913 he was traded to the St. Louis Cardinals, but after he had appeared in only two games as a pinch-hitter, the Giants purchased him back. In 1914 he jumped to the St. Louis Terriers in the new Federal League, where he enjoyed considerable success as a starting pitcher and as a second baseman. After the FL folded, Doc was acquired by the St. Louis Browns in the dispersal draft. Crandall was hit hard in his only two appearances before the Browns released him. At the age of 28 his career appeared to be over.

However, he went to the Pacific Coast League, became a starter again, and compiled an outstanding record over the next 13 years. With the Los Angeles Angels he won 224 games, lost 147, and posted an earned run average of 2.92. In 1917 he won 26 games for the Angels. The next year he was working on a no-hit game with two outs in the ninth inning when his brother Karl, playing for the Salt Lake City Bees, spoiled his bid. Because of the war the PCL suspended play in July, and Doc joined the Boston Braves for the remainder of the season, making his final big league appearance at the age of 30.

Doc owned the Wichita club in the Western League for two years, served as pitching coach for the Pittsburgh Pirates for four seasons, and managed the Des Moines Demons of the Western League in 1935. He returned to the PCL to coach at Seattle in 1937 and Sacramento in 1938.

In his later years, Crandall suffered a series of strokes that left him paralyzed. He died in Bell, California, on August 17, 1951, at the age of 63. His biography appears in *Deadball Stars of the National League* and in the SABR Biography Project. Rating: Faber System 21st; *Total Baseball* 12th.

Dave Davenport

Born: David W. Davenport, February 20, 1890, Alexandria, LA
Debut: April 17, 1914; age 24
Last Game: September 1, 1919; age 29
Record: 73–83   .468   2.93   4844   217
Clubs: Cincinnati NL; St. Louis FL; St. Louis AL

At 6'6" the man they called "Big Dave" towered over his teammates. By leading the Texas League with 204 strikeouts for the San Antonio Broncos in 1913, he earned his way to the major leagues. After getting off to an inauspicious start for the Cincinnati Reds in 1914, he jumped to St. Louis in the new Federal League where he hit his stride in 1915. He won 22 games for the Terriers and led the league in complete games, shutouts, and strikeouts. Once he pitched both ends of a doubleheader, winning one game, 1–0, and losing the other by the same score. After that season he jumped again, this time across town to the St. Louis Browns. Manager Fielder Jones called him the best pitching prospect with whom he had ever worked. For a time it appeared Big Dave might live up to his manager's expectations. He pitched and won two complete games in one day in 1916 against the New York Yankees. For two years he enjoyed moderate success with the Browns, winning 17 games in 1917 despite leading the league with 11 wild pitches. When the "fight or work" order was issued by Secretary of War Newton Baker in 1918, Davenport secured a job in Alameda and pitched in the very strong semi-pro Shipbuilders League in the San Francisco Bay area.

He had two problems — a violent temper and a fondness for alcohol — that got him in trouble in 1919. In late August he was suspended for breaking training rules. When he returned from suspension, he pulled a knife on manager Sunset Jimmy Burke, who had succeeded Jones as skipper in 1918. That was the end of Big Dave's major league career. He was through with the big leagues at the age of 29, but he was not through with baseball. In the summer of 1921 he joined the Ogden club of the Northern Utah League. He became a sensation in northern Utah. Fans jammed the ballpark to watch him pitch, and hundreds signed petitions asking that he be permitted to stay with the club, but directors of the other clubs voted to expel him from the league. The reason for his expulsion was not given, but an Ogden sportswriter said it was because he was "too darn good."[15] As if to prove the scribe correct, Big Dave pitched a perfect game in his final appearance in the league, allowing nary a base runner in Odgen's 5–0 victory. After his Utah experience Davenport played semi-pro ball in various places around the country, most notably Beloit, Wisconsin.

Dave Davenport died in El Dorado, Arkansas, on October 16, 1954. Few newspapers reported his death, but one sportswriter in Ogden, Utah, remembered him as "the finest hurler ever to pitch in this section of the nation."[16]

Ranking: Faber System 54th; *Total Baseball* tie for 64th.

Ed Doheny

Born: Edwin Richard Doheny, November 24, 1873, Northfield, VT
Debut: September 16, 1895; age 21
Last Game: September 7, 1903; age 29
Record: 75–83   .475   3.75   -9002   198
Clubs: New York NL; Pittsburgh NL

Ed was a sandlot star at the age of 14. Before he reached the age of majority he had pitched professionally for Farnham, Quebec, and St. Albans in his home state. Making his major league debut near the end of the 1895 season, the young man got off to a poor start, losing all three decisions that fall. Over the next few seasons he improved slightly, but never posted a winning season with the Giants. In 1897 he logged an earned run average of 2.12, which would have led the league except he pitched too few innings to qualify for the title. He was suspended several games for "breaches of discipline." His biographers wrote that Doheny's behavior could be as wild as his pitching often was.[17] (He twice led the league in wild pitches.)

In mid-season 1901 he was released by the Giants and signed 10 days later with the Pittsburgh Pirates. Suddenly the man who could not win in New York became a star in Pittsburgh. He went 6–2 for the Pirates in the later part of 1902, and 16–4 in 1903, followed by 16–8 in 1904, helping the Corsairs win the National League pennant in all three of his seasons in the Steel City.

In the middle of the 1904 season, with 12 wins already to his credit, Doheny began exhibiting strange behavior, especially when he had been drinking. He had a few unpleasant confrontations with teammates and then he began believing he was being followed by detectives. Probably suffering from paranoia and exhaustion, toward the end of July he left the team without permission, going to his home in Massachusetts to rest. He rejoined the Pirates in Boston during an August road trip and pitched well, winning six of eight decisions.

But another series of misbehaviors caused his sanity to be questioned. In September he was taken home by his brother and placed under the care of a physician. His sympathetic teammates sent him a gift of his Pirate uniform, an action he misinterpreted. On October 10 while the Pirates were playing the Boston Americans in the first modern World Series, Doheny suffered a breakdown. He threw his doctor headfirst out the door and warned him not to return. The next morning he knocked his male nurse down with a cast-iron stove leg. His wife hurried to the neighbors for help. For an hour Ed held a score of neighbors and several policemen at bay, threatening to kill the first man who touched him. Eventually two policemen overpowered him. After an examination by doctors, he was declared insane and committed to an asylum in Danvers, Massachusetts, where his condition worsened. He lived another 13 tragic years and died in the Medfield State Asylum, on December 29, 1916, at the age of 43.

The story of Ed Doheny's life is told in SABR's *Baseball Biography Project*. Ranking: Faber System 65th; *Total Baseball* tie for 76th.

Red Ehret

Born: Philip Sydney Ehret, August 31, 1868, Louisville, KY
Debut: July 7, 1888; age 19

Last Game: June 25, 1898; age 29
Record: 139–167   .454   4.02   -12,609   248
Clubs: Kansas City AA; Louisville AA; Pittsburgh NL; St. Louis NL; Cincinnati NL; Louisville NL

Red Ehret was one of a surprisingly large number of baseball players who grew up in Louisville in the years following America's Civil War. At the age of 19 he signed with the Kansas City Cowboys, who sold him to the Louisville Colonels the next year for $500, the first of many moves the pitcher made. All in all he toiled for six different major league clubs, never spending more than three seasons with any. His only 20-win season came for the AA champion Colonels in 1890. In the post-season World Series against the National League champion Brooklyn Bridegrooms, he won two games and saved another, thus having a hand in all three victories by the Colonels. In 1893 Ehret led the league in shutouts, one of five seasons in which he was among the top ten in his league in that category. An excellent control pitcher, he was also among the ten leaders five times in fewest-walks-plus hits per inning, five times in fewest bases on balls per nine innings; and four times in lowest earned run average. Despite these good numbers Red lost more games than he won. After his major league career ended, he continued in the minors. In the 1900 census Ehret was listed as a ball player living in Minneapolis. In 1901 he played with Matthews and Ft. Wayne in the Western Association; in 1902–04 he was with Memphis of the Southern Association. In 1906 he pitched one game for Montgomery before he turned to umpiring. He officiated in the Northwestern League in 1907. Red died in Cincinnati on July 28, 1940, at the age of 71.

Ranking: Faber System tied for 42nd; *Total Baseball* also tied for 42nd. The two systems agree perfectly on his ranking.

Duke Esper

Born: Charles H. Esbacher, July 28, 1868, Salem, NJ
Debut: April 18, 1890; age 21
Last Game: July 12, 1898; age 29
Record: 101–100   .502   4.39   5837   286
Clubs: Philadelphia AA; Pittsburgh NL; Philadelphia NL; Washington NL; Baltimore NL; St. Louis NL

He played baseball as Charlie or Duke Esper but kept his legal name Esbacher for all other purposes. It has been written, probably inaccurately, that the term charley horse for a leg cramp was introduced because Charlie Esper walked like a lame horse. He is said to have been one of the first pitchers ever to have a three-pitch inning. In 1891 he was a 20-game winner, and three times finished in his league's top ten in won-lost percentage. In 1896 he won 14 of 19 decisions for Baltimore's league champions. After the season Connie Mack, manager of the Milwaukee Brewers in the Western League, announced that he had purchased Esper for $1000. National League owners were shocked that Duke was sent to the minors. Chris von der Ahe of the St. Louis Browns protested that the Browns had put in a waiver claim. Nick Young, president of the National League, ruled in von der Ahe's favor, and Charlie became a Brown, albeit an unhappy and unsuccessful one. He was out of the major leagues in less than two years, having won only four games on the banks of the Mississippi. In 1900 Charles Esbacher was a bartender in Philadelphia. He tried to make a comeback with the Toronto Maple Leafs in 1902 but won only five games against eight losses for one of the best minor league teams of the era. After that experience he returned to Philadelphia where he died of Bright's disease on August 11, 1910, at the age of 42.

Ranking: Faber System: 32nd; *Total Baseball* 63rd.

Pete Falcone

Born: Peter Frank Falcone, October 1, 1953, Brooklyn, NY
Debut: April 13, 1975; age 21
Last Game: September 17, 1984; age 30
Record: 70–90 .438 4.07 -1055 144
Clubs: San Francisco NL; St. Louis NL; New York NL; Atlanta NL

As a schoolboy in Brooklyn, Pete attracted the attention of major league scouts. Twice he was drafted and twice he turned down the offers while waiting for a better bid. It paid off, for the third time was the charm. After rejecting a 13th-round offer by Minnesota in 1972 and a second-round selection by Atlanta in January 1973, he was drafted in the first round by the San Francisco Giants in June 1973, the fourth pick overall. Assigned to Great Falls of the Pioneer League, he got his professional career off to a blazing start, winning eight games, losing one, and posting a 1.50 earned run average. In 1974 he split the season between Fresno and Amarillo, winning a combined 12 games against eight losses and allowing fewer than two earned runs per game. In his first major league season he won 12 games for the Giants and finished second to teammate John Montefusco for NL Rookie Pitcher of the Year. After only one year in San Francisco, he was traded to the St. Louis Cardinals. Following three years in St. Louis he was traded to the New York Mets. On May 1, 1980, pitching against the Philadelphia Phillies, Pete tied a major league record by striking out the first six batters of the game. With the Mets he was known not only for his fastball and his knuckle-curve but also for his habit of saying his successes and failures were the Lord's doing. A born-again Christian, he frequently said such things as, "If God wanted me to throw strikes, He would let me." He spent four years with the Mets, his longest tenure with any club. When he was granted free agency, he signed with the Atlanta Braves but had little success down South. Only 30 years old, he told an Atlanta sportswriter that he intended to retire after the 1984 season. "I'm just tired of baseball," he said. "I'm tired of the lifestyle, and I can't see any reason to go on doing it. The game is a game, and a certain part of it is enjoyable, but everything else, forget it."[18]

He did find some joy in baseball at a different level. In 1989 he pitched for the Orlando Juice of the Senior Professional Baseball Association and compiled a 10–3 record. In 2007 he was said to have been operating a catering business in Louisiana.

Ranking: Faber System 80th; *Total Baseball* 85th.

Jack Fisher

Born: John Howard Fisher, March 4, 1939, Frostburg, MD
Debut: April 14, 1959; age 20
Last Game: September 26, 1959; age 30
Record: 86–139 .382 4.06 -12,831 167
Major League Clubs: Baltimore AL; San Francisco NL; New York NL; Chicago AL; Cincinnati NL

The first year Frostburg hosted a Little League, young Jack Fisher pitched his club to the championship. From there he went to Richmond Academy in Augusta, Georgia, where he had a sensational record of twenty wins and only one loss. Eighteen major league clubs eyed the youngster during his senior year of high school. On June 24, 1957, the Baltimore Orioles signed Jack to a major league contract. (The 18-year-old was not yet called "Fat Jack," for at 6'2", he sported 205 pounds on a well-built frame.) He was assigned to the Knoxville Smokies of the Class AA Sally League. He divided the 1958 season between the Smokies and Wilson of the Carolina League. After only two years in the minors, Jack advanced to the big leagues but was sent down to Miami of the Class AAA International League for furthering seasoning. Called back up in 1960 he was one of a quartet of pitchers, along with Chuck Estrada, Steve Barber, and Milt Pappas, all under 23 years of age, who were known as the "Baby Birds" or the "Kiddie Korps." For the first time since the club moved from St. Louis in 1954, Baltimore fielded a pennant contender. Fisher did his part to keep the Orioles competitive. From late August through mid-September he pitched 29⅔ consecutive innings without giving up a run. Despite this start he never quite lived up to his promise. He never won more than 12 games in a season, and while with the Mets he twice led the National League in losses. In the first game ever played at Shea Stadium, he was the starting pitcher for the home team and thus threw the first pitch at the new park. Prior to this time, pitchers had warmed up on the mound before the game. Because of all the pomp and ceremony and crowd noise, Jack asked Mets manager Casey Stengel if he could warm up in the bullpen instead of on the field, thus starting a custom that has endured for more than 45 years. During his big league career he gave up several historic home runs: the 521st and final homer by Ted Williams in the latter's farewell game; the 60th round-tripper by Roger Maris in 1961 to tie Babe Ruth's 1927 record; and in 1964 Willie Stargell took him out of the yard for the first home run ever hit in Shea Stadium. At card shows the milestone home runs he gave up were sometimes listed instead of positive accomplishments. Fat Jack said, "I gave up some epic gopher balls."

In 2009 he was the owner and operator of Fat Jack's Sports Bar in Easton, Pennsylvania. He told a reporter that he hoped the Mets would invite him to throw out the ceremonial first pitch at the opening of Citi Field. The honor instead went to Tom Seaver. Given the difference in the records of the two hurlers, the choice of Seaver is understandable. However, it is another disappointment for Jack Fisher in a career that had once been so promising.

Ranking: Faber System tied for 71st; *Total Baseball* 88th.

Scott Garrelts

Born: Scott William Garrelts, October 30, 1961, Urbana, IL
Debut: October 2, 1982; Age 20
Last Game: June 10, 1991; Age 29
Record: 69–53   .566   3.29   10240   265
Club: San Francisco NL

Scott grew up in Buckley, a small town in eastern Illinois. While pitching for Buckley-Loda High School, he once struck out 22 batters in a seven-inning game. (Two batters reached base on dropped third strikes.) The 17-year-old pitcher was drafted by the San Francisco Giants in the first round of the 1979 amateur draft, the 15th pick overall. After pitching that summer for Great Falls in the Pioneer League, he was promoted to Clinton in the Class A Midwest League in 1980 and to Shreveport in the AA Texas League the following season. Near the end of the 1982 season he was called up to the big club and spent his entire major league career with San Francisco, although he was sent down to Phoenix twice in his first seasons with the Giants. He had a blazing fastball, reportedly clocked at more than 100 miles per hour, and occasionally threw a knuckler. In 1985 he was selected for the National League All-Star team. His best season came in 1989 when he led the league in won-lost percentage, earned run average, and WHIP while pitching the Giants into the World Series. In 1990 he had a no-hitter going with two outs in the ninth inning, but Paul O'Neill ruined the bid with a single over the shortstop's head. Early in his career he had been plagued by wildness, but he solved this by pitching from the stretch rather than using a full windup. With the Giants he was used both as a starter and as a reliever and posted double digit saves four times.

In 1991 Garrelts had a sore arm and pitched his last major league game in midseason. In 1992, the Giants sent him to minor league clubs in San Jose and Phoenix, but as his sore arm did not heal, he was released at the end of the season. The San Diego Padres decided to take a chance and signed Scott as a free agent, but he never pitched for the Padres in the big leagues. In the spring of 1993 San Diego sent him on a rehab assignment to Rancho Cucamonga, but he did not make it back to the majors. He pitched for the Las Vegas Stars later that season and concluded his baseball career with the Omaha Royals in 1995. Although there is a sign on the outskirts of Buckley proclaiming it the home of Scott Garrelts, at last report he was living in Shreveport, Louisiana.

Ranking: Faber System 38th; *Total Baseball* tied for 42nd.

Virgil Garvin

Born: Virgil Lee Garvin, January 1, 1874, Navasota, TX
Debut: July 13, 1896; Age 22
Last Game: September 16, 1904; Age 30
Record: 57–97 .370 2.72 -13176 103
Clubs: Philadelphia NL; Chicago NL; Milwaukee AL; Chicago AL; Brooklyn NL; New York AL

Although modern record books list him as Ned, almost all contemporary accounts refer to him by his given name of Virgil. The young man from rural Texas made his professional debut with the Sherman Orphans of the Texas Southern League in 1895. The next year he started the season with New Haven of the Atlantic Association, pitched in two mid-season games for the Philadelphia Phillies, and finished the season with Newark in the Atlantic League. He was with the Reading Coal Heavers in that league and leading the circuit in won-lost percentage with .824 on a 14–3 record, when he got a second shot at the big leagues, this time with the Chicago Orphans. Virgil was a young man on the move. After two years he went to Milwaukee for one year, then back to the Windy City with the White Sox for part of a season, and on to Brooklyn.

The Milwaukee American League franchise shifted to St. Louis after the 1902 season, forcing the city to settle for a minor league club in the American Association. Milwaukee manager Joe Cantillon signed Garvin to pitch for the Brewers. A newspaper account of the signing shows, with a candor unusual in that time, some of the baggage that Virgil would bring with him.

> Joe Cantillon believes that he can manage Pitcher Virgil Garvin. For that reason the lanky ex–Brewer will be seen in a Milwaukee uniform. Yesterday Cantillon signed Garvin for the local association team and the fellow who dislikes the colored population will start south with the Brewers next month. In securing the former big leaguer, Cantillon made a good move, as Garvin can pitch excellent ball when he is inclined to.... Garvin occasionally remembers he is from Texas, and when that moment comes upon him he cannot avoid flourishing a revolver. Garvin was booked to play with Brooklyn, but a difference of financial matters made it necessary for the pitcher to decline.... Garvin had some advance money from the Brooklyn manager, but this will be returned by Cantillon.[19]

Despite the offer to return the advance, Brooklyn would not release Garvin from his contract, and back to the Superbas went the Texan. But he did not stay there long. He spent parts of seven seasons with five different clubs in the majors.

With tongue in cheek, one San Antonio scribe wrote that Navasota Ned, the Demon Texan, must have help from the supernatural world in order to throw such a wickedly breaking curve.[20] Although Garvin had a world of talent, including a devastating curveball, he never had a winning record in the Show. Bill James and Rob Neyer wrote that he may have been the unluckiest pitcher in major league history.[21] The numbers support that conclusion. For example, in 1904 he won five games and lost 16, despite having an earned run average of 1.72. Anyone can have an unlucky year, but for Virgil it went on season after season. Over his seven-year major league career he won 57 games and lost 97 while posting a 2.72 ERA compared to the league's 3.48. With that differential, James and Neyer posit he should have had an 86–68 won-lost record. Was it all bad luck? Someone was unkind enough to suggest that Garvin was so disliked by his teammates that they purposely lost some games he pitched, hoping the team would get rid of him. That sounds preposterous, but newspapers of the day were replete with references to Virgil's troublemaking.

Garvin's problem was drinking and losing control of himself. In 1903 he was jailed for taking a shot at a bartender in Chicago. In mid–August 1904 as Brooklyn traveled by train to St. Louis, Garvin and a few teammates got roaring drunk, and as the club secretary tried to calm him down, Virgil "beat him to a pulp" then continued destroying the Pullman car. The Brooklyn club released him, but the management of the New York Highlanders thought they could control the erratic pitcher. They were locked in a tight pennant race with the Boston Americans and needed another hurler. In a crucial mid–September encounter between the two challengers, Garvin lost to Cy Young, 4–2. Going into the last week of the season, the Highlanders were only one-half game behind Boston and needed to sweep a four-game series to clinch the pennant. Manager Clark Griffith did not trust Garvin and did not use him in this series. Boston defeated the overworked Jack Chesbro to take the flag. (Chesbro made eight starts in the final fifteen days of the season.) That mid–September loss was Virgil's final major league appearance.

The Texan went to the northwest to ply his trade in Portland, Seattle, and Butte. He won 25 games for Portland in 1905 but got in trouble with the management. A newspaper reporter maintained that when he is right, he is one of the best pitchers in the United States, but that no manager wants him. "Garvin had pitched some wonderful games," the scribe wrote, "and when he was right he was practically unbeatable. But his old failing came to the surface. He could not leave the joy water alone and kept his manager in trouble all the time.... He is now piling lumber in a little sawmill on the Columbia River."[22] However, the reporter wrote him off too quickly. Garvin was back in the PCL in 1906 and won 20 games for Portland and Seattle. In 1907 he pitched for Butte in the Northwestern League and again won 20 games. Wherever he pitched, sportswriters praised the ex–major leaguer's ability but condemned his conduct.

Virgil's bad luck extended to his family. His wife was hospitalized at least three times for mental illness. In the winter of 1907 Garvin became ill with consumption (now called tuberculosis). Thinking the warmer weather of his native Texas would improve his health, he wanted to return to Navasota. As he was then in Seattle and low on funds, his former manager and teammates raised enough money to pay for his transportation back to the Lone Star State. His health did not improve, so he decided to try the drier climate of interior California. Two weeks after his arrival in Fresno he succumbed in the county hospital on June 16, 1908, at the age of 34. Even the newspapers reporting his death could not resist making snide remarks about his character. A Nevada gazette stated: "The passing of Garvin marks the end of a career than began with great promise. Gifted with the highest ability of a baseball pitcher, Garvin was a very reckless sort and scattered to the winds his natural endowments. The Texan was a rather eccentric character and failing to find companionship among the players he sought and wooed the flowing bowl."[23]

Despite a losing record, bad luck, and troubling relationships, Garvin showed a great deal of ability. Ranking: Faber System 85th; *Total Baseball* ninth. This is by far the greatest difference in rankings by the two analyses. The Faber System penalizes him for all his losses, whether caused by bad luck or not, whereas *Total Baseball* rewards him for well-pitched games even in a losing cause.

Les German

Born: Lester Stanley German, June 1, 1869, Baltimore, MD
Debut: August 27, 1890; age 21
Last Game: August 6, 1897; age 28
Record: 34–63 .351 5.49 -19,122 20
Clubs: Baltimore AA; New York NL; Washington NL

Les German grew up in Aberdeen, a small city in northeastern Maryland. As a teenager he started his professional baseball career. After pitching well for Lowell in the Atlantic Association in 1889, he received his chance in the big leagues with the old Baltimore Orioles. After failing to achieve much success at that level, he went back to the minors. In 1891 he led the Eastern Association with 35 victories for the Buffalo Bisons. After a stint in the Southern League, where he threw a no-hitter for the Augusta club, he returned to the majors with the New York Giants, where he broke even in 16 decisions in 1893 and posted his only winning season with a 9–8 record in 1894. In all of his other major league seasons he had a losing record, including a 2–20 mark for Washington in 1896. After the Senators released him in 1897, he was offered a contract by Buffalo but held out for $50 a month more than the Bisons had proposed. Buffalo refused to up the ante, so German signed the next spring with Rochester, where he played third base. An unverified account has him playing in the San Francisco Bay area, where the cold wind and dampness gave him a sore arm, leading to his retirement from baseball.

At any rate he was back in Aberdeen in 1900, working as a clerk in a sporting goods store, selling guns and ammunition. An expert trap shooter, Les was employed by the DuPont Powder Company to give trap shooting exhibitions, sometimes performing with the famous Annie Oakley. In 1915 he established a world record by breaking 499 of 500 targets at a shoot in Atlantic City. He won far more trap shoots than baseball games. Even in his major league playing days he was probably much better at shooting than at pitching. On his very first trip to Florida in 1895 he killed a panther, and the cat's skin was displayed behind the catcher's box at the Polo Grounds.

Les died in Germantown, Maryland, on June 10, 1965, a few days after his 65th birthday. Les German is commemorated in the Aberdeen Room Archives and Museum in his hometown. By major league standards, German was not a very good pitcher. *Baseball Ratings* rates all 877 pitchers having five or more eligible seasons. Les ranks at the very bottom, 877th in the list. Among the 89 hurlers profiled in this book, the Faber System ranks him 89th; *Total Baseball* has him 83rd.

Charlie Getzien

Born: Charles H. Goetzien, February 14, 1864, in Germany
Debut: August 13, 1884; age 20
Last Game: July 19, 1892; age 28
Record: 145–139   .511   3.46   9177   298
Clubs: Detroit NL; Indianapolis NL; Boston NL; Cleveland NL; St. Louis NL

Born in Germany, Charlie as an infant came to the United States with his parents in 1865. He became a naturalized citizen and spelled his surname Getzien, although most newspapers of the day had it as Getzein. As a lad he took quickly to baseball and made a name for himself in the Chicago amateur ranks. At the age of 19 he began his professional career with Grand Rapids in the Northwestern League. When that club folded, he was sold to the Detroit Wolverines of the National League. A weak team when Charlie joined them, the Wolverines improved and soon became pennant contenders. The young man had his best two seasons for Detroit in 1886 and 1887, winning 30 games and 29 games in those two seasons, respectively, and posting winning percentages of .732 and a league-leading .690. Year after year he ranked among the top ten leaders in important pitching categories, such as wins, strikeouts, and fewest bases on balls per nine innings pitched. Twice he ranked fifth in shutouts. On October 1, 1884, he held the Philadelphia Phillies hitless in a 1–0 triumph. It is not considered an official no-hitter since the game was called because of rain after six innings. He almost got another no-hitter. In 1887 the Wolverines won the National League pennant and competed in a post-season showdown against the American Association champion St. Louis Browns. In Game 6 of the series Charlie had a 9–0 lead with two outs in the ninth inning and had not allowed a hit. Getzien was one out away from a no-hit game, facing batting champion Tip O'Neill. O'Neill swung and the ball streaked toward right field, falling a few feet short of the outstretched glove of the fielder.

Getzien had a straight-armed back swing and a little skip in his delivery. He had a good fastball, a fine drop, and he excelled at mixing speeds. Because of his peculiar curveballs, he was called "the Pretzel Twirler." Actually the term pretzel was used more often in another nickname. He and catcher Charlie Ganzel were called "the Pretzel Battery" because both were of German descent. In 1886 he and his left-handed teammate, Lady Baldwin, set an all-time record for wins by a righty-lefty duo by posting a combined 72 wins.

When Detroit dropped out of the National League after the 1888 season, Getzien was purchased by the Indianapolis Hoosiers. In 1891 he was transferred to Boston, where he was released in July. Charlie failed in a one-day trial with Cleveland, then pitched a few games for St. Louis before he was released for the final time in July 1892.

Getzien returned to Chicago and worked briefly for the *Tribune* as a typesetter and as a pitcher for the company baseball team. The 1900 and 1910 censuses both showed him as an inspector for a grain elevator. He died of a heart attack in 1932 at the age of 68. He is profiled in *Nineteenth Century Stars*. Ranking: Faber System 26th; *Total Baseball* tied for 45th.

Ted Gray

Born: Ted Glenn Gray, December 31, 1924, Detroit, MI
Debut: May 15, 1946; age 21
Last Game: September 8, 1955; age 30
Record: 59–74 .444 4.37 -1977 151
Clubs: Detroit AL; Chicago AL; Cleveland AL; New York AL; Baltimore AL

Ted was a star pitcher for suburban Highland Park High School and on Detroit sandlots. Only 17 when he was signed by the Tigers in 1942, he was assigned to Winston-Salem in the Piedmont League. Near the end of the season he was called up to the big club but did not play. On a major league bench at the age of 17, his official debut had to wait until after the end of World War II. Ted turned 18 on New Year's Eve and soon enlisted in the U.S. Navy. He pitched for the Great Lakes Naval Training Station team and was then sent to the South Pacific, where he pitched for a navy team based on New Hebrides. His success in pitching for naval teams led to unrealistic comparisons to Lefty Grove, Carl Hubbell, Hal Newhouser, and other great left-handers.

After the war Ted was assigned to Buffalo of the Class AAA International League. With the exception of three games with the Tigers in the spring of 1946, Gray spent two years in the minors before returning to Detroit in 1948. He had his most successful major league experience in the first half of the 1950 season. With 10 victories already to his credit, he was named to the American League All-Star team. By giving up a game-winning home run to

Red Schoendienst in the 14th inning, he became the losing pitcher of the All-Star Game. He never won another game that year, and never had another winning season in his entire major league career, but he ranked among the top ten American League pitchers in strikeouts for four consecutive years, 1950–54. His repertoire featured a fastball and a forkball. It is said that chronic blisters limited his success. At the end of the 1954 season he was traded to the Chicago White Sox. In 1955 he tied a league record by appearing with four different AL clubs in one season before his major league career came to an end in September.

Ranking: Faber System 78th; *Total Baseball* tied for 64th.

Don Gullett

Born: Donald Edward Gullett, January 6, 1951, Lynn, KY
Debut: April 10, 1970; age 19
Last Game: July 9, 1978; age 27
Record: 109–50   .686   3.11   11475   348
Clubs: Cincinnati NL; New York AL

A native of rural Greenup County in northeastern Kentucky, Gullett attended McKell High School in South Shore, where he compiled an amazing athletic record. As a high school senior he was honorable mention all-state in basketball and had a 9–2 record as a baseball pitcher, striking out 120 batters in 52 innings and once throwing a perfect game. But his exploits on the gridiron made him a schoolboy legend. In one game against Wurtland High School, he scored an unbelievable 72 points as he ran for 11 touchdowns and kicked six extra points. During the season the all-state phenom scored 240 points, rushed for 2,112 yards, averaged 40 yards per kick as a punter, and kicked 24 extra points.

Don was selected in the first round of the 1969 amateur draft by the Cincinnati Reds. The teenager pitched for the Sioux Falls Packers that summer and led the Northern League with a 1.96 ERA. Starting in 1970 he spent his first seven major league seasons with the Reds. After becoming a free agent he signed with the New York Yankees and closed out his pitching career with the Bronx Bombers. Gullett had the good fortune of spending his career with powerful teams, playing in the World Series during six of his nine seasons in the majors. He is one of the few players in major league history to have pitched for four consecutive world champions — Cincinnati's Big Red Machine in 1975 and 1976 and the Bronx Bombers in 1977 and 1978. Three times he led his league in won-lost percentage — 1971 and 1975 in the NL and 1977 in the AL. His .686 winning percentage in the 1970s was the best of any pitcher for the decade and the sixth best of all time. He finished among the top ten in his league in major pitching categories ten times.

Shoulder and rotator cuff problems brought his pitching career to a halt in 1978, when at the age of 27 he should have been at the peak of his game. He sat out the 1979 and 1980 seasons trying to get his shoulder back in shape but finally gave up, and the Yankees released him. He retired to his Kentucky farm and was out of baseball for several years. In 1990 he accepted a position as pitching coach for the Reds' Double A farm club in Chattanooga. His season was cut short by a heart attack. After undergoing triple bypass surgery, he was put on a strict diet and exercise program. The exercise program was difficult because he developed tendonitis in his knees. He gave up running before he eventually resumed it. A year later he was promoted to Nashville. In 1993 he was brought up to the big club and was the pitching coach for the Reds until he and manager Dave Miley were fired by the last-place club in June 2005. Soon he was back in the club's good graces and has worked in various capacities for the Reds, notably in their player development program. In 1993 Don Gullett was inducted into the Dawahares-Kentucky High School Athletic Association Sports Hall of Fame. Could another Hall of Fame — perhaps the one in Cooperstown — have beckoned him had his rotator cuff not torn?

Ranking: Faber System 17th; *Total Baseball* 34th.

Ad Gumbert

Born: Addison Courtney Gumbert, October 10, 1868, Pittsburgh, PA
Debut: September 15, 1888; age 19
Last Game: August 28, 1896; age 27
Record: 123–103 .547 4.27 1846 288
Clubs: Chicago NL; Boston PL; Pittsburgh NL; Brooklyn NL; Philadelphia NL

Ad started his professional baseball career with Zanesville of the Tri-State League when he was still a teenager. After a 27–9 start for the Kickapoos, including two no-hitters, he was acquired by the Chicago White Stockings. After a good rookie season, he jumped to Boston of the Players League, where his 23 wins helped the Reds win the PL pennant. When the PL folded Gumbert returned to Chicago for two seasons. In 1893 he held out against a salary cut and was traded to Pittsburgh well after the season had started. Although the new pitching distance instituted in 1893 caused his earned run average to skyrocket, he managed winning seasons in 1893 and 1894. In 1895 and part of 1896 he pitched for Brooklyn and ended his career with Philadelphia at the age of 27. He was primarily a finesse pitcher with good control and not a lot of strikeouts. For a pitcher he was a good hitter. The five home runs he hit as a pitcher in 1889 stood as a National League record until it was broken by Hal Schumacher in 1934. On Labor Day in 1890, pitching in relief, he won the game with a ninth-inning grand slam.

After retiring from baseball Addison returned to Pittsburgh and entered politics. In the 1900 census he is listed as a clerk; in 1910 as Allegheny County Sheriff; and in 1920 as a county commissioner. A popular speaker, the stocky, red-faced politico liked to tell the story of his almost no-hitter. According to Ad, one day in 1890 while pitching for Boston against Cleveland in the Players League, he had held the opponents hitless for eight innings. The first man up in the ninth struck out. The second man popped out to third baseman Billy Nash. There was only one more out to get to complete the no-hitter. The next man up was Pete Browning. As Gumbert was pitching to the Gladiator, the ball slipped and plunked the batter in the ribs. After shaking his bat at Ad and calling him a variety of vile names, Browning trotted down to first base. With a runner on first base because of the hit batsman, the no-hitter was still intact. The next batter hit a weak roller toward second base. Browning, running down the line, purposely stuck his foot in front of the bounding ball. He was called out, of course, but under the rules the batter was credited with a hit. Gumbert lost his no-hit bid, and Browning got his revenge for having been struck in the ribs.

Addison Gumbert died in his native Pittsburgh on April 23, 1925. He is profiled in *Baseball's First Stars*. Ranking: Faber System 31st; *Total Baseball* 50th.

George Haddock

Born: George Silas Haddock, December 25, 1866, Portsmouth, NH
Debut: September 27, 1888; age 21
Last Game: September 20, 1894; age 27
Record: 95–87   5.22   4.07   6651   215
Clubs: Washington NL; Buffalo PL; Boston AA; Brooklyn NL; Philadelphia NL

George started his professional career at the age of 20 in the Western League with the Emporia and Kansas City teams. Even though he won only three games while losing 25 for Troy of the International Association in 1888, Washington brought him up to the big leagues at the end of the season, where he lost the only two games he started. He had a losing record for the Senators again in 1889. In 1890 he jumped to the Buffalo Bisons of the Players League and led that circuit with 26 losses against nine wins. At this point he had never had a winning season, but things turned around the next year. He joined the Boston Red Stockings and led them to the American Association pennant with 34 victories. He tied for the league lead in wins and shutouts and was second in winning percentage, earned run average, and opponents' on-base percentage. In 1892 he had another good year, winning 29 games for the Brooklyn Bridegrooms. Injuries limited his performance the next season and he was out of baseball in 1894 at the age of 27. A Washington reporter wrote that Haddock had excellent control and was elusive in his twists and drops.[24] His nickname was "Gentleman George," but it was not meant as a compliment. The rougher element in the game apparently used it to express scorn for his more decorous demeanor.

After he retired from baseball Haddock lived in Boston with his widowed mother. According to the 1910 census he was in the retail hay and grain business, and in 1920 he was a Christian Science practitioner. He died at his home in the Roxbury section of Boston on April 18, 1926, at the age of 59.

A biographical sketch of Haddock appears in *Baseball's First Stars*. Ranking: Faber System tied for 55th; *Total Baseball* 59th.

Noodles Hahn

Born: Frank George Hahn, April 29, 1879, Nashville, TN
Debut: April 18, 1899; age 19
Last Game: June 7, 1906; age 27
Record: 130–94   .580   2.55   23,394   422
Clubs: Cincinnati NL; New York AL

As a lad growing up in Nashville, Frank acquired the nickname "Noodles," and it stuck with him his entire life. Several explanations for the origin of the appellation exist, all of them involving noodle soup in one way or another. At the age of 16 the precocious youngster turned pro in 1895, joining the Chattanooga Warriors of the Southern League and moving to Mobile when the franchise was transferred there in midseason. After a good year with Mobile in 1896 he was acquired by the Detroit Wolverines of the Western League. After two years with Detroit he was purchased by the Cincinnati Reds in 1899, making his major league debut a few days shy of his 20th birthday. He had terrific speed, a good curve, and what *The Sporting News* described as "the best control ever displayed by a green southpaw."[25] Noodles had an outstanding rookie season, winning 23 games against eight losses and leading the NL in strikeouts. He attributed his success to swearing off drink, saying, "This year shows me what I can do when I am not drinking. I'll never again indulge in any kind of strong drink."[26] In 1900 he pitched a no-hitter and again led the league in strikeouts. In 1901 he was the NL strikeout king for the third consecutive year and started a string of three straight years in which he won more than 20 games. On May 22 he became the first man since the introduction of the modern pitching distance to strike out 16 batters in a game, a mark that stood for more than 30 years until Dizzy Dean posted 17 strikeouts one day in 1933. Hahn's 1901 season was also remarkable in that he won 22 games for a last-place club, winning 42 percent of Cincinnati's victories, the second highest percentage of a team's wins by a pitcher during the twentieth century, trailing only Steve Carlton's 46 percent for the Phillies in 1972. He was the Faber System Pitcher of the Year in 1901.[27] In 1903 he pitched 34 complete games in 34 starts. Always a workhorse, he may have shortened his career by overwork. During the 1905 season Noodles hurt his arm and was released by the Reds. In November the New York Highlanders signed him as a free agent, but he pitched only six games in the Bronx, retiring at the age of 27 in June 1906.

During his offseasons Hahn had studied at the Cincinnati Veterinary College. Upon retirement he became a veterinary inspector for the United States Government in the Queen City. To keep active in baseball, Noodles played semi-pro ball in the Cincinnati area and kept a locker at Crosley Field. Frequently he donned a uniform and pitched batting practice for the Reds until 1946, when he was 67 years old. In the early 1950s he and his wife moved to the mountains of western North Carolina to a tiny town called Candler. He died February 6, 1960, in Candler at the age of 80.

Hahn is profiled in *Deadball Stars of the National League* and in the SABR *Baseball Biography Project*. He was inducted into the Cincinnati Reds Hall of Fame in 1963. Had he not developed arm trouble at the age of 27, he might be enshrined in Cooperstown today. Ranking: Faber System eighth; *Total Baseball* sixth.

Harry Harper

Born: Harry Clayton Harper, April 24, 1895, Hackensack, NJ
Debut: June 27, 1913; age 18
Last Game: May 8, 1923; age 28
Record: 57–76   .429   2.87   -8618   107
Clubs: Washington AL; Boston AL; Brooklyn NL

Pitching for the Minneapolis Millers of the American Association in 1915, Harper logged two notable performances. On May 19 he pitched a no-hitter against the St. Paul Saints. On July 5 he issued an incredible 20 bases on balls in a game at St. Paul. Harry was more successful after he retired from baseball than he was on the mound. Despite a decent earned run average, he lost far more games than he won. He had the misfortune of pitching most of his career for the Washington Senators at a time when the Nats were not very good. In 1920 he was traded to the Boston Red Sox, who swapped him to the Yankees at the end of the season. Harry led the league twice—neither time in a positive way. He topped the circuit with 13 wild pitches in 1918 and with 21 losses the following year. Although he got his share of strikeouts (four times in the league's top ten in K's per nine innings), he was better known for his lack of control. Five times he was among the top five in wild pitches, four times in bases on balls, and three times in hit batsmen.

One time his lack of control almost sparked a riot. On August 25, 1921, Harper was pitching for the Yankees, who were locked in a pennant race with the defending world champion Cleveland Indians. Going into the game the Yanks had a half-game lead, but the Tribe was well on its way to knocking the New Yorkers out of first place, leading 15–1 in the eighth inning. Either from lack of control or out of frustration, Harper hit three consecutive batters—Charlie Jamieson in the ribs, Larry Gardner on the arm, and Steve O'Neill in the middle of his back. O'Neill took umbrage, picked up the ball, threw it at Harry, then walked over and swatted him with a right to the jaw and a left to the ribs. Players and umpires separated the combatants and Steve was ejected from the game. At the end of the season Harper was out of the majors but came back and appeared for his final game with the Brooklyn Dodgers in 1923 at the age of 28.

While he was pitching in the big leagues, Harry set up an off-season junk business that grew into a major trucking firm. He also owned a road construction contracting company, a large self-service supermarket, a fuel company, a beverage business, and a farm. He became a multimillionaire and a force in New Jersey politics. His career may have been helped by the fact that he married Bessie Brewster, daughter of a prominent road contractor and lived in his father-in-law's home for some time. A Republican, he was an unsuccessful candidate for the U.S. Senate, and settled for such posts as Bergen County sheriff, state labor commissioner, and state civil service commissioner.

Harry Harper died in St. Vincent's Hospital in New York City on April 23, 1926, the day before his 68th birthday.

Ranking: Faber System 84th; *Total Baseball* tied for 56th.

Jack Harper

Born: Charles William Harper, April 2, 1878, Galloway, PA
Debut: September 18, 1899; age 21
Last Game: June 6, 1906; age 28

Record: 80–64 .556 3.55 6710 252
Clubs: Cleveland NL; St. Louis NL; Cincinnati NL; Chicago NL

Although his given name was Charles, Harper was known as Jack throughout his career. He was born in Sugar Creek Township in the oil country of Venango County, Pennsylvania. As a teenager he played semi-pro ball for clubs in western Pennsylvania and eastern Ohio that were supported mainly by men in the oil business. His professional start was with Montgomery in the Southern League in 1898. When that loop disbanded due to the Spanish-American War, Jack caught on with the Grand Rapids Cabinetmakers in the Interstate League. Although he made his major league debut in 1899, he was used so sparingly his first two seasons that he was considered a rookie in 1901. What a rookie year it was! His 23 wins for St. Louis rank among the top ten in victories by a freshman since 1893, as do his numbers of games, innings pitched, and wild pitches thrown. After a trade to Cincinnati he had another 20-plus-win season in 1904, when he recorded an impressive 23–9 record. That was his last really good year.

A story has been published to the effect that he hit Chicago Cubs playing manager Frank Chance with a pitch. To get revenge, Chance persuaded the Cubs' owner to purchase Harper, then cut his salary and allowed him to pitch only one inning the next summer. This account is inaccurate. According to contemporary newspapers, Harper had a series of misfortunes that prevented him from pitching. His thumb was split when struck by a ball off the bat of Dan McGann. When he tried to return to action, the thumb was split again. This was followed by an attack of stomach trouble that threatened to keep him out for several more weeks. Thinking that he could recuperate faster at home than in Chicago, he requested and was granted time off without pay and went home to Oil City.[28] He recovered enough to pitch in the American Association in 1907, dividing the season between Columbus and St. Paul, but never made it back to the majors.

After retiring from baseball Harper entered the business world, first with a shoe store and later with a small community grocery store near Chautauqua, New York. He died in Jamestown, New York, on September 30, 1950, at the age of 51.

Ranking: Faber System 41st; *Total Baseball* 80th.

Pink Hawley

Born: Emerson P. Hawley, December 5, 1872, Beaver Dam, WI
Debut: August 13, 1892; age 19
Last Game: August 20, 1901; age 28

Record: 167–179   .483   3.96   2976   407
Clubs: St. Louis NL; Pittsburgh NL; Cincinnati NL; New York NL; Milwaukee AL

When identical twins were born to Camille and Franc Hawley in 1872, the music store owner could not tell them apart. Camille solved his problem by marking one baby with a pink ribbon, the other with a blue. Emerson received the pink ribbon, his brother Elmer the blue. As they grew into baseball-playing age, the twins became famous in amateur circles throughout the Badger State as "the Pink and Blue Battery," with Pink pitching and Blue catching. Tragically, Blue died of pneumonia in 1891, and Pink tried to make it professionally.

At a Chicago training camp, Cap Anson was impressed with the youngster but had no need for another pitcher. However, he recommended Pink to the Fort Smith club and the lad headed for Arkansas. It is reported that in one game for Fort Smith against a team from Krebs, Indian Territory, Hawley lost 1–0 to Iron Man Joe McGinnity on a catcher's error, despite allowing no hits and striking out 21 batters. A different account of the same game said Pink struck out 27 and lost on a scratch infield single, a passed ball, and an error. Either way, it was an impressive performance. Soon Hawley was signed by the St. Louis Browns and pitched in the Mound City for three years. In 1895 he was traded to Pittsburgh for Red Ehret and $3000. In his first year with the Pirates, he won 31 games and led the league in shutouts and innings pitched. He reduced his wild pitches from a league-leading 21 to a more-acceptable 10 that year. Over his career he made 210 wild pitches, the third most of any hurler in major league history. A good hitter and fielder, he hit .308 with five home runs and 42 RBIs in 1905.

In Pittsburgh the handsome young man became an athletic idol. With his diamonds, stovepipe hats, frock coat, morning trousers, and fastidious dress, he became known as "the Duke of Pittsburgh." A cigar was named the Duke of Pittsburgh in his honor. After the 1897 season he was traded to Cincinnati and had a fine year for the Reds in 1898, winning 27 games against 11 losses for a winning percentage of .711. For his career, though, he was below the break-even mark with a dozen more losses than wins. After two years in Cincinnati and one season each in New York and Milwaukee, Pink pitched for a year for Buffalo in the Eastern League, then retired and opened a cigar store in La Crosse, Wisconsin.

However, he was not quite ready to leave baseball completely behind. After two years away from the game, he was pitching for La Crosse in the Wisconsin State League. He helped organize the Wisconsin-Illinois League and managed the La Crosse Pinks through 1908. In 1909 he moved to Oshkosh and managed the Indians that season. In 1910 he was still living in Oshkosh and listed his occupation as baseball manager. The 1920 census named him as a bowling alley manager.

After several years of illness, Emerson Hawley died at his home in Beaver Dam on September 19, 1938, at the age of 65.

He is profiled in *Nineteenth Century Stars*. Ranking: Faber System twelfth; *Total Baseball* thirteenth.

Long John "Egyptian" Healy

Born: John J. Healy, October 27, 1866, Cairo, IL
Debut: September 11, 1885; age 18
Last Game: July 6, 1892; age 25
Record: 78–136 .364 3.84 -3468 138
Clubs: St. Louis NL; Indianapolis NL; Washington NL; Chicago NL; Baltimore AA; Brooklyn NL; Louisville NL

Healy was born in Cairo in the section of Illinois known as Little Egypt, hence his nickname "Egyptian." At 6'2" he was most often called "Long John" during his playing career. His father died while John was a child, and his brother Frank, 17 years older and a druggist, was the chief support of his mother and siblings. Long John made his major league debut at the age of 18. He pitched for seven different clubs in his eight-year career, compiling a losing record with every team except Louisville, where he broke even in two decisions his final season. He ranked in the top ten in his league three times in shutouts and twice each in strikeouts and earned run average. On the negative side he was in the top ten four times each in bases on balls, wild pitches, and losses. His 29 losses in 1887 led the league. His .310 winning percentage in the 1880s was the lowest posted by any major leaguer for the decade. With those kinds of numbers, how was he able to survive the '80s and pitch into the '90s? Because year after year he pitched for weak teams that gave him little run support.

The highlight of his career came in 1887 when he joined a group managed by Albert Spalding for a trip around the world, playing baseball on several continents. He pitched in the gold fields of Australia, in the capital of India, in the sands of the Sahara, under the shadow of the Pyramids, in Rome, Paris, London, and Dublin. Long John retired from baseball at the tender age of 25 to become a policeman in St. Louis. He rose rapidly in the ranks, being promoted to detective in a short time. However, the lure of the game was strong, and he unsuccessfully attempted a comeback with the Minneapolis Millers in 1895–96. Returning to the police force, he made his last appearance as a ball player when he pitched the policemen to a win over the city's firemen in a

game at Sportsman's Park. After contracting consumption (tuberculosis), he took a leave of absence and went to Nebraska in a vain hope that the drier climate would improve his health. He lost more than 100 pounds before succumbing to the disease in St. Louis on March 16, 1898, at the age of 31.
Ranking: Faber System 81st; *Total Baseball* 82nd.

George Hemming

Born: George Earl Hemming, December 15, 1868, Carrollton, OH
Debut: April 21, 1890; age 21
Last Game: June 12, 1897; age 28
Record: 91–82 .526 4.53 13,852 279
Clubs: Cleveland PL; Brooklyn PL; Brooklyn NL; Cincinnati NL; Louisville NL; Baltimore NL

George Hemming was called "Ole Wax Figger" presumably because of some fancied resemblance to a wax figure. He made his major league debut at the age of 21 and pitched for six different teams in his eight-year career. In 1893 and again in 1894 he pitched a complete game every time he started, a total of 66 complete games in two years. In 1895 he won 20 games for the Baltimore Orioles and had his best winning percentage the following season with a 15–6 (.714) record. However, he had problems the next year and was out of the majors by midseason. Hemming tried to continue pitching in the minor leagues. He retired from the Springfield Ponies of the Connecticut League in 1904. After being out of the game for a year, he announced he was going to "bust back into baseball"[29] with Wilkes-Barre of the New York League in 1906. However, an article on the famous old Orioles in a 1913 newspaper reported that "George Hemming has not done much for baseball in recent years."[30] Accounts of his life after baseball are very sparse. The 1920 census showed him as married but living apart from his family in a rented room in Springfield, Massachusetts. His occupation was listed as "none." He died June 3, 1930, in Springfield at the age of 61.
Ranking: Faber System 33rd; *Total Baseball* tied for 68th.

Glenn Hobbie

Born: Glenn Frederick Hobbie, April 24, 1936, Witt, IL
Debut: September 20, 1957; age 21
Last Game: July 25, 1964; age 28
Record: 62–81 .434 4.20 2442 206
Clubs: Chicago NL; St. Louis NL

A native of Montgomery County in downstate Illinois, 18-year-old Glenn signed with the Chicago Cubs as an amateur free agent in the spring of 1955. During the next three years he pitched for three different clubs in the Northern League, for the Dubuque Packers of the Midwest League, and for the Memphis Chickasaws of the Southern Association. Near the end of the 1957 season he was called up to the majors and pitched for the Cubs until he was traded to St. Louis on June 2, 1964. A badly strained shoulder shelved him for most of the season. He won only one game for the Cardinals before ending his major league career on July 25 at the age of 28. During the offseason he was traded to Detroit but never appeared in a game for the Tigers. He pitched for the Syracuse Chiefs of the International League in 1965 but was unable to make the club during spring training in 1966. Glenn had only two winning seasons in the majors (1958 and 1959) and led the National League with 20 losses in 1960. Hobbie was a better pitcher than would appear from his won-lost record, for the Cubs were a second-division club every year he was with them. After his retirement from baseball Glenn returned to Montgomery County. He settled in Hillsboro, the county seat, and worked as the plant supervisor of the Roller Derby Skate Company. For a time he served as president of the Bottomley-Ruffing-Schalk Baseball Museum in nearby Nokomis, a shrine to three Hall of Famers from the area.

Ranking: Faber System 60th; *Total Baseball* tied for 76th.

Art Houtteman

Born: Arthur Joseph Houtteman, Jr., August 7, 1927, Detroit, MI
Debut: April 29, 1945; age 17
Last Game: September 22, 1957; age 30
Record: 87–91   .489   4.14   -11,387   193
Clubs: Detroit AL; Cleveland AL; Baltimore AL

Art seemed destined for the big leagues from childhood. His father vowed his son would reach the majors by the time he was 17. Amazingly, the father's wish came true. The lad became a star on the sandlots, at Central Catholic High School, and in American Legion ball. The Tigers signed him as an amateur free agent a few days after his 17th birthday and assigned him to Detroit's top farm club at Buffalo in the International League. He was promoted to the big club late in the 1945 season. When most of the World War II veterans returned in 1946, Art was again sent to Buffalo, where he led the league in strikeouts. Back in the big leagues in 1948, Art lost game after game in which he pitched well but the club scored few runs in his support. That is when he first acquired the nickname "Hard Luck Houtteman." However, he soon had worse luck off the diamond than on it.

During spring training in Florida his convertible collided with a fruit truck, fracturing his skull. He was able to return to the mound and was honored by a sportswriters association as the year's most courageous athlete. In 1950 he made the American League all-star team and pitched a one-hitter in which he faced the minimum 27 batters; the only man to record a safe hit was caught stealing and both hitters whom he walked were erased in double plays. He made the American League all-star team that year. The day after the season ended Art married Shelagh Marie Kelly. Immediately after returning from their honeymoon the groom was drafted into the army. When he reported to camp, he was declared unfit for combat because the noise of gunfire gave him severe headaches, probably the result of his skull fracture. He spent the next 11 months pitching for the camp baseball team. After his discharge he rejoined the Tigers. Returning from spring training in 1952 with her first child and Art's mother, Shelagh ran her new Cadillac off a mountain road in Tennessee. The seven-month-old baby, Sheryl, was thrown from the car and killed.

After this tragedy, Hard Luck Houtteman was back on the mound again. He was one out away from a no-hitter against Cleveland on April 26 when he shook off his catcher's sign for a curve and threw a fastball that cost him the no-no. He had an excellent fastball, a good curve, and a slider, but he just could not win consistently. He lost 20 games that year. In 1954 he was traded to Cleveland and had one of his better seasons with 15 wins and only seven losses for the pennant-winning Indians. He pitched in only two innings in the World Series that fall against the New York Giants. In 1957 he was sold to Baltimore and shipped down to Vancouver of the Pacific Coast League. Late in the season the Orioles called him up and he made his last major league appearance with the Birds that fall at the age of 30.

In 1958 Houtteman pitched for the Charleston Senators, Detroit's farm club in the American Association. The next year he joined the Portland Beavers of the Pacific Coast League. He hung up his spikes at the age of 32 after the end of the 1959 season. That winter he became a sports reporter for a Detroit television station, and later became a sales executive with Paragon Steel in Detroit until he reached retirement age. On May 6, 2003, at the age of 75, he died of an apparent heart attack at his home in suburban Rochester Hills.

His life is reviewed in the *SABR Biography Project*. Ranking: Faber System 67th; *Total Baseball* 54th.

Charles Hudson

Born: Charles Lynn Hudson, March 16, 1959, Ennis, TX
Debut: May 31, 1983; age 24

Last Game: August 11, 1989; Age 30
Record: 50–60   .455   4.14   -4221   136
Clubs: Philadelphia NL; New York AL; Detroit AL

At South Oak Cliff High School in Dallas, Charlie played shortstop on the baseball team but he was not a star. He thought he could not afford to go to college, but at the urging of his civics teacher he applied to and was accepted by Prairie View A&M. His college coach converted him into a pitcher, a position at which he was much more adept and where his mediocre hitting was less of a handicap. Hudson helped take Prairie View to two NAIA playoffs and became the school's first alumnus to reach the major leagues as a pitcher. He had unusually long fingers with which to grip the baseball and a "buggy whip" arm. He was drafted by the Philadelphia Phillies in the 12th round of the 1981 amateur draft. The Phils sent him to Helena in the Pioneer League and then to Venezuela for winter ball. In 1982 he was assigned to the Peninsula Pilots, where he led the Carolina League in ERA and tied for the lead in wins. He climbed all the way from Class A ball to the majors the next spring, making his big league debut with the Phillies in May. He pitched a complete-game victory over the Los Angles Dodgers that October to help get the Phillies into the World Series. In the Fall Classic, though, he lost both games he pitched. He never had a winning season in the City of Brotherly Love. Following the 1986 season he was traded to the New York Yankees and got off to a great start, winning his first six games. It was thought that he had become a better balanced pitcher, not simply a hard thrower. But his newfound success did not last. A month-long slump led to a brief demotion to Columbus, but he rebounded and 1987 turned out to be his only winning season in the major leagues. In 1988 he started losing again, and the Yankees traded him to Detroit in the spring of 1989.

Hudson was having a miserable season with the Tigers when in the depths of a month-long depression he got drunk and climbed into his mother-in-law's Mercury Cougar. He woke up at 2:12 A.M. on August 11, pinned inside the car wrapped around a telephone pole in the Detroit suburb of Farmington Hills. He spent a day and a half in intensive care. He had surgery to insert two rods into his left leg, which was broken clear through. His right knee needed reconstruction; his right ankle was broken. A month later he was sentenced to one year's probation after pleading guilty to driving while impaired. "The only good thing was nobody else was involved and my arm wasn't hurt," he said. "I was going through a time when I wasn't pitching.... I was just trying to drink my problems away when all I ended up doing was hurting myself."[31] The accident was just the start of a series of troubles for Hudson. His mother died. A cousin committed suicide. His wife divorced him. The city of Farmington Hills sent him a $2500 bill for the broken telephone pole. The Tigers put him on the 60-day disabled list, and then granted him free agency. No team signed him.

A half-dozen years later he thought things were getting better. He said he had been sober for two years and God was watching over him. For half of the past six years he had been in a wheelchair, on crutches, or with a cane, but now he had recovered. In the spring of 1995 the Chicago Cubs invited him to spring training. Inspired by George Foreman's comeback at the age of 40, he said he could make it back at the age of 35 "if the Good Lord wills it."[32] Unfortunately, the Cubs used him in only one spring training game and released him before the season started. There would be no comeback at the age of 35 for Charlie Hudson.

Ranking: Faber System 83rd; *Total Baseball* 74th.

Percy Jones

Born: Percy Lee Jones, October 28, 1899, Harwood, TX
Debut: August 6, 1920; age 20
Last Game: June 11, 1930; age 30
Record: 53   57   .482   4.34   -759   166
Clubs: Chicago NL; Boston NL; Pittsburgh NL

Jones made his major league debut before playing a game in the minors. After three years with the Cubs he was sent down to the Pacific Coast League. He won 16 games for Los Angeles in 1923 and 13 for Seattle in 1924 before being called back to Chicago in 1925. He was a lefty who relieved more often than he started. During nine seasons in the majors, he never led the league in any pitching category. He won 12 games in 1926, his best year. In midseason 1928 Percy inherited a half-million dollars from his grandmother's estate but continued pitching. After his major league career ended, he finished the 1930 season with the Columbus Redbirds in the American Association. In 1931 he opened the season with two wins, and then fell from a third-story window and broke his back, requiring him to spend the rest of his life in a wheelchair. Jones died in Dallas, Texas, on March 18, 1979, at the age of 79.

Ranking: Faber System 73rd; *Total Baseball* 75th.

Addie Joss

Born: Adrian Joss, April 12, 1880, Woodland, WI
Debut: April 26, 1902; age 22
Last Game: July 11, 1910; age 30

Record: 160   97   .623   1.89   27,658   541
Club: Cleveland AL

See the entry on Addie Joss in Part Two of this book.

He is profiled in *Deadball Stars of the American League*, in the *SABR Biography Project*, and is the subject of a book-length biography by Scott Longert, *Addie Joss: King of the Pitchers*. Cleveland: Society for American Baseball Research, 1998.

Ranking: Faber System fourth; *Total Baseball* fifth; Bill James third.

Joe Kennedy

Born: Joseph Darley Kennedy, May 24, 1979, La Mesa, CA
Debut: June 6, 2001; age 22
Last Game: September 29, 2007; age 28
Record: 43   61   .413   4.79   807   140
Clubs: Tampa Bay AL; Colorado NL; Oakland AL; Arizona NL; Toronto AL

Joe played baseball, basketball, football and volleyball at El Cajon Valley High School. He was drafted out of Grossmont Community College by the Tampa Bay Devil Rays in the eighth round (252nd overall pick) of the 1998 amateur draft. He worked his way up the Tampa Bay system from Princeton in 1998, to Hudson Valley, Charleston, and Durham before making the big leagues in 2001. For three seasons Joe was a starting pitcher for the Devil Rays, with an occasional trip back down to the minors. After the 2003 season he was traded to the Colorado Rockies, where he had his best major league season with a 9–7 won-lost record and an ERA of 3.66 in 2004. In 2005 he was traded to the Oakland Athletics. From that point on he was used mainly in the bullpen, with only a few starts mixed in. He suffered shoulder and biceps injuries and was released by the A's in 2007. Afterwards he played briefly for Arizona and Toronto. During his last few years he also had some minor league stints in Orlando, Colorado Springs, Sacramento, and Syracuse. On November 23, 2007, he collapsed at the home of his in-laws in Florida. He was taken to Brandon Hospital, where he was pronounced dead at the age of 28. The cause of death was ruled to be hypertensive heart disease with degeneration of the mitral valve.

Frank Killen

Born: Frank Bissell Killen, November 30, 1870, Pittsburgh, PA
Debut: August 27, 1891; age 20
Last Game: June 27, 1900; age 29

Record: 164 131 .556 3.78 28,049 423
Clubs: Milwaukee AA; Washington NL; Pittsburgh NL; Boston NL; Chicago NL

Lefty Killen was one of the outstanding pitchers of the 1890s. As a teenager in 1890 he pitched for three different minor league clubs, tossing a no-hitter for Minneapolis in the Western Association. He broke into the majors in 1891 at the age of 20. He pitched a few games for Milwaukee late that season, and then won 29 games for Washington in 1892. Traded to Pittsburgh the next spring, he came into his own by winning a league-leading 36 games for the Pirates that season. No left-handed pitcher has won that many games in a year since then. He was slowed by injuries in both 1894 and 1895. In July 1894 his arm was broken by a line drive hit by Patsy Tebeau. In June 1895, he was spiked on his leg by Parke Wilson while covering home plate. Thinking Wilson had intentionally tried to injure him, Killen slugged the perpetrator and was ejected from the game. A few days later Frank came down with blood poisoning from the wound and was hospitalized for almost two months. He bounced back with a terrific year in 1896, leading the league with 30 wins, in complete games with 44, and in shutouts with five. After that he tapered off and was out of the majors by mid-season 1900. However, he pitched in the minors for the next three years, notching another 37 victories in Wheeling, Indianapolis, and Atlanta to bring his professional total to more than 200 wins. He umpired for a while in 1906. After his retirement he operated a hotel and a tavern in Pittsburgh. He died of a heart attack at the age of 69 in 1939.

Killen is the subject of a biographical sketch in *Nineteenth Century Stars*. Ranking: Faber System tied for seventh; *Total Baseball* eighth.

Eric King

Born: Eric Steven King, April 10, 1964, Oxnard, CA
Debut: May 15, 1986; age 22
Last Game: October 4, 1992; age 28
Record: 52 45 .536 3.97 3844 200
Clubs: Detroit AL; Chicago AL; Cleveland AL

Eric was signed as a 19-year-old amateur free agent by the San Francisco Giants in 1983 and assigned to Great Falls in the Pioneer League, the first of ten minor league clubs for whom he pitched between 1983 and 1998. His entire baseball career was marked by transfers from one club to another, back and forth between the big leagues and the minors. In 1984 he pitched for Clinton in the Midwest League. In 1985 he pitched in the Texas League All-Star game for the Shreveport Captains, a Giants farm club. At the end of the season he was traded to the Detroit Tigers. As a rookie he went 11–4 for the

Tigers in 1986, but the Tigers put him in the bullpen for the next two years and sent him down to Nashville and Toledo for parts of 1986 and 1988 before trading him to the Chicago White Sox in 1989. The Sox sent him to Sarasota for parts of the 1989 and 1990 seasons before returning him to the starting rotation. Eric had his best season in 1990 when he won 12 games and lost four. However, the Sox traded him to Cleveland, where he was unable to duplicate that success. The Indians sent him to Colorado Springs and then granted him free agency after the 1991 season. King signed with Detroit for another campaign and divided the 1992 season between the Tigers and their farm clubs in London (Ontario) and Toledo. After the Tigers released him, Eric came back and played for the Pacific Suns in the Western League in 1998. What an odyssey — fourteen teams in eleven seasons. Only once (1987) did he spend an entire season with a single major league club. Ranking: Faber System 64th; *Total Baseball* 51st.

Silver King

Born: Charles Frederick Koenig, January 11, 1868, St. Louis, MO
Debut: September 28, 1886; age 18
Last Game: August 19, 1897; age 29
Record: 203   154   .569   3.18   5992   421
Clubs: Kansas City NL; St. Louis AA; Chicago PL; New York NL; Washington NL

Known also as Charley King, he was dubbed "Silver" because of his white hair; King was a translation of the German name Koenig. He started his professional career with St. Joseph of the Western League at the age of 17 and appeared in a few games for the Kansas City Cowboys near the end of the season. In 1887 Charley had an impressive rookie year with 32 victories, the first of four consecutive seasons in which he won at least 30 games. In 1888 he had a sensational year, perhaps the best pitching performance ever by a 20 year old. Silver led the league with 45 wins, a 1.64 earned run average, six shutouts, a WHIP of 0.876, and 64 complete games in 65 starts. He lacked 14 strikeouts of winning the pitching Triple Crown. In 1890 he again led the league with a 2.69 ERA and four shutouts. Using no windup, he started his pitching motion in the back left corner of the pitcher's box and stepped across to the right side while releasing the ball. The introduction of the pitching rubber in 1893 hampered his delivery, and he never again won more than 10 games in a season. Throughout much of his career, King was involved in disputes with management over his salary. After the 1893 season he temporarily quit baseball to join his father's bricklaying business. He came back in 1896 for two more years before leaving the game for good and becoming a very

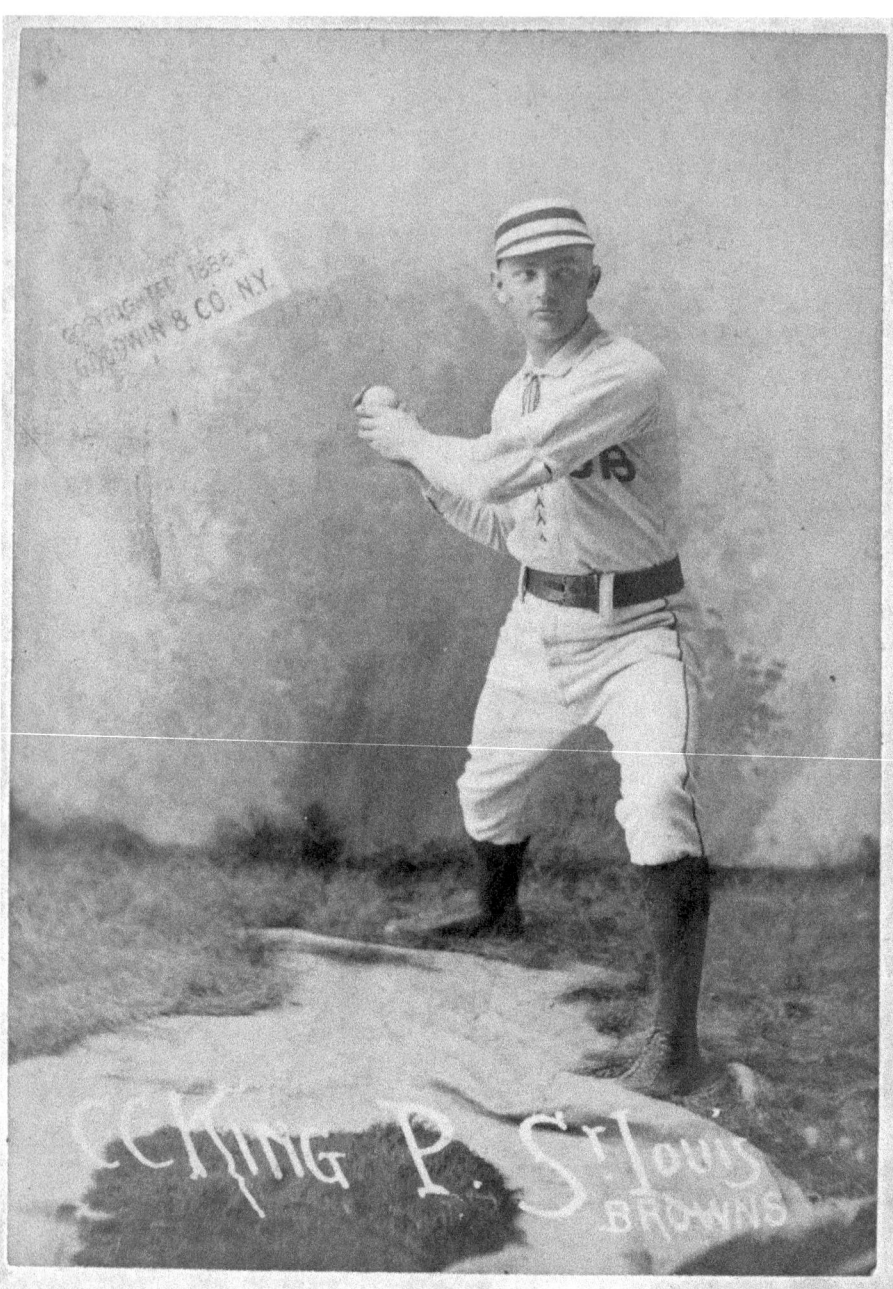

successful brick contractor. He died in St. Louis on May 21, 1938, at the age of 70.

Silver King is profiled in *Nineteenth Century Stars*. Ranking: Faber System tenth; *Total Baseball* fourth.

Clay Kirby

Born: Clayton Laws Kirby, Jr., June 25, 1948, Washington, DC
Debut: April 11, 1969; Age 20
Last Game: September 28, 1976; Age 28
Record: 75   104   .419   3.84   -60   230
Clubs: San Diego NL; Cincinnati NL; Montreal NL

At the age of 12 Clay was a star Little League pitcher in Arlington, Virginia. After attracting attention nationally for his exploits at Washington-Lee High School, he was selected by the St. Louis Cardinals in the third round of the 1966 amateur draft. Following three seasons in the minors, he was taken by the San Diego Padres in the 1968 expansion draft. In his rookie season with the weak-hitting Padres he led the National League with 20 losses. His most notable performance came on July 21, 1970. In a game against the New York Mets, Kirby walked Tommie Agee in the first inning. The speedster stole second, then third, and scored on a groundout by Art Shamsky. The Mets had a 1–0 lead on no hits. Clay held them hitless through eight innings, but the Padres were unable to score. With two outs in the bottom of the eighth, Kirby was due to bat. Although Clay was only three outs away from a no-hitter, manager Preston Gomez chose to take him out for a pinch-hitter. The pinch-hitter struck out; the relief pitcher ruined the no-hitter by giving up two hits in the top of the ninth, and Kirby lost the game as well as the no-hitter.

In November 1973 Clay was traded to Cincinnati and enjoyed two winning seasons with the Big Red Machine before being sent to another weak team, the Montreal Expos. After a losing season, he was released by the Expos and tried to make a comeback with San Diego. The Padres sent him to their farm club in Hawaii, but he won only one game for the Islanders. After retiring, Kirby returned to Arlington. For several years he was tournament chairman for the Major League Baseball Players Alumni in golfing events to benefit

Opposite: Silver King won at least 30 games in each of his first four big league seasons. In 1888 he had perhaps the best year ever by a 20-year-old pitcher, leading the league with 45 wins, a 1.64 ERA, a WHIP of 0.876, and 64 complete games in 65 starts. The introduction of the pitching rubber in 1893 hampered his delivery, and his productivity declined (Library of Congress).

the American Lung Association. He died in Arlington of a heart attack on October 11, 1991, at the age of 43. Ranking: Faber System 50th; *Total Baseball* 84th.

Phil Knell

Born: Philip H. Knell, March 12, 1865, San Francisco, CA
Debut: July 6, 1888; age 23
Last Game: September 29, 1895; age 30
Record: 79 90 .467 4.05 8525 197
Clubs: Pittsburgh NL; Philadelphia PL; Columbus AA; Washington NL; Philadelphia NL; Louisville NL; Cleveland NL

As a young man Knell played semi-pro ball in California and professional baseball in the California League. When he broke a contract to go east, the league blacklisted him. In 1889 he threw a no-hitter for St. Joseph in the Western Association. Phil pitched for seven different clubs in six seasons. He holds an all-time record — 54 batters hit by pitches in the 1891 season. He won a career-high 28 games that year for Columbus and led the American Association with five shutouts. He gave up the fewest hits per nine innings of any AA pitcher that season. His only other winning season in the majors came one year earlier when he posted 22 wins and 11 losses for the Philadelphia Quakers in the Players League. After his major league career ended, he played for the Ft. Wayne Farmers in the Inter-State League until the club released him to cut payroll. He then returned to California, played semi-pro or independent league ball, and umpired for a while in the Pacific Coast League. For more than 30 years he was a gas company employee, working as inspector, machinist, and foreman. Phil died June 5, 1944, in Santa Monica at the age of 79. Ranking: Faber System 66th; *Total Baseball* tied for 68th.

Sandy Koufax

Born: Sanford Braun, December 30, 1935, Brooklyn, NY
Debut: June 24, 1955; age 19
Last Game: October 2, 1966; age 30
Record: 165 87 .655 28,699 563
Clubs: Brooklyn NL; Los Angeles NL

See the entry on Sandy Koufax in Part Two of this book.

With Ed Linn, he wrote an autobiography, *Koufax*, New York: Viking Press, 1966. A book-length biography was written by Jane Leavy, *Sandy Koufax: A Lefty's Legacy*, New York: Harper Collins, 2002.

Ranking: Faber System second; *Total Baseball* third; Bill James first.

Johnny Kucks

Born: John Charles Kucks, July 27, 1933, Hoboken, NJ
Debut: April 17, 1955; age 21
Last Game: September 25, 1960; age 27
Record: 54 56 .491 4.10 -6640 147
Clubs: New York AL; Kansas City AL

In February 1952 the New York Yankees signed 18-year-old Johnny Kucks out of Jersey City's Dickinson High School for a reported $13,500. Assigned to the Norfolk Tars of the Piedmont League, the teenager went 19–6 with a 2.55 ERA. He spent the next two years in military service. Upon his discharge, he went straight to the big leagues. In 1956 he had his best season for the Yankees, going 18–9 in the regular season and winning the decisive seventh game of the World Series with a three-hit shutout of the Brooklyn Dodgers. He never had another winning season in the majors. In 1959 he was traded to Kansas City and had two losing seasons with the A's. He had an especially bad year in 1960 with a 4–10 record and an ERA of 6.00. He blamed his lack of success on poor handling by manager Bob Elliott and bad luck. "There's nothing wrong with my arm," he told reporters. "I just haven't had any luck. No breaks. That's not an alibi. I don't care what anybody says, you've got to be lucky."[33] There were rumors that the Yankees wanted him back, but instead he was purchased by Baltimore, which then traded him to St. Louis. He never got into any games with either the Orioles or Cardinals, and was sent down to the International League. In 1961 he pitched for the Rochester Red Wings. In 1962 and 1963 he was with the Atlanta Crackers, winning 14 games each year. After his retirement he signed with Lerner Sports Marketing and announced his availability for fundraisers, giving motivational talks, and signing memorabilia.

Ranking: Faber System 79th; *Total Baseball* 81st.

Ted Lewis

Born: Edward Morgan Lewis, December 25, 1872, Machynlleth, Wales
Debut: July 6, 1896; age 23
Last Game: September 26, 1901; age 28
Record: 94 64 .595 3.53 5383 270
Clubs: Boston NL; Boston AL

Lewis was a ballplayer, good enough to win nearly 60 percent of his games in a six-year major league career. But he was much more than a ballplayer. Rory Costello wrote that like Sir Thomas More, Lewis was a man for all seasons. Educator, elocutionist, natural leader, he embodied an array of talents but always retained a winning humility. Costello said that Horatio Alger could not have conjured up a life story like this, which has the power to make the most hardened cynic believe in ideals again.[34]

The first major leaguer ever born in Wales, Ted came to the United States with his parents at the age of eight. Immediately he got a job delivering groceries and found other odd jobs to help with the family budget. He worked in a department store and as a surveyor's helper, studied borrowed textbooks and saved enough ($50) to travel to Ohio, where he was able to survive his freshman year at Marietta College by working as a letter carrier, hotel clerk, and janitor. In his sophomore year he transferred to Williams College, where he became the star pitcher on the baseball team. In order to earn money to go to graduate school, he joined the Boston Beaneaters in 1896. Two years later he had his best season with a 26–8 record, a league-leading .765 percentage, and an ERA of 2.90. His teammates gave him the nickname of "Parson," as he did not drink, refused to play ball on Sundays, and read his Bible daily. Among the rowdy players of the time, such a nickname might have been uttered with a sneer, but because of Ted's humility and sincerity it was a mark of respect, not of derision.

He earned a master's degree at Williams in 1899 and decided in 1901 to retire from baseball and devote full time to teaching. From 1901 to 1903 he taught elocution at Columbia, then he returned to his alma mater and taught oratory for eight years. In 1910 he ran for Congress as a Democrat in a strongly Republican district and lost by only a few hundred votes. In 1911 he moved to the Massachusetts Agricultural College at Amherst (now the University of Massachusetts), where he served as professor, dean, acting president, and president. In 1927 he accepted the presidency of the University of New Hampshire and established its first graduate school.

For two years Lewis suffered from liver cancer and died on May 23, 1936, at the age of 63. Today the "Pitching Professor" is remembered chiefly as an educator, but according to Tim Murnane, in his youth he was known as "a superb pitcher, with great curves and fine speed, both of which he used with rare judgment."[35]

Ben McDonald

Born: Larry Benard McDonald, November 24, 1967, Baton Rouge, LA
Debut: September 6, 1989; age 21
Last Game: July 16, 1997; age 29
Record: 78   70   .527   3.91   1874   205
Clubs: Baltimore AL; Milwaukee AL

An all-state performer in three sports at Denham Springs (Louisiana) High School, Ben was selected by the Atlanta Braves in the 27th round of the 1986 amateur draft. He did not sign with the Braves, opting instead to attend Louisiana State University, where he played varsity basketball as well as baseball. During his three years at LSU, Ben became one of the most highly touted college baseball players of all time. In 1988 he led the U.S. Olympic team to a gold medal, winning complete games against both South Korea and Puerto Rico. Twice he helped LSU reach the College World Series. In 1989 he went 14–4, set a Southeastern Conference record with 202 strikeouts, was named to the All-American team, and won the Golden Spikes Award, given annually to the nation's best amateur player. Following this, his junior year at LSU, Ben was chosen by the Baltimore Orioles as the first pick in the first round of the 1989 amateur draft. Represented by hard-nosed agent Scott Boras, he engaged in tough negotiations with the Orioles before signing for a record bonus of $350,000 and a guaranteed salary of nearly one million dollars.

The high-priced youngster did not join the Orioles immediately. During the summer he pitched in the Cape Cod League, a showcase for premier college players. Ben made two starts for the Frederick Keys in the Carolina League before being called up to the majors. Because of injuries he never lived up to his early promise, never leading the league in any pitching category. Throughout most of his career he suffered from shoulder problems and underwent three rotator cuff surgeries. He was on the disabled list six times in eight years.

After retiring, McDonald returned to Denham Springs. Never one to spend his money on luxury automobiles or extravagant living, Ben resides in 2009 on a six-acre plot with a ranch house and a fishing pond. He is still married to his college sweetheart, enjoys hunting, fishing, and coaching the youth teams on which his son and daughter play. "Baseball was good to me," he says. "The sport allowed me to travel around the world, compete at the highest level possible and make a very good living. I have no regrets. I won a high school championship and an Olympic gold medal, pitched in a College World Series and played in the big leagues for nine years. Some people say I ran into a lot of hard luck, but I feel extremely lucky to accomplish what I did."[36]

In 2008 Ben McDonald was inducted into the College Baseball Hall of Fame. Ranking: Faber System tied for 61st; *Total Baseball* 25th.

Willie McGill

Born: William Vaness McGill, November 10, 1873, Atlanta, GA
Debut: May 8, 1890; age 16

Last Game: June 12, 1896; age 22
Record: 72   74   .493   4.59   -2049   161
Clubs: Cleveland PL; Cincinnati AA; St. Louis AA; Cincinnati NL; Chicago NL; Philadelphia NL

Willie was not the youngest player ever to pitch in the major leagues. (Joe Nuxhall and perhaps others were younger.) He was, however, the youngest to hurl a complete game, the youngest to pitch a shutout, and the youngest to win 20 games in a season. He was probably the youngest ever to pitch a no-hit game in the minor leagues. He made his professional debut at the age of 15 for Evansville in the Central Inter-State League and was more than four months shy of his 16th birthday when he tossed his no-hitter. He reached the major leagues at the age of 16 and was a 20-game winner his rookie season. He never matched that victory total again. A heavy drinker, he liked the high life, broke training rules, and frequently was out of condition, causing him occasionally to be absent from his team. In 1892 he missed most of the season because of arm trouble. As he was not pitching professionally at the time, Notre Dame recruited him to pitch in a game against Michigan, claiming he had been a student there years before and therefore was eligible. Despite protests by the Wolverines, Willie pitched the Irish to a win in the first baseball game ever played between the rival universities. Before returning to the majors Willie won 14 games for Menominee of the Michigan-Wisconsin League that season.

McGill was out of the majors at the age of 22, the youngest exit ever by a player with five or more eligible seasons. Apparently, he overcame his conditioning problems and pitched in the minor leagues for eight years after leaving the big leagues and in semi-pro circuits after that. Among the minor league clubs for which he pitched were St. Paul, Grand Rapids, and Peoria of the Western League; Evansville of the Three I; Milwaukee, Toledo, and Indianapolis of the AA; Worcester and Norwich of the Connecticut League; and Freeport of the Wisconsin State League. The young man did get around! Later he became a coach and an athletic trainer, callings that few would have predicted for the fast-living youngster of the Gay Nineties. Willie died at the age of 70 on August 29, 1944, in Indianapolis.

He is profiled in *Baseball's First Stars*. Ranking: Faber System 74th; *Total Baseball* 49th.

Jim McGlothlin

Born: James Milton McGlothlin, October 6, 1943, Los Angeles, CA
Debut: September 20, 1965; age 21

Last Game: September 28, 1973; age 29
Record: 67 77 .465 3.61 -6605 170
Clubs: California AL; Cincinnati NL; Chicago AL

Jim McGlothlin was signed out of Reseda High School in California's San Fernando Valley as a free agent in 1962. The Angels assigned him to farm clubs and brought him along slowly. He was with the Hawaii Islanders in 1964 and the Seattle Angels in 1965 before joining the big club late in the season. In his best year in California, he won 12 and lost eight with a 2.96 ERA in 1967. He led the American League with six shutouts that season. Three years later he was traded to Cincinnati and helped the Reds win pennants in 1970 and 1972. His 14 wins in 1970 represent his season-high in victories. He appeared in two World Series games with the Reds but had no decisions. Late in the 1973 season Cincinnati traded him to the White Sox but he won no games in Chicago and was released by the Sox during spring training in 1974. He was ill at the time, but the severity of his illness was not known. Actually, he had leukemia and died from the disease at the age of 32 on December 23, 1975, at his home in Union, Kentucky, a suburb of Cincinnati. His death at an early age was a loss for baseball but a greater loss for his young wife and three children. Ranking: Faber System 68th; *Total Baseball* 79th.

Denny McLain

Born: Dennis Dale McLain, March 29, 1944, Chicago, IL
Debut: September 21, 1963; age 19
Last Game: September 12, 1972; age 28
Record: 131 91 .590 21,858 412
Clubs: Detroit AL; Washington AL; Oakland AL; Atlanta NL

Seldom has a pitcher risen so high or fallen so low as Denny McLain. At Mt. Carmel High School he led his team to three Chicago championships, with a 38–7 record. Upon graduation in 1962 he signed with the Chicago White Sox for a $10,000 bonus. Assigned to the Harlan Smokies in the Appalachian League, Denny made a spectacular professional debut by pitching a no-hitter in his first start. After just two games he was promoted to Clinton, Iowa, in the Midwest League. At both minor league stops Denny assumed his pitching prowess empowered him to disregard team rules, an assumption he carried with him to the major leagues. At the time players with a year in the minors were susceptible to a draft if not promoted to the majors. The Sox chose not to promote Denny and lost him to the Detroit Tigers in 1963. The Tigers sent him to Duluth-Superior in the Northern League and then to

Knoxville in the Sally before calling him up in September. Although he got off to a good start with the Tigers, he was sent down to Syracuse in the International League at the beginning of the 1964 season, but he was soon back up in the big leagues. He went 16–6 in 1965 and had his first 20-win season in 1966, when he was selected to start the All-Star Game. In 1968 he was the best pitcher in baseball, as he became the American League's first 30-game winner since Lefty Grove in 1931. No major leaguer has reached that number since. Denny's 1968 record was 31–6 with a league-leading .838 winning percentage and a 1.96 ERA. He won the first of two consecutive Cy Young awards and was named the AL Most Valuable Player. His pitching was largely responsible for the Tigers winning their first pennant since 1945. He was the Faber System AL Pitcher of the Year in both 1968 and 1969, when he again led the league in wins.[37]

With his baseball salary, money from commercial endorsements, and performing as a headliner in Las Vegas, McLain was probably making more money than anyone else in the game in the late 1960s. He was perhaps the best and most famous pitcher in baseball in 1968 and 1969. Suddenly his world came crashing down. In 1970 he was suspended for half the season for his participation in a bookmaking operation. Financial problems forced him to file for bankruptcy, despite his six-figure income. Later in the season he was suspended again for dousing two sportswriters with ice water and again for carrying a gun on a team flight. In the entire year he won only three games. Never popular with his teammates for his erratic behavior and ill-chosen words, he was traded to the Washington Senators after the end of the season. In 1971 he led the league with 22 losses. He never had another winning season after his last award-winning season of 1969. He concluded his professional career in Des Moines in 1973, washed up before the age of 30.

Off the field his misadventures continued. Several legitimate business ventures failed. He turned to loan sharking, bookmaking, and smuggling. In 1984 he was convicted of racketeering, extortion, and cocaine trafficking. Sentenced to 23 years in prison, he was freed when the verdict was overturned on procedural grounds. He apparently went straight for a few years, but in 1995 he was convicted on charges of embezzlement, money laundering, mail fraud, and conspiracy. He spent seven more years in prison.

A biography of Denny McLain appears in SABR's *Baseball Biography Project*. Ranking: Faber System eleventh; *Total Baseball* tied for 52nd.

Sadie McMahon

Born: John Joseph McMahon, September 19, 1867, Wilmington, DE
Debut: July 5, 1889; age 21

Last Game: July 12, 1897; age 29
Record: 173 127 .577 3.51 38,776 546
Clubs: Philadelphia AA; Baltimore AA; Brooklyn NL; Baltimore NL

See the entry on Sadie McMahon in Part Two of this book. He is profiled in *Nineteenth Century Stars*. Ranking: Faber System third; *Total Baseball* seventh.

Erskine Mayer

Born: James Erskine Mayer, January 16, 1890, Atlanta, GA
Debut: September 4, 1912; age 22
Last Game: September 27, 1919; age 29
Record: 91 70 .565 2.96 7065 261
Clubs: Philadelphia NL; Pittsburgh NL; Chicago AL

While studying engineering at Georgia Tech, Mayer became a star pitcher for the Yellow Jackets baseball team. In his senior year (1910), he left school to start his professional career with Fayetteville of the East Carolina League. He went 15-2, led the league in winning percentage, and helped the Highlanders win the circuit's championship. In 1911 he pitched for Albany in the Sally League and threw a no-hitter. The next year, while pitching for Portsmouth, his 26-9 record led the Virginia League in both wins and percentage and earned him a promotion to the big leagues. In 1914 he had the first of two 21-win seasons for the Phillies and posted an excellent 2.58 ERA. His best outing was a one-hit, 2-0 shutout of the Cardinals. Between them, he and Grover Cleveland Alexander accounted for 48 of the club's 74 wins. Both Mayer and Alexander had great seasons in 1915, as they pitched the Phillies to their first National League pennant. Mayer's record was 21-15, with an ERA of 2.36. He started two games in the World Series against the Boston Red Sox that fall, going the route in a 2-1 loss in the second game of the Series. President Woodrow Wilson threw out the first pitch in this game, the first one ever attended by a president of the United States. Mayer started the fifth game but was taken out with the score tied 2-2 in the third inning.

Erskine never had another 20-win season, although he continued to pitch well. After he was traded to Pittsburgh in 1918, he and Art Nehf of the Boston Braves engaged in one of the great pitching duels in major league history. Both moundsmen hurled scoreless ball for 15 innings. In the 16th inning Wilbur Cooper relieved Mayer and got the win when the Pirates scored two runs in the 21st inning. In 1919 the Chicago White Sox claimed Erskine on waivers. He pitched only one inning in the subsequent World Series, allowing one unearned run. He was completely unaware that some of his teammates were conspiring with gamblers to throw the Series.

In 1920 Mayer returned to the minor leagues but pitched only one game for the Atlanta Crackers before retiring. Later he umpired briefly in the South Georgia League. While operating a cigar store in downtown Los Angeles, he died of a heart attack on March 10, 1957, at the age of 67. He is profiled in *Deadball Stars of the National League* and in SABR's *Baseball Biography Project*. Ranking: Faber System 39th; *Total Baseball* 47th.

Al Mays

Born: Albert C. Mays, May 17, 1865, Canal Dover, OH
Debut: May 10, 1885; age 19
Last Game: May 2, 1890; age 24
Record: 53   90   .371   3.91   -7983   97
Clubs: Louisville AA; New York AA; Brooklyn AA; Columbus AA

Al Mays was born in Dover, on the Tuscarawas River in eastern Ohio, in May 1865. The town of his birth was on the Ohio-Erie Canal and sometimes was called Canal Dover to distinguish it from other Dovers in Ohio. May was an important month in Al's life. He was born in May, made his big league debut in May, pitched his final game in May, and lost his life in that month. In five and a fraction seasons in the majors, he pitched for four different clubs and had little success with any of them. During his two years with the New York Metropolitans he lost a total of 62 games, leading the American Association with 34 losses in 1887. His only winning season was in 1889 when he had a 10–7 record with Columbus. The next spring he made only one start. Although he pitched a complete game, he gave up fourteen hits, eight bases on balls, and thirteen runs, eight of them earned. That ended his major league career.

One day in May 1905 Mays and his friend Frank Huff were in a small boat on the Ohio River near historic Blannerhassett Island when a strong storm hit the area and overturned the boat. Mays was thrown from the boat into the river. Although the water was only three feet deep at this point, he was unable to get to his feet because of the strong current. Clinging to the boat for dear life, Huff watched his friend drown, unable to come to his rescue. The death of Al Mays at the age of 39 was ruled an accidental drowning. Ranking: Faber System tied for 86th; *Total Baseball* tied for 70th.

Win Mercer

Born: George Barclay Mercer, June 20, 1874, Chester, WV
Debut: April 21, 1894; age 19

Last Game: September 27, 1902; age 28
Record: 131   164   .444   3.99   20,650   429
Clubs: Washington NL; New York NL; Washington AL; Detroit AL

See the entry on Win Mercer in Part Two of this book. Mercer's life and death are reported in *Baseball's First Stars* and the SABR Baseball Biography Project. Ranking: Faber System sixth; *Total Baseball* fifteenth.

Willie Mitchell

Born: William Mitchell, December 1, 1889, Pleasant Grove, MS
Debut: September 22, 1909; age 19
Last Game: May 31, 1919; age 29
Record: 84   92   .477   2.88   8269   309
Clubs: Cleveland AL; Detroit AL

Willie played baseball at Mississippi State University from 1905 to 1909. In 1909 he became the first of 41 former MSU players to play in the big leagues. Before making it to the majors, he pitched part of a season with San Antonio in the Texas League, where he threw a no-hitter. From 1910 to 1916 he was a leading pitcher for Cleveland, which was never in serious contention for a pennant during those years. He was the Opening Day pitcher in 1912, 1914, 1915, and 1916. His best season was 1913, when he was 14–8 (.636) with a 1.91 ERA, the fifth best in the AL. That season he ranked second in strikeouts per nine innings and also in the top ten in win-loss percentage, WHIP, and shutouts. Mitchell missed part of the 1918 season due to military service in World War I. He closed out his major league career with the Detroit Tigers in 1919, then pitched in the minors for six years. In his best minor league season he won 25 games for Vernon of the Pacific Coast League in 1920. His final season in professional baseball came at the age of 34 with Topeka of the Western Association in 1924. He returned to the Magnolia State and died at Sardis on November 23, 1973, at 83 years of age. Willie Mitchell is a member of the Mississippi State University Hall of Fame.

Ranking: Faber System 22nd; *Total Baseball* tied for 52nd.

Bob Moose

Born: Robert Ralph Moose, Jr., October 9, 1947, Export, PA
Debut: September 19, 1967; age 19
Last Game: September 25, 1976; age 28
Record: 76   71   .517   3.50   891   244
Club: Pittsburgh NL

When he was only seven years old Bob Moose began playing baseball for the White Valley Pirates in the Franklin Township Little League. After six years of Little League ball, he continued through Pony League, American Legion, and high school baseball, becoming one of the most respected pitchers in the area. He threw three no-hitters for Franklin Area High School and also played varsity basketball and football, once scoring four touchdowns in a game. Seventeen-year-old Bob Moose was selected by the Pittsburgh Pirates in the 18th round of the 1965 amateur draft, the 342nd pick overall. The same week he graduated from high school, he started his professional career in the Appalachian League in Salem, Virginia. He made the rookie all-star team. In 1966 he played for Gastonia and Raleigh. In 1967 he was at Columbus in the IL and Macon in the Southern League. Bob's childhood dream came true when he made his first major league start for the Pirates that September. A native of the Pittsburgh area, he spent his entire major league career with the team he had idolized as a boy. In 1968 Moose was named the Pirate Rookie of the Year. His best season came in 1969 when he led the National League with a percentage of .824, based on 14 wins and three losses. He pitched a no-hitter against the New York Mets that September. In 1972 his pitching helped the Pirates win the NL East crown. Facing the Cincinnati Reds, champions of the West, the teams were tied at two games each in the best-of-five series. The Bucs had a 3–2 lead going into the last of the ninth. Johnny Bench led off the frame with a game-tying homer. Tony Perez and Denis Menke followed with singles. With the count two balls and no strikes on Cesar Geronimo, the Pittsburgh manager summoned Moose from the bullpen. What a difficult spot for the reliever! Sparky Anderson brought George Foster in to pinch-run for Perez. Moose induced Geronimo to fly to deep right, with Foster advancing to third base. Then Darrel Chaney popped out. Moose was almost out of the inning — there were two outs as the righty faced Hal McRae. Moose unleashed a hard slider in the dirt in front of the plate. It bounced off catcher Manny Sanguillen's arm, and Foster sprinted home with the winning run. Moose had lost the game on a wild pitch, and the Reds — not the Pirates — went to the 1972 World Series. From that point on, injuries hampered the career of the hard-throwing right-hander. In 1973 he had a knee operation to remove some cartilage. The next year a blood clot sidelined him for most of the season. When he recovered from two operations necessitated by the clot, he was moved from the starting rotation to the bullpen, where he expected to become the closer.

However, tragedy struck. Several of his teammates were hosting a birthday party for Moose at a golf course and restaurant owned by Bill Mazeroski. Driving on State Route 7, a narrow, twisting road near Martins Ferry, Ohio,

Moose lost control of his car on the rain-slickened road. Considering the conditions, he was probably driving too fast. After swerving onto the bank of the road, he veered back to the left of the center line and crashed head-on into another car. The other driver and Moose's passengers escaped with minor injuries. Moose, however, was pronounced dead at the scene. His life ended on his 29th birthday.

Ranking: Faber System 45th; *Total Baseball* 60th.

Ed "Cannonball" Morris

Born: Edward Morris, September 28, 1862, Brooklyn, NY
Debut: May 1, 1884; age 21
Last Game: October 1, 1890; age 28
Record: 171   122   .584   29,902   423
Clubs: Columbus AA; Pittsburgh AA; Pittsburgh NL; Pittsburgh PL

He was called "Cannonball" because of the speed with which he threw his fastball, but he also had a good curve and an effective change-up. Although he was born in Brooklyn, Ed moved with his family to California and grew up on the sandlots of San Francisco. He was a member of the St. Mary's College team in 1881 and 1882, one of 62 alumni from that small institution to play in the major leagues. Morris joined the Actives of Reading, Pennsylvania, in the Inter-State Association in June 1883 and moved up to the major leagues with Columbus in the American Association in 1884. On May 24 of that year, Ed pitched a no-hitter against the Pittsburgh Alleghenies, one base on balls preventing a perfect game.

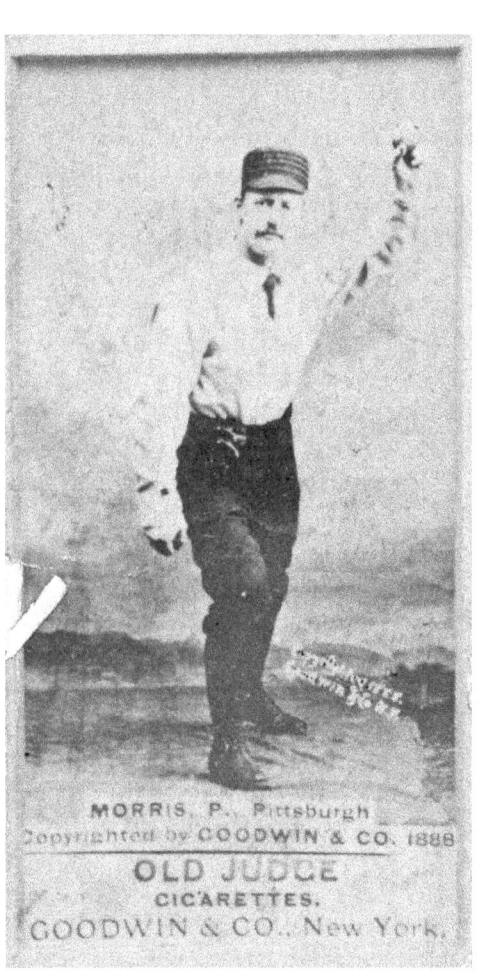

Ed "Cannonball" Morris won 30 or more games for three consecutive years, with a high of 41 victories in 1886. In 1887 a rule change outlawed his hop-skip-jump style of pitching and he lost effectiveness. He was out of the majors at the age of 28 (Library of Congress).

At the end of the season he was purchased by the Alleghenies and spent the rest of his major league career with Pittsburgh. For three consecutive years, 1884 through 1886, he won at least 30 games, with a high of 41 victories in 1886.

In 1887 a rule change restricted a pitcher to just one forward step in his delivery. As Morris had used a hop-skip-jump style of pitching, the adjustment caused him to develop a sore arm. He won only 14 games that season, as he was in trouble with his manager for his drinking and was often fined for carousing. During the winter he joined the YMCA, cut down on his drinking, and worked on the new delivery. He bounced back with 29 wins in 1888. In 1889 he started out with a sore arm and later pulled a muscle. He resumed some of his former habits and was released for excessive drinking but was later reinstated. In 1890 he pitched a few games for the Pittsburgh entry in the Players League before ending his major league pitching career at the age of 28. In 1892 he tried to make a comeback with Memphis of the Southern League but soon gave it up. Returning to Pittsburgh he opened a saloon and later served as deputy warden at the Western Pennsylvania Penitentiary and worked as a county employee. He died in Pittsburgh on April 12, 1937, at the age of 74.

Cannonball Morris is profiled in *Nineteenth Century Stars*. Ranking: Faber System seventh; *Total Baseball* sixteenth.

Elmer Myers

Born: Elmer Glenn Myers, March 2, 1894, York Springs, PA
Debut: October 6, 1915; age 21
Last Game: April 19, 1922; age 28
Record: 55   72   .433   4.06   5273   214
Clubs: Philadelphia AL; Cleveland AL; Boston AL

While pitching for the York Springs Social Club, Myers acquired the nickname "Big Jim." Scouted by Connie Mack, manager of the Philadelphia Athletics, Elmer was signed to a professional contract in the fall of 1913. The next spring Mack sent Myers to the Raleigh club managed by his son Earl in the North Carolina State League. In 1915 Elmer won the league's Triple Crown for pitchers, leading the circuit in wins, percentage, and strikeouts with a 29–10 (.744) record and 268 punchouts. Earl Mack notified his father that Big Jim was ready for the big time. In his major league debut the lanky right-hander pitched a complete game two-hitter and struck out a dozen batters. In 1916, pitching for the last-place A's, Myers lost 23 games. He had a losing record in 1917 as the Mackmen were again cellar dwellers.

During the 1918 season Elmer was drafted into the army. A stretcher-bearer attached to a unit near Verdun, Myers was a victim of a mustard gas attack by the Germans two months after he was sent to the frontlines. After spending weeks in hospitals recuperating from effects of the gas, he was discharged and sent home. Mack traded him to Cleveland. Although he had lost 40 pounds and the hop off his fastball during his illness, he had a decent season with the Indians, posting an 8–7 record. In 1920 Cleveland traded him to the Boston Red Sox. He got off to a sensational start in Fenway, winning nine straight games. However, the effects of the gassing continued to bother him. In 1922 Elmer asked the Sox to send him out west in the hopes that a high altitude and dry climate might help him. During the next six years he pitched for various minor league clubs in Salt Lake City, Los Angeles, and Knoxville before pitching his last game for Columbus in the American Association in 1928.

After retiring from baseball Big Jim moved to New Jersey, where he drove a truck and sold meat products for a packing house, ran a concession stand on the Boardwalk in Atlantic City, and finally operated a tavern on Black Horse Pike in Collingswood, where he died on July 29, 1976, at the age of 82. Ranking: Faber System 57th; *Total Baseball* 86th.

Jim Nash

Born: James Edwin Nash, February 9, 1945, Hawthorne, NV
Debut: July 3, 1966; age 21
Last Game: September 30, 1972; age 27
Record: 68   64   .515   3.58   4175   205
Clubs: Kansas City AL; Oakland AL; Atlanta NL; Philadelphia NL

Although he was born in Nevada, Nash considers Georgia his home state. Called "Jumbo Jim" because of his size (6'5", 230 pounds), Nash was signed in 1963 by the Kansas City Athletics as a free agent out of the University of Georgia. In 1964 he was assigned to the Burlington (Iowa) Bees of the Midwest League and was a starting pitcher in the loop's all-star game. Near the end of the season he was promoted to Birmingham in the Southern League. In 1965 he pitched for the Lewiston Broncs in the Northwest League and led the circuit in strikeouts. The next year he was back in the Southern League again, this time with the Mobile Athletics, but he was called up to the parent club in midseason.

He got off to a great start in Kansas City, winning his first seven decisions and winding up with a 12–1 (.923) record and a 2.06 ERA. He was named the AL Rookie Pitcher of the Year by *The Sporting News*. He continued to pitch well for the A's but never again had such gaudy numbers. He was traded to Atlanta after the 1969 season and then to Philadelphia in midseason 1972. He lost all eight games he pitched for the Phillies and was released during spring training the next year. He tried pitching for Birmingham but gave it up because of a torn rotator cuff. Jim moved to Marietta, Georgia, and took a position with Bell South, where for many years he ordered, activated, and maintained Integrated Services Digital Networks (ISDN). He coached youth teams and started the baseball program at Kennesaw State College.

Ranking: Faber System tied for 61st; *Total Baseball* 62nd.

Gary Nolan

Born: Gary Lynn Nolan, May 27, 1948, Herlong, CA
Debut: April 15, 1967; age 18
Last Game: September 18, 1977; age 29
Record: 110 70 .611 3.08 4687 335
Clubs: Cincinnati NL; California AL

The Cincinnati Reds selected Gary out of Oroville (California) High School in the first round of the 1966 amateur draft, the 13th pick overall. They assigned him to Sioux Falls of the Northern League, where he went 7–3 with a 1.82 ERA. That was the extent of his minor league experience except for brief rehabilitation stints with Tampa in 1968 and Indianapolis in 1969 and 1974. Called up to the Reds in 1967, Nolan got off to a great start, striking out the side against the Houston Astros in the first inning of his major league debut. He had a 14–8 record in his rookie season, good enough to finish second to Tom Seaver in the voting for the NL Rookie of the Year. His 206 strikeouts set an NL record for teenaged rookies, since broken by Dwight Gooden. Almost immediately he was hampered by arm problems, which reduced his playing time in 1968 and 1969. Healthy in 1970, he won 18 games against seven losses and helped the Reds win the NL pennant. In the first game of the playoffs he pitched nine innings of shutout baseball to defeat the Pittsburgh Pirates, but he lost the first game of the ensuing World Series to the Baltimore Orioles. In 1972 he had a 15–5 (.750) record with a 1.99 ERA, despite having neck and shoulder problems that caused him to miss at least ten starts. He led the league in won-lost percentage and was second to Steve Carlton in ERA, as he helped the Reds win another pennant. In the NLCS he was leading the Pirates, 2–1, after six innings when his arm tightened, forcing him to leave the game. In the World Series he lost to Oakland in his only decision.

Arm problems sidelined Gary during the 1973 and 1974 seasons. In 1975 he came back strong, winning the Hutch Award, which is given to the major league player who best exemplifies fighting spirit and competitive desire to win. In 1975 and 1976 Nolan had identical 15–9 records as the Big Red Machine won two consecutive World Series, the first NL team to accomplish that feat in more than a half-century. Gary finally got a World Series victory, defeating the Yankees, 7–2, in the fourth game as the Reds swept the Bronx Bombers. Arm troubles struck again in 1977, ending Gary's stay with the Reds. Traded to California, he failed to win a game for the Angels and was released. In 1978 the Milwaukee Brewers invited him to spring training, signed him as a free agent, but released him before the start of the season. Gary had pitched in one game and knew his shoulder problems were not over. He considered having another operation. "It's not a tough operation," he said. "They just have to scrape the calcium deposits off." The problem is not the operation, but the rehabilitation. "For 30 days, you don't know if you can raise your arm up, let alone throw the ball. I don't know if I want to go through the same ordeal again."[38] Out of baseball at the age of 29, Gary Nolan accepted a job at the MGM Grand Hotel in Las Vegas. He was elected to the Cincinnati Reds Hall of Fame in 1984. Ranking: Faber System nineteenth; *Total Baseball* eighteenth.

Hank O'Day

Born: Henry Francis O'Day, July 8, 1862, Chicago, IL
Debut: May 2, 1884; age 21
Last Game: October 3, 1890; age 28
Record: 73   110   .399   3.74
-8741   97
Clubs: Toledo AA; Pittsburgh AA; Washington NL; New York NL; New York PL

Hank O'Day was the only man in the history of baseball to be a National League player, manager, and umpire. As a pitcher he did not enjoy a great deal of success, winning as many as 20 games in a season only once. After a sore arm ended his pitching career, he umpired in the National League from 1895 to 1927 and was acclaimed as one of the best arbiters in the game (Library of Congress).

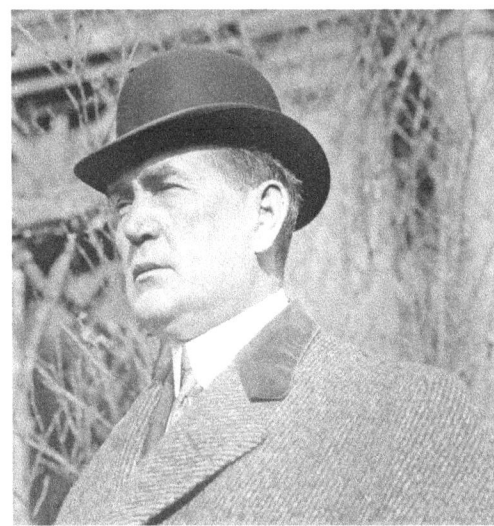

Hank O'Day was the only man in the history of baseball to be a National League player, manager, and umpire. He was probably a better umpire than he was a pitcher or a manager. The lad grew up in the stockyards district of Chicago and played ball on the prairie at Western Avenue and Madison Street. St. Mary's College, in faraway California, lists him as one of four alumni, along with Ed "Cannonball" Morris, Charlie Geggus, and Jim McElroy, who attended the school from 1881 to 1883 and later pitched in the major leagues. None of his biographies mention this. His professional career began with Bay City and Toledo in the Northwestern League in 1883. For the next ten years he was back and forth between the majors and the minors. Three times he lost 20 or more games in a season, with his 29 losses in 1888 leading the league. His best season came in his last year, 1890, when he won 20 games in the Players League. However, he developed arm trouble and ended his pitching career in the minor leagues in 1893.

O'Day umpired in the National League from 1895 to 1927 and was universally acclaimed as one of the best umpires in the game. He was the umpire who called Fred Merkle out for failing to touch second base in the 1908 game that cost the Giants the pennant. This remains one of the most controversial calls in baseball history, but according to the rules the play was a force-out at second base. In 1920 Hank was the second base umpire when Bill Wambsganss made the first unassisted triple play in World Series history. O'Day took two years off from umpiring to manage the Cincinnati Reds in 1912 and the Chicago Cubs in 1914. Under his leadership both clubs finished in fourth place. O'Day retired from umpiring following the 1927 season and became the National League's scout for new umpires. He died of bronchial pneumonia in a Chicago hospital on July 2, 1935, at the age of 72.

Biographies of Hank O'Day are presented in *Baseball's First Stars, Deadball Stars of the National League*, and SABR's *Baseball Biography Project*. In 2009 he was on the ballot for selection to the National Baseball Hall of Fame as an umpire, but fell four votes short of election. Ranking: Faber System 86th; *Total Baseball* tied for 70th.

Phil Ortega

Born: Filomeno Coronada Ortega, October 7, 1939, Gilbert, AZ
Debut: September 10, 1960; age 20
Last Game: May 4, 1969; age 29
Record: 46 62 .426 4.43 -553 153
Clubs: Los Angeles NL; Washington AL; California AL

As a 17-year-old schoolboy, Phil pitched the Casa Grande Cotton Kings to the 1958 Arizona state semi-pro championship and to a seventh-place finish in the national tournament in Wichita. He was named to the All-America Semi-Pro team by the National Baseball Congress. The next year he was signed out of Mesa High School by the Los Angeles Dodgers. He was assigned to the Spokane club in the Pacific Coast League. In 1960 Ortega pitched for Spokane and for Green Bay of the Three-I League before being called up to the majors. For the next three years he shuffled back and forth between Spokane and Los Angeles without collecting a major league victory. His first big league win came in 1964 when he shut out Milwaukee on a four-hitter. As the game was against the Braves, sportswriters had a field day linking the victory to Ortega's Indian ancestry. In the offseason the Dodgers traded Phil to Washington. The highlight of his stay with the Senators came on May 29, 1966, when he struck out seven consecutive Red Sox batters. The California Angels purchased him in April 1969, but he appeared in only five games for them. In May Ortega was involved in an early-morning fight outside an Anaheim restaurant and was hospitalized with a broken jaw and cuts and bruises. He was placed on the 60-day disabled list. In July, shortly before he was scheduled to come off the DL, he was fined $500 by the Angels manager for appearing in a hotel lobby clad only in his underwear. The Angels sent him down to the Hawaii Islanders of the Pacific Coast League. Phil never pitched in the majors again. In 1970 he hurled for Hawaii. The next season he was with Monterrey in the Mexican League.

Ranking: Faber System tied for 76th; *Total Baseball* 87th.

Jim O'Toole

Born: James Jerome O'Toole, January 10, 1937, Chicago, IL
Debut: September 26, 1958; age 21
Last Game: July 22, 1967; age 30
Record: 98   84   .538   3.57   7150   266
Clubs: Cincinnati NL; Chicago AL

Jim was signed as an amateur free agent out of the University of Wisconsin-Milwaukee by the Cincinnati Reds in 1957. He was assigned to Nashville, where he led the Southern Association in wins and strikeouts. At the end of the season he was promoted to the big club. The lefty soon became the ace of the staff. In 1961 he had a 19-9 (.679) record with an ERA of 3.10. The ERA was second-best in the NL; he ranked third in wins, percentage, and shutouts, and fourth in strikeouts. He helped the Reds win the NL pennant, but lost both of his decisions in the World Series because Cincinnati was shut out by Yankee pitchers in the two games O'Toole started. After winning 16 games in 1962 and 17 in 1963, Jim had another outstanding year in

1964, posting a 17–7 (.708) mark with an ERA of 2.66. His record slipped after that, and he was traded to the Chicago White Sox in 1967. In July while racing his brother, who was given a trial with the Sox, he crashed into an outfield wall at Comiskey Park, tearing ligaments in his left shoulder. That fall the Sox sent him to Indianapolis of the Pacific Coast League. Jim tried out with the Pale Hose again the next spring but was released before the season began. He was picked up by the Columbus Jets and spent about three months in the International League before being released on June 27, 1968. In 1969 he tried out with the Seattle Pilots but did not make the team. Jim Bouton reported that O'Toole was pitching for the Ross Eversoles in the Kentucky Industrial League in 1970.[39] He was inducted into the Cincinnati Reds Hall of Fame that same year. During the 2008 and 2009 seasons Jim O'Toole provided color commentary on telecasts of the home games of the Dayton Dragons of the Midwest League.

Ranking: Faber System 37th; *Total Baseball* 39th.

Pol Perritt

Born: William Dayton Perritt, August 30, 1891, Arcadia, LA
Debut: September 7, 1912; age 21
Last Game: July 3, 1921; age 29
Record: 92   78   .541   2.89   2495   257
Clubs: St. Louis NL; New York NL; Detroit AL

Because his surname sounded like parrot, he was nicknamed "Pol." As a young man he pitched for the Los Angeles Angels in the Pacific Coast League. He divided the seasons of 1912 and 1913 between the Angels and the St. Louis Cardinals. After winning 16 games for the Cards in 1914, he was traded to the New York Giants. In 1915 Pol decided to jump to the Federal League, but McGraw, with the help of a pay raise, persuaded the pitcher to stay with the Giants. Twice he won 18 games for the McGrawmen. His best season was 1917, when he had a record of 17–7 (.708) and an ERA of 1.88, finishing third in the NL in both percentage and ERA. He appeared as a reliever in three games of the World Series that fall against the Chicago White Sox. In 1918, on his 27th birthday, he was the winning pitcher in the second-fastest game ever played in the NL, as he shut out Brooklyn, 1–0, in a 57-minute contest. In the spring of 1919 Perritt announced that oil had been discovered on land he owned in Houma, Louisiana, and he was retiring from baseball to devote himself to the oil business. He leased some 3,000 acres near Shreveport and became a director in several big companies that were sinking wells in the area. One of his partners was Harry Sinclair, who was later implicated in the Teapot

Dome scandal. The lure of the diamond was too much for Pol to resist and he returned to baseball on a part-time basis, never being involved in more than three big league decisions in any year from 1919 through 1921. He also pitched a few games for Minneapolis of the American Association in 1921, going 3–1 for the Millers. Perritt returned to his Louisiana oil businesses and died in Shreveport on October 15, 1947, at the age of 56.

Ranking: Faber System 40th; *Total Baseball* 78th.

Wiley Piatt

Born: Wiley Harold Piatt, July 13, 1874, Blue Creek, OH
Debut: April 22, 1898; age 23
Last Game: August 1, 1903; age 29
Record: 86 79 .521 3.61 -3685 211
Clubs: Philadelphia NL; Philadelphia AL; Chicago AL; Boston NL

Growing up in Adams and Scioto counties in southern Ohio, Wiley played baseball with area amateur and semi-pro clubs. A Portsmouth sportswriter wrote that the youngster had large words printed on both sides of his grip: "Wiley Piatt, Star Pitcher of Otway Team, Scioto."[40] In 1897 the name Piatt became celebrated outside Scioto County. Pitching for the Dayton Old Soldiers in the Inter-State League, he threw three straight shutouts and established a league record with 11 strikeouts in a game. This attracted the attention of the Philadelphia Phillies, who drafted him. He had an outstanding rookie season, with a 24–14 (.652) record, an ERA of 3.18, and a league-leading six shutouts. Newspapers described him as a sensational southpaw. He followed this with 23 wins in his sophomore season. Those were to be his only two winning seasons in the big leagues. He slumped to nine wins in 1900. When the Phillies did not pay him what he thought he was worth, he announced he was quitting baseball to enter law school at Ohio State University. However, another major league club came to Philadelphia in 1901—the Athletics in the American League. Connie Mack, manager of the new club, said the lefty had as much speed as Amos Rusie and offered a contract that was acceptable to the Ohioan. Mack soon lost confidence in his new acquisition and released the pitcher in July. In August he signed as a free agent with the Chicago White Sox and stayed with the Sox through the rest of 1901 and 1902. Before the 1903 season began, Wiley jumped back to the National League to join the Boston Beaneaters. On June 25, 1903, Wiley became the only twentieth century pitcher to pitch and lose two complete games in one day. He did not pitch badly that day, losing 1–0 and 5–3. After one year in Boston, Piatt was out of the majors. A Portsmouth scribe wrote that the bright lights had dimmed Wiley's career.[41]

Although his major league career was over, Piatt was not through with baseball. He played four more years with four minor league clubs — Nashville, Toledo, Paducah, and Charlotte — before his professional career ended. Then it was back to Ohio and more semi-pro baseball for Wiley Piatt. He died in Cincinnati on September 20, 1946, at the age of 72. Ranking: Faber System 58th; *Total Baseball* 55th.

Toad Ramsey

Born: Thomas A. Ramsey, August 8, 1864, Indianapolis, IN
Debut: September 5, 1885; age 21
Last Game: September 17, 1890; age 26
Record: 114 124 .479 3.29 5436 204
Clubs: Louisville AA; St. Louis AA

While working as a bricklayer before his professional baseball career began, Ramsey severed the tendon on the index finger of his left (pitching) hand with a trowel. Throwing with a fastball motion, he held the ball with his index finger retracted, as he could not straighten it, and with just his finger tip on the ball. Some baseball writers say Toad invented the knuckleball. Actually, his pitch moved like a modern knuckle-curve. While pitching for Chattanooga in the Southern League in 1885, he was purchased by the Louisville Colonels. In his first full major league season in 1886, he led the majors with 38 wins and struck out 499 batters, the second-highest total in major league history. On August 11 he became the first big league pitcher to pitch an extra-inning one-hitter when he went 12 innings against Baltimore while giving up one lone safety. He led the league in 1886 with 66 complete games in 67 starts. In 1887 he won 37 games and led the league with 355 strikeouts, despite the four-strike rule in effect that year. He struck out 17 batters in one game that season; he had accomplished the feat twice in 1886. During his career he had 15 or more strikeouts in a game seven times.

After those two outstanding seasons, Toad's career went downhill rapidly. He lost 30 games in 1888. After winning only one of his first 17 decisions in 1889, he was traded to St. Louis. He rebounded in 1890, winning 24 games against 17 losses for the Browns, but was released in September. It was reported that his habitual drunkenness ruined his career.[42] After he was released by the Browns, Toad tried pitching in the minor leagues. He was with the Denver and St. Joseph clubs of the Western Association and Savannah of the Southern League over the next five years without having much success with any of them.

Toad Ramsey died in Indianapolis on March 27, 1906, at the age of 41.

Although the cause of his death was listed as pneumonia, one of his former teammates said, "Drink laid him under the sod."[43]

Ramsey is profiled in *Nineteenth Century Stars*. Ranking: Faber System 63rd; *Total Baseball* 14th. This is one of the larger differences between the two rankings.

Billy Rhines

Born: William Pearl Rhines, March 14, 1869, Ridgway, PA
Debut: April 22, 1890; age 21
Last Game: June 22, 1899; age 30
Record: 114 103 .525 3.47 6906 248
Clubs: Cincinnati NL; Pittsburgh NL

While a student at Bucknell University, Billy Rhines became a professional baseball player, starting his career in 1888 at Binghamton and Jersey City. In 1889 he won 27 games for Davenport and Monmouth in the Central Inter-State League, earning him a promotion to the majors. Billy was a side-armed right-hander who developed a pitch called an upcurve because his delivery appeared to break up instead of down. In his rookie season he won 28 games for the Cincinnati Reds and led the NL with an ERA of 1.95. The *Baseball Encyclopedia* named him the NL Rookie of the Year for 1890.[44] In 1891 he lost 24 games. Things went terribly wrong for Rhines in 1892. In March, on a bet, he wrestled Walter Norman and suffered a broken collar bone. In May he was involved in another fight and was expelled from the team for drunkenness. Although he was reinstated in July, Billy won only five games in 1892 and 1893 combined. In 1894 he was back in the minors with the Grand Rapids Rustlers of the Western League, where he won 25 games. Back with Cincinnati he posted 19 wins in 1895. In 1896 he led the league in ERA despite having a broken third finger on his pitching hand. He is the only man ever to lead the NL in ERA at both the 50' pitching distance and the current 60'6" distance. In a game in which Rhines pitched against the New York Giants on July 12, 1897, the Reds carried the home field advantage to an extreme. As the opposition lineup featured six left-handed batters and the home team batted mainly from the starboard side, the Cincinnati groundskeepers dug the dirt out of the left-side batter's box and filled it with loose sand. Despite these shenanigans, the Reds lost to Amos Rusie. In 1897 Rhines won 21 games but was traded to Pittsburgh in the offseason. He did not have much success with the Pirates and was released on June 23, 1899. After his major league career ended, he pitched one season for Grand Rapids in the Western Association. He returned to Ridgway, worked as a lumberman, managed an independent team, and ran taxi and bus businesses.

Billy Rhines died of heart trouble in his hometown on January 30, 1922, at the age of 52. Rhines is profiled in *Baseball's First Stars*. Ranking: Faber System tied for 42nd; *Total Baseball* 28th.

J. R. Richard

Born: James Rodney Richard, March 7, 1950, Vienna, LA
Debut: September 5, 1971; age 21
Last Game: July 14, 1980; age 30
Record: 107   71   .601   18,174   327
Club: Houston NL

During his senior year at Lincoln High School in Rustin, Louisiana, J. R. was the school's dominant athlete. At 6'8" and 220 pounds, he was a star in both basketball and baseball. A right-handed pitcher, he allowed no runs during the entire baseball season and hit four consecutive home runs in one game. In the 1969 amateur draft the Houston Astros made him their first-round pick, second choice overall. He turned down 200 basketball scholarship offers to sign with the Astros. He started his professional career with Covington in the Appalachian League. In 1970 he was promoted to Cocoa in the Florida State League and threw a no-hitter against Daytona Beach. In 1971 he moved up to the Class AAA American Association with the Oklahoma City 89ers. In September the Astros called him up to the majors. In his first start he struck out 15 San Francisco Giants to tie the record for the most strikeouts in a major league debut. In his second start he pitched a two-hitter against the Cincinnati Reds. After that fine beginning his control problems held him back for years, as he was shifted back and forth between Houston and their minor league affiliates in Oklahoma City and Denver. It was not until 1976 that he had his first 20-win season. Although he never mastered his control (leading the league in bases on balls and wild pitches three times each), he won 18 games in each of his seasons after 1976. His great stuff compensated for his wildness. In 1978 he led the league with 303 strikeouts, the first NL right-hander to strike out more than 300 batters in a year since 1892. The next year he struck out 313. More than a strikeout artist, Richard led the league in ERA in 1979 and in fewest hits per nine innings three times.

In 1980 J. R. got off to a great start. During the first half of the season he won 10 games and lost only four while compiling a 1.90 ERA. He was selected to start the All-Star game. Despite this success, he complained of discomfort in his shoulder and forearm. On July 14 he had trouble seeing the catcher's signs, experienced numbness in his fingers, and felt his arm go dead. It was the last major league game he ever pitched. Placed on the disabled list, he checked into a Houston hospital for a series of physical and psychological tests. Although an angiogram revealed a completely obstructed artery in his right arm, doctors concluded that no surgery was needed. On July 30 he suffered a major stroke and collapsed on the field before a game. A massive blockage in his right carotid artery made immediate surgery necessary. Later examinations revealed he had suffered three separate previous strokes.

In 1981 J. R. underwent a rehabilitation program. The following year he went to spring training with the Astros and pitched a few minor league games for Daytona Beach and Tucson. In 1983 he had a surgical bypass in his left leg. The Astros finally released him on April 27, 1984.

After his baseball career ended Richard returned to Louisiana, invested in some business deals, and lost more than $300,000 in an oil business scam. A divorce cost him most of the rest of his money. In 1989 he tried out with the Orlando Juice of the Senior Professional Baseball Association but failed to make the team. By 1994 Richard was homeless and destitute, living under a bridge in Houston. After spending many nights under an overpass, he turned to the New Testament Church. The minister, Reverend Floyd Lewis, helped J. R. get back on his feet. The ex-ballplayer overcame a drug problem, started working for an asphalt company, and later became a minister at the church, working with homeless people and troubled youth. He became involved in the Houston community and started working with donors to establish baseball programs for children. In 2005 a low-budget movie called *Resurrection: The J. R. Richard Story* was released but received little acclaim.

His former teammate, Hall of Famer Joe Morgan, said, "He had the greatest stuff I have ever seen and it still gives me goosebumps to think of what he might have become."[45]

Ranking: Faber System 20th; *Total Baseball* 26th.

Lew Richie

Born: Elwood Lewis Richie, August 23, 1883, Ambler, PA
Debut: May 8, 1906; age 22
Last Game: August 8, 1913; age 29
Record: 74   65   .532   2.54   1605   237
Clubs: Philadelphia NL; Boston NL; Chicago NL

As a teenager Lew pitched for independent and semi-pro teams in the area around Williamsport, Pennsylvania. From 1903 through 1905 he played with independent teams in Wilmington (Delaware), Oxford (Pennsylvania) and Williamsport. In August 1905 he was the property of the Holyoke Paperweights in the Connecticut League. The Brooklyn Superbas purchased him but the sale was voided, and Lew became a free agent. He signed with Philadelphia in 1906 and made his major league debut with the Phillies. He enjoyed modest success with Philadelphia and later with Boston, but it was not until he was traded to Chicago in 1910 that he hit his stride. In his first three years with the Cubs the right-hander won 42 games against only 23 losses and turned in excellent ERAs each year. While Richie was with the Cubs Damon Runyon traveled with the team and engaged in many pranks with the talented pantomimist, whom he dubbed "Lurid Lew." Richie earned a more savory nickname, "Lew the Giant Killer," when he defeated the Bruins' greatest rival, the New York Giants, three times in one week. Although Richie never led the league in any pitching category, he established a good reputation by pitching shutouts in more than one-eighth of his starts. In 1913 his skills declined and he was traded to Kansas City of the American Association. He started the 1914 season with the Blues but finished the year in Sioux City, where he went 9–1 for the Western League Indians. When he registered for the draft in 1918, Lew was a plumber for the Pennsylvania Railroad, living in Erie. He died at South Mountain on August 15, 1936, a few days before his 53rd birthday.

Ranking: Faber System 47th; *Total Baseball* 36th.

Amos Rusie

Born: Amos Wilson Rusie, May 30, 1871, Mooresville, IN
Debut: May 9, 1889; age 17
Last Game: June 9, 1901; age 30
Record: 245 174 .585 3.07 32,408 631
Clubs: Indianapolis NL; New York NL; Cincinnati NL

See the entry on Amos Rusie in Part Two of this book.

He is profiled in *Baseball's First Stars* and in SABR's *Baseball Biography Project*. Rusie is a member of the National Baseball Hall of Fame in Cooperstown. Ranking: Faber System first; *Total Baseball* first; Bill James second.

Ben Sanders

Born: Alexander Bennett Sanders, February 16, 1865, Catharpin, VA
Debut: June 6, 1888; age 23
Last Game: October 14, 1892; age 27
Record: 80 70 .533 3.24 8400 218
Clubs: Philadelphia NL; Philadelphia PL; Philadelphia AA; Louisville NL

After playing some amateur ball in his native Prince William County, Ben pitched at Roanoke College, where he caught the attention of professional clubs. He spent two seasons in the minor leagues, one year with Nashville and one season divided between Altoona and Canton. In 1888 Harry Wright signed him for the Philadelphia club in the National League as a pitcher/outfielder. Throughout his career Ben played occasionally in the field and had a lifetime batting average of .271. As a pitcher he was noted for his excellent control. He had an unorthodox delivery, ending up with his back to the plate after hurling the ball, making it difficult for him to field bunts and other balls hit toward the pitcher's box. In each of his first three major league seasons he won 19 games. In his rookie year he led the league in fewest walks per game and tied for the lead in shutouts with eight. Since then no pitcher has had more shutouts in his rookie season. Ben carried a perfect game into the ninth inning against Chicago before giving up a scratch single. He finally pitched a no-hitter against Baltimore in 1892.

At the end of the 1890 season Ben announced his retirement from baseball to pursue an engineering degree at Vanderbilt University. The Phillies released him, but the Athletics signed him by offering an unusual deal: he need not report until the college semester was over; his contract would run only until the end of the season; and he would be paid a full season's salary. He reported to the A's in mid–June and pitched well until his arm went lame in late August, causing him to finish the season in the outfield. Sanders graduated from Vanderbilt in the spring of 1892, and signed with Louisville for the same conditions the A's had offered the previous year. At the end of the season he went to work for the firm that was building Chicago's elevated railway. In 1894 he started his own engineering firm in Louisville. Later he said he was willing to return to baseball if the Louisville club made him its manager, but his proposal was declined. Ben Sanders died in Memphis on August 29, 1930, at the age of 65.

Sanders is profiled in *Baseball's First Stars*. Ranking: Faber System 53rd; *Total Baseball* tenth. The high ranking in the encyclopedia was given because points for his hitting prowess were included in his rating.

Doc Scanlan

Born: William Dennis Scanlan, March 7, 1881, Syracuse, NY
Debut: September 24, 1903; age 22
Last Game: September 1, 1911; age 30
Record: 65   71   .478   3.00   16,918   272
Clubs: Pittsburgh NL; Brooklyn NL

Apparently Doc Scanlan had a great talent for multi-tasking. It seems he was often doing two entirely different things at the same time, occasionally in two different places. After pitching for the strong St. Cecilia's School in his native Syracuse, he went into college ball. Various records show he was on the team at Manhattanville College in 1899–1900, at Fordham in 1900–01, and at Syracuse University in 1902–03. During the two years he played for Syracuse, he also pitched professionally for the Ilion Typewriters in the New York State League. As the college and professional clubs played different schedules and college eligibility rules were not enforced stringently, these seemingly exclusive events could very well have occurred. He broke into the majors with Pittsburgh in 1901 and was traded to Brooklyn during the 1904 season. He won 14 games for the Superbas in 1905 and 18 games in 1906. In both seasons he compiled a winning record for a woefully weak Brooklyn club. While he was pitching for the Superbas, Scanlan acquired his nickname "Doc" by studying medicine. Demonstrating his mastery of multi-tasking, Scanlan earned his medical degree from the Long Island Medical College in 1907. He continued pitching professionally through the 1911 season. Even after he became a prominent Brooklyn physician, he played semi-pro ball each summer for one of the strongest teams in New York City. Later he started taking summer vacations in the Berkshires or Adirondacks and pitching for semi-pro teams in those resort areas. In order to surprise fans in his hometown, he secured permission to pitch one game for the Syracuse Stars of the International League in 1918. At the time the physician was 37 years old and had been out of professional baseball for nearly seven years but was in excellent physical condition. He shut out Jersey City on three hits for five innings and got credit for the victory.

Dr. William D. Scanlan died at his home in Brooklyn on May 29, 1949, at the age of 68. He was buried at one of his favorite vacations spots, Stockbridge, in the Berkshires of Massachusetts. In 2006 he was inducted into the Syracuse Baseball Wall of Fame.

Ranking: Faber System 35th; *Total Baseball* 58th.

Pete Schneider

Born: Peter Joseph Schneider, August 20, 1895, Los Angeles, CA
Debut: June 20, 1914; age 18
Last Game: August 2, 1919; age 23
Record: 59 86 .407 2.66 -9254 117
Clubs: Cincinnati NL; New York AL

At the age of 16 Pete started his professional career as a pitcher with the Seattle Giants of the Northwestern League. In his third season in the Northwest he got off to a 12–2 start, earning him a spot in the major leagues with the Cincinnati Reds. The young man spent five years in the Queen City, posting good ERAs but losing many more games than he won, except for the 1917 season when he won 20 games and lost 19 and turned in an ERA of 2.10. Following the 1918 season he was purchased by the New York Yankees but hurt his arm and never won a game for the Yanks. He was out of the majors at the age of 23, having recorded the lowest winning percentage of any pitcher of the decade. Schneider then joined the Vernon Tigers of the Pacific Coast League, where he became a hard-hitting outfielder. He spent part of 1920 with Beaumont in the Texas League, then returned to Vernon. In seven seasons in the PCL, he hit for an average of .333. On May 11, 1923, he had the greatest day at the plate ever achieved by a player at that level. In a game against the Salt Lake City Bees, he hit five home runs, including two grand slams, plus a double, scored six runs and had 14 RBIs. His last year in the Pacific Coast League was 1925, when he played for Vernon and Sacramento. In 1926 he joined the Salt Lake club, which had moved down to the Utah-Idaho League. Before finally retiring he also played for Oklahoma City, Wichita, Little Rock, and Springfield.

None of the baseball reference books or on-line sites mentions one of the most critical incidents of his life, although it was widely reported in newspapers across the country. In February 1935 he engaged in a fistfight with Gustav Schnabel in a Los Angeles beer parlor. The fight reportedly started when Schnabel said some disrespectful things to Schneider's wife. Schnabel was killed in the fight. Schneider was convicted of manslaughter and sentenced to seven years in prison. While in prison Pete managed the San Quentin baseball team. An Oakland columnist wrote that Schneider was a very good manager.[46] Pete Schneider died on June 1, 1957, in Los Angeles at the age of 61.

Ranking: Faber System 82rd; *Total Baseball* 44th.

Jim Scott

Born: James Scott; April 23, 1888; Deadwood, SD
Debut: April 25, 1909; age 21
Last Game: August 17, 1917: age 29
Record: 107   113   .486   2.30   -6451   245
Club: Chicago AL

Although he was born in South Dakota, Jim grew up in Lander, Wyoming. He planned to attend Nebraska Wesleyan University and become a physician. (Some sources report he played baseball at the school in 1908–09, but he almost certainly did not.) In 1907 the youngster made his professional debut with the Oskaloosa Quakers of the Iowa State League and moved up rapidly. In 1908 he won a league-leading 30 games for Wichita in the Western Association and set a league record with 16 strikeouts in a game. The right-handed hurler used a hard curveball and a tricky spitball. He made his major league debut with the Chicago White Sox two days after his 21st birthday. He was given the nickname "Death Valley Jim" because he arrived in the Windy City on the same train as another Scott, the notorious Death Valley Scotty. The moniker was perhaps pinned on him by Ring Lardner, who frequently referred to Scott in his baseball novel, *You Know Me Al*.[47] Perhaps a more fitting nickname would have been "Hard Luck Jim." In nine big league seasons he compiled an ERA of 2.30 and yet lost more games than he won. In 1913 Jim had an ERA of 1.90, the only pitcher in major league history to lose 20 games while having an ERA of less than 2.00. He also won 20 games that season for a rare 20-win 20-loss season. Another example of his luck came on May 14, 1914. Pitching against Doc Ayers, Jim held the Washington Senators hitless for nine innings. However, the Sox were unable to score and the game went into extra innings tied at zero. In the tenth inning Chick Gandil led off with a single and Howie Shanks followed with a base hit that took a bad hop and allowed the winning run to score. For 75 years Scott was credited with a no-hitter before the criteria for a no-hitter were changed.

After the United States entered World War I, Scott enlisted in the army and left the White Sox late in the 1917 season. He served in France during the summer of 1918. After the war he went to work in a foundry in Beloit, Wisconsin. He turned down an offer to try out for the White Sox again in 1919 but headed west to join the San Francisco Seals. In the spring of 1920 he showed up with a full beard, which caused quite a controversy. The league voted to ban facial hair among all Pacific Coast League players. Scott won 25 games and led the PCL in ERA. In 1923 he pitched another no-hitter, winning the game this time. From 1919 through 1924 he won 96

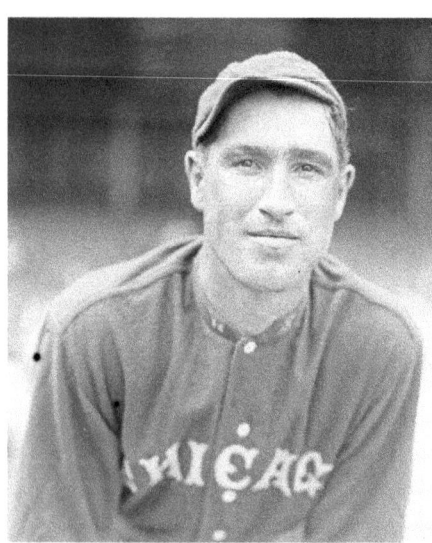

"Death Valley" Jim Scott was a hard-luck pitcher who lost more major league games than he won despite having a career earned run average of 2.30. In 1913 he became the only pitcher in major league history to lose 20 games while having an ERA of less than 2.00 (Library of Congress).

games for the Seals, then joined the New Orleans Pelicans in the Southern Association, where he won 31 games in three years. He retired as an active player at the age of 39 after the 1927 season. He umpired in the Southern Association in 1928, 1929, and 1932 and in the National League in the 1930 and 1931 seasons.

For several years he had worked part-time in the movie industry during offseasons. After leaving baseball he worked full-time for RKO and Republic, as chief electrician and head property man. After he retired in 1953 he began experiencing heart trouble and had a heart attack in 1956. Thinking the desert air would be beneficial, he traveled to Jacumba, California, where he suffered a fatal heart attack on April 7, 1957. He was not quite 69 years old.

Biographical sketches of Death Valley Jim are given in *Deadball Stars of the American League* and in SABR's *Baseball Biography Project*. Ranking: Faber System 44th; *Total Baseball* 17th.

Dupee Shaw

Born: Frederick Lander Shaw, May 31, 1859, Charlestown, MA
Debut: June 18, 1883; age 24
Last Game: July 17, 1888; age 29
Record: 83   121   .407   3.10   816   129
Clubs: Detroit NL; Boston UA; Providence NL; Washington NL

How Shaw acquired the nickname "Dupee" is not well known, but it was strictly a baseball cognomen. In all references to him outside the game, he is called Frederick. He broke into the major leagues with the Detroit Wolverines in 1883 and jumped to the Boston Reds of the rebel Union Association in mid-season 1884. Combining his record from the two clubs would give him 30 wins and 33 losses in 1884. On July 19 he struck out 18 St. Louis Maroons in one game and had a season total of 451 punchouts. After the UA folded, Shaw paid a $1000 fine and was reinstated in the National League. In 1885 he won 23 games and pitched a no-hitter for the Providence Grays, but his performance deteriorated after he was obtained by Washington the following year.

Shaw claimed he was the first pitcher to windup prior to delivering the ball. His behavior in the pitcher's box may not have started the calumny that left-handed pitchers are eccentric, but it gave credibility to that view. "Yes, I know I'm nutty," he said, "but I'm getting away with it."[48] One writer described Dupee's antics thusly:

> After considerable swinging and scratching around with his feet, during which he would deliver a lengthy speech to the batter, to the effect that he was the best

pitcher on earth and the batter a dud, he would stretch both arms at full length over his head. Then after gazing fixedly at the first baseman for a moment he would wheel half around and both arms would fly apart like magic. He would wind his left arm around again and let the ball fly, running at the same time all the way from the box to the home plate.[49]

After retiring from baseball, Shaw returned to the Boston area. In 1900 he was a bartender in Beantown and a grocer there in 1910. In 1920 he may have been a "municipal contractor" for the city of Providence, Rhode Island. In 1930 he was back in Massachusetts, living in the household of his cousin, Edward Lyons, who operated a billiard parlor in Everett. Shaw died in Wakefield, a Boston suburb, at the age of 78 on January 12, 1938.

Ranking: Faber System 83rd; *Total Baseball* 61st.

Harry Staley

Born: Henry Eli Staley, November 3, 1866, Jacksonville, IL
Debut: June 23, 1888; age 21
Last Game: July 30, 1895; age 28
Record: 136 119 .533 3.80 -387 306
Clubs: Pittsburgh NL; Pittsburg PL; Boston NL; St. Louis NL

A long-time resident of Springfield, Harry started his professional career with independent clubs in central Illinois. In 1885 and 1887 he pitched for Decatur. In 1886 his right-handed tosses were for his hometown Springfield team. Several clubs in the area were bidding for his services in 1888, but he signed with the St. Louis Whites of the Western Association. *The Sporting News* called him "one of the most promising pitchers of the west. He has remarkable speed and throws a very puzzling ball," the paper reported. "He is quick and active and altogether a model ball player, as he always enters into a game with a determination to win and never loses faith or gives up hope." In June he was sold to the Pittsburgh Alleghenys and his major league career was underway. In 1889 he had the first of four consecutive 20-win seasons in the majors. In 1890 he jumped to the Players League and led the circuit in WHIP and was second in ERA and shutouts. Back in the National League in 1891, he led the senior circuit in WHIP and had 24 victories as he divided the season between Pittsburgh and Boston. In 1892 he helped the Beaneaters win the pennant. A good hitter, Staley also played in the outfield. In 1893 he had nine RBIs in one game. After that year his skills declined and he had only two more years in the majors. However, he continued pitching in the minor leagues with such teams as Wheeling in the Iron and Oil League and Springfield of the Southern Illinois League. Staley's health deteriorated and he entered

a sanitarium in Battle Creek, Michigan, where he died after an operation on January 12, 1910, at the age of 43.
Ranking: Faber System 23rd; *Total Baseball* 37th.

Ed Stein

Born: Edward F. Stein, September 5, 1869, Detroit, MI
Debut: July 24, 1890; age 20
Last Game: June 27, 1898; age 28
Record: 109   78   .583 3.97   11338   290
Clubs: Chicago NL; Brooklyn NL

A right-handed pitcher, Stein got his professional start with the Saginaw–Bay City Hyphens of the International Association in 1890. Cap Anson signed him in July and he was in the big leagues with the Chicago Colts at the age of 20. Possessing a good fastball, he had a good first season, pitching two two-hit games. In 1891 he got off to another good start but his lack of control led to many bases on balls. In midseason Stein was sold to Omaha of the Western Association. In 1892 he was picked up by Brooklyn and had an excellent season with 27 wins, an ERA of 2.84 and six shutouts. In 1893 he won 19 games. In 1894 he posted a 26–14 record for a club that won only 70 games all year. On June 2 he pitched a rain-shortened six-inning no-hitter against Chicago, winning, 1–0, as he limited his free passes to five. However, he had not overcome his control problems. Ed lost a game to Boston, 7–1, despite allowing only two hits, as he walked nine and threw two wild pitches. He was seriously injured in a bicycle accident in October 1896 and missed the entire 1897 season. He tried to come back in 1898 but could not make the grade.

Stein returned to Detroit and went into business and politics. In the 1920 census he was listed as the proprietor of an iron business. Not long after that he was elected Wayne County sheriff. At that time, Prohibition was the law of the land. Many Detroit officials, including the county sheriff, did not enforce the dry laws. Detroiters openly frequented speakeasies and "blind pigs" (establishments that illegally sold alcoholic beverages). In a raid on one such place, the Deutsches Haus, the state police arrested the mayor, a congressman, and Sheriff Stein. Later Stein was implicated in a financial scandal. Apparently these events did not turn the populace against him. He was still sheriff when he died on May 10, 1928, at the age of 58. The voters elected Ed's wife, Margaret, to fill the remainder of his term.

Ed Stein is profiled in *Baseball's First Stars*. Ranking: Faber System 30th; *Total Baseball* 41st.

Scott Stratton

Born: Chilton Scott Stratton, October 2, 1869, Campbellsville, KY
Debut: April 21, 1888; age 18
Last Game: July 2, 1895; age 25
Record: 97   114   .460   3.87   5673   231
Clubs: Louisville AA; Pittsburgh NL; Louisville NL; Chicago NL

As a boy in Taylorsville, Kentucky, Scott earned the nickname "Taylorsville Wonder" for his exploits on the diamond. Batting left-handed, he played first base and the outfield, but it was as a right-handed pitcher that he gained his greatest fame. After he broke into the major leagues at the age of 18, hundreds of Taylorsville residents would take the train to Louisville to watch their hometown hero pitch. After two losing seasons, the youngster had a great year in 1890, pitching the Colonels to their only major league pennant. He led the league in ERA, win-loss percentage, WHIP, and ratio of strikeouts to bases on balls. He was second in wins with 34, second in shutouts, third in complete games, and sixth in strikeouts. Between June 28 and August 28 he won 16 straight games (a number since reduced to 15 by a change in the method of naming the winning pitcher). It was by far his best season in the majors; he had only one other winning season, with a 21–19 record in 1892. In 1893 he established a record that endured for 20 years by giving up 12 hits while pitching a shutout. Stratton was released by Chicago in mid-season 1895 at the age of 25. Although he never pitched another game in the major leagues, he immediately caught on as an outfielder with the St. Paul Saints of the Western League. He played six seasons in the minors for teams in St. Paul, Reading, Bristol, Wilkes-Barre, and Hartford before winding up his career at the age of 30 in 1900. He hit .324 in 537 minor league games. After he retired from baseball Stratton returned to his native Kentucky. In 1920 he was living on a farm in Nelson County. By 1930 he was back in Louisville, where he died from a heart attack March 8, 1939, at the age of 68.

Scott Stratton is profiled in *Baseball's First Stars*. Ranking: Faber System 49th; *Total Baseball* 29th.

Jack Taylor

Born: John Besson Taylor, May 23, 1873, Sandy Hill, MD
Debut: September 16, 1891; age 18
Last Game: September 12, 1899; age 26
Record: 120   117   .506   9494   355
Clubs: New York NL; Philadelphia NL; St. Louis NL; Cincinnati NL

In the closing years of the nineteenth century there were two right-handed pitchers named John Taylor in the National League. Both were called Jack. To distinguish them, sportswriters dubbed John B. Taylor "Brewery Jack" for his heavy drinking and John W. Taylor "The Brakeman" for allegedly throwing games. Long before he acquired the "Brewery" tag, young Jack moved with his widowed mother and his siblings to Staten Island. Growing up in the West New Brighton section of the island, Jack played amateur ball with four neighborhood boys (Jack Sharrott, George Sharrott, Tuck Turner, and Jack Cronin), all of whom eventually made it to the National League, although none of them became stars. Jack started his professional career at the age of 17 with the Lebanon Cedars of the Eastern Association in April 1891 and was traded to Troy in midseason. In September he made his major league debut for the New York Giants. He pitched a four-hitter and allowed only one earned run, but it was not enough as the Giants were shut out. He never pitched another game for New York. He spent the 1892 season with Albany in the Eastern League but made it back to the majors with Philadelphia that September. He pitched for the Phillies the next five years and was a 20-game winner three times. However, his drinking made him unreliable. During 1897 he was frequently cited for imbibing and was at odds with his manager. After the 1897 season he was traded to the St. Louis Browns. He led the NL with 42 complete games the next year. He also led the loop with 29 losses. After one season, the Browns traded him to Cincinnati. After a game in the Polo Grounds on Memorial Day, Taylor received permission to visit his mother on Staten Island. He did not return as scheduled and was missing for several days. It was discovered that he had gone on a fishing (and drinking) trip with some buddies. He was suspended for five weeks without pay, costing him $500, and fined $700 for violating a temperance clause in his contract. This amounted to a loss of nearly half of his season's pay of $2500.

Jack made his last start for the Reds in September 1899. In the fourth inning of the game he was stricken by a severe pain in his right side. He could not lift his pitching arm or maintain a grip on the ball. He was sent home for the remainder of the season. That winter he appeared to recover and was hoping to pitch again. However, in late January he became ill and died at an infirmary on Staten Island on February 7, 1900, at the age of 26. The official cause of death was acute nephritis, commonly referred to as Bright's disease.

An account of Jack Taylor's life by Peter Mancuso is included in SABR's *Baseball Biography Project*. Ranking: Faber System 16th; *Total Baseball* 27th.

Jeff Tesreau

Born: Charles Monroe Tesreau, March 5, 1888, near Ironton, MO
Debut: April 12, 1912; age 24
Last Game: June 11, 1918; age 30
Record: 115   72   .615   2.43   11,054   358
Club: New York NL

Born on a farm in southeastern Missouri, Tesreau left school after the eighth grade to work in a lead mine and pitch for the company team. His blazing fastball earned him a spot on the Perryville club of the independent Trolley League, where he won 37 of the 43 games he pitched in 1908. He signed with Austin of the Texas League but was released and spent the 1909 season trying out with various clubs. His fastball was impressive, but his inability to control it cost him a chance to advance. In 1910 he pitched for Shreveport in the Texas League and compiled a respectable 15–14 record with 179 strikeouts and only 71 walks, indicating he was gaining control of his pitches. The New York Giants purchased him and brought him to the big city in September, but he did not appear in any major league games that year. A sportswriter noticed Tesreau's resemblance to heavyweight boxer Jim Jeffries and nicknamed him "Jeff."[50] For the rest of his career he was known as Jeff Tesreau. At the suggestion of a New York pitching instructor, Jeff experimented with the spitball and used it successfully for Toronto of the Eastern League in 1911. He made his major league debut the next spring and had an outstanding rookie year. He won 17 games against

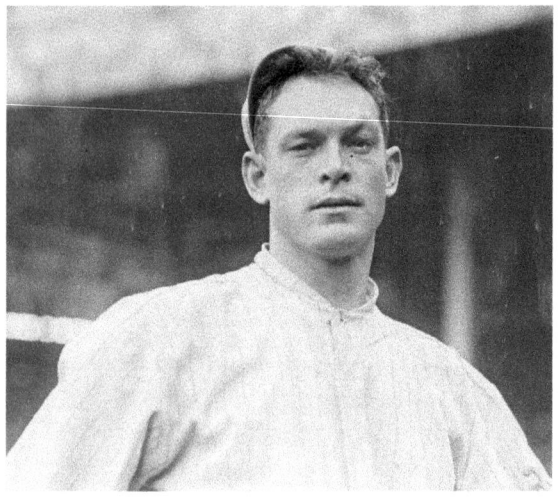

Jeff Tesreau was one of the best pitchers of the Deadball Era. As a rookie he led the league in earned run average and pitched a no-hitter. In each of his first three National League seasons, he led the loop in allowing the fewest hits per innings pitched. In 1914 he led the league in shutouts. Twice he won more than 20 games in a season. Following a dispute with manager John McGraw, Tesreau left the major leagues at the age of 30 and spent the rest of his life coaching the Dartmouth College baseball team (Library of Congress).

only seven losses and led the league with an ERA of 1.96. He pitched a no-hitter and allowed the fewest hits per nine innings of any NL pitcher. He led the league in that category each of his first three seasons. He won 22 games in 1913 and 26 games in 1914. In the latter year he led the league with eight shutouts. A New York sportswriter wrote that the right-hander had "curves which bend like barrel hoops and speed like lightning."[51] Jeff helped the Giants win the NL pennant in 1912, 1913, and 1917 but did not fare very well in the World Series, winning only one game against three losses.

John McGraw, manager of the Giants, put Tesreau in charge of a contingent of players needing extra work prior to spring training in 1918. When Mac asked Jeff to report on the evening activities of the players, the pitcher refused, saying what the players did after hours was their own business. This caused a breach between manager and pitcher that indirectly led to Jeff's early exit from organized baseball. During World War I, Jeff left the team in July 1918 to take a job with Bethlehem Steel and pitch in the Steel League. With the war over, Jeff refused to report to the Giants in 1919, and McGraw refused to release or trade him. Tesreau accepted an offer to coach the Dartmouth College team and spent the rest of his life with Dartmouth, occasionally pitching for semi-pro teams in New England and managing teams in the Northern League, a summer league that attracted college players from across the nation.

On September 19, 1946, Big Jeff suffered a stroke during a fishing trip and died five days later in Hanover, New Hampshire, at the age of 57. He is profiled in SABR's *Baseball Biography Project*. Ranking: Faber System fifteenth; *Total Baseball* twentieth.

Lee Viau

Born: Leon A. Viau, July 5, 1866, Corinth, VT
Debut: April 22, 1888; age 21
Last Game: August 27, 1892; age 26
Record: 83   77   .519   3.33   -124   168
Clubs: Cincinnati AA; Cincinnati AL; Cleveland NL; Louisville NL; Boston NL

Soon after the boy's birth the family moved from Vermont to Hanover, New Hampshire, where Lee's father became a janitor for Dartmouth College. Perhaps the father's employment or Lee's athletic skills helped the boy gain entrance to the Ivy League school at a time when young men of humble origin seldom attended prestigious colleges. Viau played left field and pitched for the school and somehow attracted the attention of the Cincinnati Reds. He signed with a minor league club in St. Paul, where he pitched well enough in 1887 to earn a promotion to the majors in the spring of 1888. The tiny right-hander (5'4", 160 pounds) got off to a brilliant start, winning eight straight games before suffering his first loss. During his rookie season he won 27 games against 14 losses and had an ERA of 2.65. Although he won 22 games the next year, his earned run average increased by more than one run per game, and he never again matched his first-year performance. He spent parts of three seasons with Cleveland and parts of one year with Louisville and Boston, compiling losing records with all three clubs. He was out of the majors at the age of 26. Perhaps the reason for his decline was his overuse of alcohol. He hung on in the minors for several years, pitching for Fall River and Haverhill in the New England League and for Paterson of the Atlantic League before leaving organized baseball in 1898 at the age of 32. While at Paterson he arrived at the park drunk one day. Future Hall of Famer Honus Wagner chastised him. The little pitcher grabbed a water bucket and emptied it over Wagner's head, whereupon the shortstop wrapped his big hands around Lee's throat, lifting him completely off the floor. After a short while Honus released the shaken pitcher and they remained teammates until Wagner was called up to the major leagues. After his professional career was over, Viau played semi-pro ball for a while and did some umpiring, then he became manager of the game room at the Paterson Elks Club. On December 17, 1947, at the age of 81, Lee Viau died in Hopewell, New Jersey.

Viau is profiled in SABR's *Baseball Biography Project*. Ranking: Faber System tied for 69th; *Total Baseball* tied for 56th.

Don Wilson

Born: Donald Edward Wilson, February 12, 1945, Monroe, LA
Debut: September 29, 1966; age 21
Last Game: September 28, 1974; age 29
Record: 104   92   .531   3.15   8492   340
Club: Houston NL

Don was signed by the Houston Colt 45's as a free agent out of Compton Community College in the spring of 1964. The teenager was assigned to the Cocoa Colts team in the Cocoa Rookie League, promoted to the Cocoa Astros in the Florida State League in 1965 and to the Amarillo Sonics of he Texas League the following season. He posted spectacular ERAs–1.44 in 1965 and 2.21 in 1966. His 18–6 record with Amarillo earned him advancement to the big leagues. As a rookie, the hard-throwing right-hander pitched a no-hitter against the Braves, striking out Hank Aaron for the final out of the game. He pitched his second no-hitter in 1969 against Cincinnati. In 1974 he pitched eight no-hit innings against the Reds before manager Preston Gomez removed him for a pinch-hitter, depriving him of a chance for a third no-hit game. Cincinnati figured prominently in his pitching feats. In 1968 he struck out 18 Reds in one game, tying Sandy Koufax's modern NL record. In this game he struck out eight consecutive batters, tying another modern NL record. His best season may have been 1971 when he had a 16–10 record, an ERA of 2.45, and led the league with the fewest hits per nine innings pitched. He pitched in the All-Star game that July.

In the early morning of February 5, 1975, Bernice Wilson awakened to the sounds of a crying child and an engine running in the attached garage. When Bernice called for help, her husband was found dead in the front seat of his car and five-year-old Alexander dead in a bedroom above the garage. Bernice and daughter Denice were hospitalized, but both recovered. The medical examiner pronounced the deaths of Don and his son were caused by carbon monoxide poisoning. He also stated that Don's blood alcohol level was 167 on a scale where any number about 100 is considered proof of intoxication. The examiner was required to rule whether the death was a homicide, a suicide, or an accident. He delayed his finding for a month while Houston police investigated. The police found no evidence of a homicide. Friends and teammates concurred that Wilson had revealed no suicidal tendencies and was looking forward optimistically toward the next baseball season. The medical examiner eventually ruled that the death was an accident. He speculated that Wilson may have turned on the car's ignition so the heater could warm him on a cold night. The finding of accidental death was widely accepted at the time. Nevertheless, some present-day sources state flatly that the death was a suicide, without citing any evidence for their opinion. Don Wilson was 29 years old when he died at his Houston home.

Ranking: Faber System 18th; *Total Baseball* 23rd.

Jack Wilson

Born: John Francis Wilson, April 12, 1912, Portland, OR
Debut: September 9, 1934; age 22
Final Game: September 16, 1942; age 30
Record: 68　72　.486　4.59　-6165　153
Clubs: Philadelphia AL; Boston AL; Washington AL; Detroit AL

After playing for the University of Portland, Wilson got his professional start with the Portland Beavers of the Pacific Coast League from 1932 through 1934. He appeared in two games for the Philadelphia Athletics in the fall of 1934 but was returned to Portland, who traded him to the Boston Red Sox in February 1935. One of his more notable achievements came in his first game for the Sox when he hit a home run in the 11th inning to secure his first major league victory. Jack spent seven seasons with the Sox. Although he played for four different major league clubs, all but six of his big league decisions were for the Crimson Hose. His best year was in 1937, when he won 16 games and had an ERA of 3.70, the only time his ERA was below 4.00 in his major league career. Wilson never led the league in any major category, but he was second in strikeouts per nine innings in 1937 and second in shutouts in 1938. His skills declined rapidly after 1940, and his record in his last two seasons combined was five wins and 17 losses. He managed the Salem Senators in the Western International League in 1947 and 1948. His name was mostly absent from the sports pages after that. Even his induction into the Oregon Sports Hall of Fame in 1994 drew little attention from the national press. His last known residence was in Lynnwood, Washington, just north of Seattle. Jack Wilson died in nearby Edmonds on April 19, 1995, at the age of 83.

Ranking: Faber System tied for 76th; *Total Baseball* 46th.

George Winter

Born: George Lovington Winter, April 27, 1878, New Providence, PA
Debut: June 15, 1901; age 23
Last Game: September 18, 1908
Record: 83   102   .449   2.87   -12,100   167
Clubs: Boston AL; Detroit AL

Eddie Plank and George Winter were teammates at Pennsylvania College (now called Gettysburg College). Connie Mack signed Plank to a contract with the Philadelphia Athletics, and Eddie was on his way to Cooperstown. Thinking the slightly built Winter was too small to be a major league pitcher, Mack passed on George. However, Jimmy Collins, manager of the Boston Americans, had seen Winter pitch for a YMCA team in York, Pennsylvania, and signed him. The right-handed pitcher got off to a good start in Boston in 1901, winning 16 games and posting an ERA of 2.80 his rookie season. He never won more than 16 games in any subsequent year, and although he usually had a good ERA, he lost more games than he won for Boston. His effectiveness was hindered by a case of malaria, which flared up from time to time. Somewhere along the line he acquired the nickname "Sassafras," probably an allusion to the winter sassafras vine.

In 1908 Winter was the losing pitcher in a very unusual game. On June 9 Sassafras was leading Cleveland, 2–1, going into the fifth inning. Nig Clarke led off that frame for the Naps with a single, Bill Hinchman popped out, and the next seven batters hit safely. Winter was out of the game by this time, but

All Pitchers 271

the onslaught continued against reliever Ralph Glaze. Glaze got one more out, but Hinchman atoned for his first inning popup by hitting a three-run homer. In this one inning every man in the Cleveland lineup had hit safely and scored a run, perhaps for the only time in major league history. A few days later Winter was waived to Detroit. He won only one game for the Tigers but pitched in the World Series for the first time. Sassafras pitched only one inning, but that was more than he had hurled for Boston, who used him as a ticket taker instead of as a pitcher in the 1903 Series.

After leaving the major leagues, Winter pitched two years for the Montreal Royals of the Eastern League before going into the sporting goods business in Wilmington, Delaware. George Winter died May 26, 1951, in Franklin Lakes, New Jersey, at the age of 73.

Ranking: Faber System tied for 71st; *Total Baseball* 73rd.

Appendix

All-Star Teams

An all-star team of one player at each position plus five pitchers has been selected from the ratings by the Faber System, *Total Baseball*, and Bill James. In the views of the analysts these are the best players of all time who ended their major league playing careers at the age of thirty or younger.

Pos.	Faber System	Total Baseball	Bill James
1b	Dick Hoblitzell	Vic Saier	Dick Hoblitzell
2b	Rennie Stennett	Hub Collins	Jim Lefebvre
ss	Ray Chapman	Ray Chapman	Ray Chapman
3b	Freddie Lindstrom	Red Smith	Freddie Lindstrom
c	Fred Carroll	Fred Carroll	Fred Carroll
rf	Chicken Wolf	Ross Youngs	Ross Youngs
cf	Bill Lange	Bennie Kauff	Bill Lange
lf	Carlos May	Curt Blefary	Carlos May
p	Amos Rusie	Amos Rusie	Sandy Koufax
p	Sandy Koufax	Bob Caruthers	Amos Rusie
p	Sadie McMahon	Sandy Koufax	Addie Joss
p	Addie Joss	Silver King	Bob Caruthers
p	Bob Caruthers	Addie Joss	Tommy Bond

Close but No Cigar

This section of the Appendix are listed some players whom the reader might have expected to see among the 197 entries in the main parts of the book. For the reasons stated, none of them made it.

They Flamed Out Too Early

Among the hundreds of early leavers there were several who had been named Rookie of the Year but were out of the major leagues at the age of thirty or younger. Six of these men failed to attain five or more eligible seasons; they flamed out too early. Tragically, Ken Hobbs was killed in a plane crash at the age of 22. Although he tried to come back, Herb Score never overcame the effects of being hit in the eye by a line drive. Mark Fidrych succumbed to arm trouble, and Joe Charboneau was felled by a bad back. Pat Listach was hampered by a broken toe, and Butch Metzger gave in to control problems. None lived up to the brilliant future that could have been predicted from their rookie seasons.

Player	Date of Birth	Rookie Year	Final Game	Age	Eligible Years
Joe Charboneau	June 17, 1955	1980	June 1, 1982	27	1
Mark Fidrych	August 15, 1954	1976	October 1, 1980	26	1
Ken Hubbs	December 23, 1941	1962	September 29, 1963	21	2
Pat Listach	September 12, 1967	1992	June 29, 1997	29	2
Butch Metzger	May 23, 1952	1976	June 28, 1978	26	2
Herb Score	June 7, 1933	1955	May 4, 1962	28	4

He Lingered Too Long

Dave Orr played three days too many to gain an entry in this work. The good hitting first baseman turned 31 on September 29, 1890. On October 2 he played his last game before suffering a career-ending stroke. Had he met the age limit, Orr would have been ranked number one among early-leaving first sackers by both the Faber System and *Total Baseball*.

Disputed Birthdates

Sources disagree about the dates of birth of several ballplayers. Among those in dispute are two players whose inclusion in this book depends upon which date is accepted. In both of these cases the better evidence seems to indicate that the player was past his 31st birthday when he participated in his last major league contest.

Player	Date of Birth	Last Game	Age
Bill Keister	August 17, 1871 or 1874	August 25, 1903	29 or 32
Hugh McQuillan	September 15, 1895 or 1897	September 11, 1927	30 or 32

Notes

Preface

1. A regular is defined as a catcher who appeared in at least one-half of his team's games, a player at a different position who played in at least two-thirds of the schedule, or a pitcher who had 15 or more decisions.

Part One

1. Charles F. Faber, *Baseball Ratings: The All-Time Best Players at Each Position, 1876 to the Present*, 3rd ed. (Jefferson, NC: McFarland, 2008).
2. Pete Palmer and Gary Gillette (eds.), *The Baseball Encyclopedia*, 9th ed. (New York: Barnes and Noble, 2004).
3. www.Baseball-reference.com.
4. www.NewspaperArchives.com.
5. John Thorn et al., *Total Baseball: The Ultimate Baseball Encyclopedia* (Wilmington, DE: Sport Media, 2004).
6. Bill James, *The New Bill James Historical Baseball Abstract* (New York: Free Press, 2003).
7. David Nemec, *The Beer and Whiskey League: The Illustrated History of the American Association — Baseball's Renegade Major League* (New York: Lyons and Burford, 1994), p. 1.
8. Philip Von Borries, "Louis Rogers Browning (Pete, the Gladiator)" in *Nineteenth Century Stars*, ed. by Robert L. Thiemann and Mark Rucker. (Kansas City: Society for American Baseball Research, 1989), p. 19. (Hereafter cited as *Nineteenth Century Stars*.)
9. Although almost everything written about them says that John and Phil were twins, John's recently discovered death certificate indicates he was born on October 29, 1859. If so, he would have been 22 when he first played in the American Association. See Nemec, *The Beer and Whiskey League*, p. 31.
10. L. Robert Davids and Richard A. Puff, "William Van Winkle Wolf (Chicken)," in *Nineteenth Century Stars*, p. 140.
11. Faber, *Baseball Ratings*, p. 78.
12. Ibid., p. 101.
13. Davids and Puff, "William Van Winkle Wolf."
14. Bob Bailey, "Chicken Wolf," in *The Baseball Biography Project*, http://sabr.org/bioproj.
15. Davids and Puff, "William Van Winkle Wolf."
16. Nineteenth century statistics are notoriously unreliable. The 100 stolen bases figure was repeated as recently as 1970 in *One for the Book* (St. Louis: Sporting News, 1970), p. 343. Modern researchers are constantly trying to correct the old records, but total agreement has not yet been reached. For example, Pete Palmer and Gary Gillette, editors of *The Baseball Encyclopedia* (New York: Barnes and Noble, 2004), p. 375, credit Lange with 400 lifetime stolen bases, whereas the leading Internet source "Bill Lange" (*http://baseball-reference.com*, 2007) gives Big Bill 399 steals. The two sources agree that Lange stole 84 bases in 1894, but they present very slight differences in his lifetime totals in several other statistical categories.
17. Faber, *Baseball Ratings*, p. 82.
18. Cited by James, *The New Bill James*, p. 764.
19. William E. Akin, "William Alexander Lange" in *Nineteenth Century Stars*, p. 19.
20. Cited by James, *The New Bill James*, p. 763.

21. Ibid., pp. 762–3.
22. Ibid., p. 764.
23. *New York Times,* December 8, 1921.
24. The nine are Jake Beckley, Jesse Burkett, Big Ed Delahanty, Hugh Duffy, Sliding Billy Hamilton, Hughie Jennings, Wee Willie Keeler, Joe Kelley, and Bid McPhee.
25. The six are Burkett, Delahanty, Duffy, Hamilton, Keeler, and Kelley. The rankings are from Faber, *Baseball Ratings,* pp. 194, 200, 202, 206, 207.
26. *New York Times,* July 25, 1950.
27. "Ross Youngs," www.thebaseballpage.com, June 23, 2009.
28. *Kerrville Daily Times,* April 26, 1992.
29. Ibid.
30. Alan Asnen, "Ross Youngs," in *The Ballplayers,* Mike Shatzkin, ed. (New York: Arbor House, William Morrow, 1990), p. 1219.
31. Faber, *Baseball Ratings,* p. 137.
32. *Washington Post,* October 14, 1921.
33. *San Antonio Sunday Light,* December 19, 1926.
34. Blair, "Once Legendary, Young Now Nearly Forgotten," *Kerrville Daily Times,* April 26, 1992.
35. Baseball page, "Ross Youngs."
36. Faber, *Baseball Ratings,* p. 274.
37. Lawrence Ritter and Donald Honig, *The 100 Greatest Baseball Players of All Time* (New York: Crown Publishers, 1981).
38. Faber, *Baseball Ratings,* pp. 81, 142.
39. Ibid., pp. 17, 161.
40. Cited by David Jones in "Benjamin Michael Kauff," *Deadball Stars of the National League,* p. 84.
41. Ibid.
42. Faber, *Baseball Ratings,* pp. 87, 148.
43. Ibid., pp. 17, 161.
44. Cited by Jones, *Deadball Stars of the National League,* pp. 84–85.
45. Ibid., p. 85.
46. *New Castle* (Pa.) *News,* August 22, 1917.
47. Cited by Jones, *Deadball Stars of the National League,* p. 86.
48. Cited by Lawrence S. Ritter, *The Glory of Their Times* (New York: HarperCollins, 1992), p. 285.
49. Ibid., pp. 300, 305.
50. James, *The New Bill James,* p. 564.
51. Faber, *Baseball Ratings,* pp. 62, 125.
52. James, *The New Bill James,* p. 754.
53. *Hammond* (La.) *Times,* June 19, 1957.
54. *Oakland Tribune,* January 22, 1936.
55. Bill James, *The Bill James Historical Baseball Abstract* (New York: Villard Books, 1988), p. 368.
56. Faber, *Baseball Ratings,* p. 274.
57. Ibid., pp. 183–84.
58. *College World Series Record Book* (Fishers, IN: Madden Publishing, 2002), pp. 35, 36, 64.
59. "A New Kind of Orient Express," *Sports Illustrated,* May 18, 1987.
60. "No Yen to Play in Japan," *Sports Illustrated,* March 28, 1928.
61. Ibid.
62. *St. Louis Post Dispatch,* January 21, 1988.
63. *Frederick* (Md.) *New Post,* March 10, 1989.
64. *Syracuse Herald-Journal,* March 10, 1989.
65. Ibid.
66. Tim Murnane was a nineteenth-century ballplayer for the Boston Red Caps and other teams and a long-time sportswriter for the *Boston Globe.* The game between Cleveland and the Braves was a benefit for the family of the recently deceased Murnane. See John Thorn, "Tim Murnane: Heart of the Game," *Base Ball: A Journal of the Early Game* 2 (Spring 2008): 92–97.
67. Faber, *Baseball Ratings,* pp. 59, 122.
68. Russell Schneider, *The Cleveland Indians Encyclopedia* (Champaign, IL: Sports Publishing, 2001), p. 145.
69. Deveaux, *The Washington Senators, 1901–1971* (Jefferson, NC: McFarland, 2001), p. 7.
70. Charles F. Faber and Richard B. Faber, *Spitballers: The Last Legal Hurlers of the Wet One* (Jefferson, NC: McFarland, 2006), p. 6.
71. David Ziegler, "Remembering Ray Chapman," in *Simply Baseball Notebook: Forgotten in Time* (http://z.leetripod.com, 2002).
72. *Cleveland News,* April 17, 1920.
73. *Spalding's Official Baseball Guide* (New York: American Sports, 1921).
74. James, *The Bill James Historical Baseball Abstract,* pp. 378–80.
75. John Ralph, "Where Have You Gone, Carlos May?" *Baseball Digest,* September 2002, p. 64.
76. Lyle Spatz, ed. *The SABR Baseball List and Record Book* (New York: Scribner, 2007), p. 383.
77. Faber, *Baseball Ratings,* p. 154.
78. James, *The New Bill James,* pp. 949–50.

79. Richard C. Lindberg, "Carlos May," in *The Ballplayers*, p. 687.
80. Ralph, "Carlos May?" pp. 55–56.
81. Ibid., p. 66.
82. James J. Skipper, *Baseball Nicknames: A Dictionary of Origins and Meanings* (Jefferson, NC: McFarland, 1992).
83. Jim Nitz, "Happy Felsch," *The Baseball Biography Project* (*http://bioproj.sabr.org/bioproj.*, 2009).
84. Many American cities, especially those with a large population of German immigrants, had gymnastic clubs called "turnverein" (English translation: "turners") in the early twentieth century. Some of these associations still exist in the twenty-first century, featuring various physical fitness activities.
85. Nitz, "Happy Felsch."
86. Jonathan Fraser Light, *The Cultural Encyclopedia of Baseball* (Jefferson, NC: McFarland, 1997), p. 799.
87. Nitz, "Happy Felsch."
88. Richard Lindberg, *The White Sox Encyclopedia* (Philadelphia: Temple University Press, 1997), p. 25.
89. Faber, *Baseball Ratings*, p. 28.
90. This tale is probably apocryphal, but it illustrates the feelings some players had about the penuriousness of their owner.
91. Harvey Frommer, *Shoeless Joe and Ragtime Baseball* (Dallas: Taylor, 1992), p. 69. Cited by Nitz, "Happy Felsch."
92. *Chicago Evening American*, September 30, 1920, cited by Nitz, "Happy Felsch."
93. Nitz, "Happy Felsch."
94. Ibid.
95. Eliot Asinof, *Bleeding Between the Lines* (New York: Holt, Rinehart and Winston, 1979). Cited by Nitz, "Happy Felsch."
96. Eliot Asinof, *Eight Men Out* (New York: Henry Holt, 1963).
97. Nitz, "Happy Felsch."

Part Two

1. Faber, *Baseball Ratings*.
2. Thorn, *Total Baseball*.
3. James, *The New Bill James*.
4. Richard Puff, "Amos Wilson Rusie (The Hoosier Thunderbolt)," *Baseball's First Stars*, Frederick Ivor-Campbell, ed. (Cleveland: Society for American Baseball Research, 1996), p. 143. (Hereafter cited as *Baseball's First Stars*.)
5. Jack Kavanagh, "Amos Rusie (The Hoosier Thunderbolt)," *The Ballplayers*, Mike Shatzkin, ed. (New York: William Morrow, 1990), p. 947.
6. Ralph Berger, "Amos Rusie," *The Baseball Biography Project* (http://bioproj.sabr.org. 2007). (Hereafter cited as SABR.)
7. Berger, "Amos Rusie."
8. Sam Crane, cited in "Amos Rusie Facts from the Baseball Page.com." (*www.thebaseballpage.com*, 2009).
9. The practice was not limited to sportswriters of the day. The inaccurate sobriquet was recently used by respected baseball historian Jack Kavanagh.
10. "When Amos Rusie was on the Mound Catchers Didn't Get the Lead Out," *http://vault.sportsillustrated.com*, 2009.
11. Puff, "Amos Wilson Rusie."
12. Berger, "Jimmy Ryan."
13. Puff, "Amos Wilson Rusie."
14. Berger, "Amos Rusie."
15. Kavanagh, "Amos Rusie (The Hoosier Thunderbolt)."
16. *New York World*, October 7, 1894.
17. Philip J. Lowry, *Green Cathedrals* (New York: Walker, 2006), p. 150.
18. *New York World*, October 7, 1894.
19. Thorn, *Total Baseball*, p. 2470.
20. Puff, "Amos Wilson Rusie."
21. The Supreme Court of the United States held that the reserve clause was not a violation of anti-trust act because baseball was not interstate commerce (*Federal Baseball Club of Baltimore v. National League of Professional Baseball Clubs, et. al.* 259 U.S. 200, 1922). The challenge by Danny Gardella in 1946 led to his reinstatement by Commissioner Chandler after a U.S. Court of Appeals had remanded the case back to the district court for a full hearing. The heroic and costly challenge by Curt Flood led to what may be one of the worst decisions in Supreme Court history, when the court again upheld baseball's exemption from the anti-trust acts in *Flood v. Kuhn*, 407 U.S. 258, 1972. Although Flood lost the case by a vote of 5–3, the apparent unfairness of the decision turned much of public opinion against the reserve clause. Three years later the clause was renounced by Major League Baseball after an arbitrator ruled in favor of Andy Messersmith and Dave McNally.
22. Puff, "Amos Wilson Rusie."
23. *Massillon* (Ohio) *Evening Independent*, December 14, 1942.

24. Ibid., pp. 65–66.
25. Al Campanis, cited by Jane Leavy, *Sandy Koufax: A Lefty's Legacy* (New York: Harper Collins, 2002), p. 55.
26. Answers.com. "Sandy Koufax." *www. answers.com/topic/sandy-koufax.*
27. James, *The New Bill James*, p. 253.
28. Faber, *Baseball Ratings*, p. 216.
29. Bob Broeg, *Super Stars of Baseball* (St. Louis: The Sporting News, 1971), p. 148.
30. Ibid., p. 149.
31. Leavy, *Sandy Koufax*, pp. 157–60. Butazolodin is used by veterinarians to treat inflammation in horses. Its use on humans has been prohibited since the 1970s. Capsolin is an ointment derived from red hot chili peppers. If applied to the skin it normally produces a burning sensation.
32. Boeg, *Super Stars of Baseball*, p. 150.
33. Faber, *Baseball Ratings*, p. 214.
34. Ibid., p. 217.
35. David L. Fleitz, *The Irish in Baseball* (Jefferson, NC: McFarland, 2009), p. 88.
36. John Heydler, cited by Fred Lieb, *The Baltimore Orioles* (New York: G. P. Putnam's Sons, 1955), p. 68.
37. Rober L. Thiemann in *Nineteenth Century Stars*, p. 90.
38. Burt Solomon, *Where They Ain't* (New York: The Free Press, 2000), p. 97.
39. Ibid.
40. Ibid.
41. Thiemann, *Nineteenth Century Stars.*
42. Ibid.
43. *Lincoln State Journal*, January 15, 1923.
44. Ibid.
45. Ibid.
46. *Lethridge Herald*, March 31, 1943.
47. *Reno Evening Gazette*, April 10, 1941.
48. This account is taken from Scott Longert, *Addie Joss: King of the Pitchers* (Cleveland: Society for American Baseball Research, 1998), pp. 41–45.
49. James, *The New Bill James*, p. 89.
50. Alex Semchuck, "Addie Joss," in *Deadball Stars of the American League*, p. 655.
51. Ibid., pp. 655–56.
52. Ibid., p. 656.
53. Ibid.
54. Palmer and Gillette, *The Baseball Encyclopedia*, pp. 1666, 1667.
55. L. Robert Davids, ed., *Great Hitting Pitchers* (Cleveland: Society for American Baseball Research, 1979). Retrieved from SABR website August 15, 2009.

56. Palmer and Gillette, *The Baseball Encyclopedia*, p. 1380.
57. *Newark* (Ohio) *Daily Advocate*, December 15, 1887.
58. *Weekly Chronicle* (Elyria, Ohio), March 20, 1908.
59. *Cedar Rapids Evening Gazette*, April 11, 1888.
60. *Historical Statistics of the United States, 1789–1945* (Washington: Bureau of the Census, 1949), p. 68.
61. Faber, *Baseball Ratings*, p. 217.
62. Glenn Stout and Richard A. Johnson, *Red Sox Century* (Boston: Houghton Mifflin, 2000), p. 29.
63. *Waterloo Daily Times Tribune*, August 13, 1910.
64. Ibid.
65. *Logansport* (Ind.) *Pharos*, July 22, 1911.
66. James, *The New Bill James*, p. 96.
67. William Akin, "Win Mercer," in *The Baseball Biography Project*, http://sabr.org/bioproj.
68. Bruce Nash and Allan Zullo, *The Baseball Hall of Shame* (New York: Pocket Books, 1985), p. 129.
69. Akin, "Win Mercer."
70. *Hamilton* (Ohio) *Evening Sun*, January 14, 1903.
71. *Fort Wayne Daily News*, January 17, 1903.
72. *Coshocton* (Ohio) *Sun*, January 20, 1903.
73. William E. Akin, "George Barclay Mercer," in *Baseball's First Stars*, p. 111.
74. Frederick G. Lieb, *The Detroit Tigers* (New York: G. P. Putnam, 1946).
75. Longert, *Addie Joss: King of Pitchers*, p. 54.
76. Ibid., pp. 53–54.
77. Ibid., p. 54.
78. Tom Deveaux, *The Washington Senators, 1901–1971* (Jefferson, NC: McFarland, 2001), p. 7.
79. *Oakland Tribune*, January 14, 1903.

Part Three

1. Faber, *Baseball Ratings*; Thorn, *Total Baseball*; James, *The New Bill James*.
2. *Lima News*, June 5, 1970.
3. Cited by Jesus Francisco Cabrera in *The Ballplayers*.
4. Faber, *Baseball Ratings*, p. 117.
5. Ibid., p. 49.

6. Ibid., p. 61.
7. Ibid., p. 13.
8. Faber, *Baseball Ratings*.
9. Gallup (N.M.) *Independent*, February 17, 2007.
10. Faber, *Baseball Ratings*, pp. 51, 114.
11. Ibid., pp. 62–63.
12. James, *The New Bill James*, p. 541.
13. Ibid., p. 50.
14. Chuck LaMar, quoted in *Frederick Post*, April 4, 1969.
15. Faber, *Baseball Ratings*, p. 113.
16. Ibid., p. 156.
17. Ibid., pp. 53–54, 117.
18. Faber, *Baseball Ratings*, p. 118.
19. *Florence Morning News*, December 9, 1951.
20. Ibid., June 1, 1952.
21. James, *The New Bill James*, p. 44.
22. *Sporting Life*, cited in *Nineteenth Century Stars*, p. 52.
23. James, *The New Bill James*, p. 283.
24. Faber, *Baseball Ratings*, p. 120.
25. Ibid., p. 56.
26. Ibid., p. 98.
27. Irv Sanborn, quoted in *http://clearbuck.com*.
28. Faber, *Baseball Ratings*, p. 128.
20. Asinof, *Eight Men Out*.
21. Irving Stein. *The Ginger Kid: The Buck Weaver Story* (Dubuque, IA: Brown and Benchmark, 1992).
22. David Fletcher, "Buck Weaver" in *The Baseball Biography Project*.
23. Faber, *Baseball Ratings*, p. 66.
24. Ibid., p. 128.
25. Ibid., p. 62.
26. Ibid., p. 63.
27. Ibid., pp. 62, 125.
28. Cited by James, *The New Bill James*, p. 581.
29. Cited in *http://findarticles.com*.
30. Faber, *Baseball Ratings*, p. 62.
31. James, *The New Bill James*, p. 421.
32. Faber, *Baseball Ratings*, pp. 73, 135.
33. Jeffrey Katz, "Earl Williams" in *The Baseball Biography Project*.
34. Faber, *Baseball Ratings*, p. 136.
35. Rico Petrocelli and Chaz Scoggins, *Petrocelli's Tales from the Impossible Dream Red Sox* (Champaign, IL: Sports Publishing, 2007).
36. Ibid.
37. Faber, *Baseball Ratings*, p. 75.
38. Ibid., p. 137.
39. Ibid., p. 101.

40. Ibid., pp. 80, 141.
41. James, *The New Bill James*, p. 79.
42. *Kansas City Bulletin*, cited in Dan Holmes, "Braggo Roth" in *The Baseball Biography Project*.
43. Ibid.
44. Faber, *Baseball Ratings*, p. 85.
45. James, *The New Bill James*, p. 78.
46. Faber, *Baseball Ratings*, p. 88.
47. Ibid., p. 81.
48. James, *The New Bill James*, p. 299.
49. Faber, *Baseball Ratings*, p. 145.
50. James, *The New Bill James*, p. 764.
51. Peter Morris, "Homer Smoot" in *The Baseball Biography Project*.
52. *New York Times*, April 6, 1974.
53. Faber, *Baseball Ratings*, pp. 82, 143.
54. Ibid., p. 84.
55. Ibid., p. 76.
56. James, *The New Bill James*, p. 754.
57. Tom Meany, *Baseball's Greatest Teams* (New York: A. S. Barnes, 1949), pp. 203–04.
58. Ibid., p. 204.
59. Norman L. Macht, "Whitey Witt" in *The Ballplayers*, p. 1193.
60. Quoted by Joseph Schuster, "Back Door to the Big Leagues," *Sport Magazine*, June 1988.
61. *http://en.Wikipedia.org/wiki/Beals_Becker*, 2009.
62. John Henshell, "Curt Blefary" in *The Baseball Biography Project*.
63. Ibid.
64. Faber, *Baseball Ratings*, p. 88.
65. Ibid., pp. 88, 90.
66. Ibid., p. 137.

Part Four

1. Cited by Bill James and Rob Neyer. *The Neyer/James Guide to Pitching* (New York: Simon & Shuster, 2004), p. 136.
2. James, *The New Bill James*, p. 14.
3. Faber, *Baseball Ratings*, pp. 214, 215.
4. Palmer and Gillette, *The Baseball Encyclopedia*, p. 1667.
5. David Nemec, *The Official Rules of Baseball Illustrated* (Guilford, CT: Globe Pequot, 2006), pp. 33–34.
6. Faber, *Baseball Ratings*, p. 216.
7. *Anaconda Standard*, September 9, 1900.
8. *Cedar Rapids Evening Gazette*, July 21, 1913.
9. Cited in Joseph M. Overfield, "Elton B. Chamberlain (Ice Box)" in *Nineteenth Century Stars*, p. 27.

10. Faber, *Baseball Ratings*, p. 217.
11. *Syracuse Herald*, July 3, 1913.
12. *Oneonta Star*, February 17, 1955.
13. Palmer and Gillette, *The Baseball Encyclopedia*, p. 1667.
14. Cited by R. J. Lesch, "James Otis 'Doc' Crandall" in *Deadball Stars of the National League*, p. 67.
15. *Ogden Standard-Examiner*, October 15, 1994.
16. Ibid.
17. Seamus Kearney and Tom Simon, "Ed Doheny," *The Baseball Biography Project*.
18. *Atlanta Journal*, September 17, 1984.
19. *Mansfield* (Ohio) *News*, February 16, 1903.
20. *San Antonio Gazette*, April 6, 1907.
21. James and Neyer, *The Neyer/James Guide*, p. 474.
22. *Oakland Tribune*, February 7, 1906.
23. *Reno Evening Gazette*, June 19, 1908.
24. *Washington Post*, September 5, 1894.
25. Cited by Dan Levitt, "Noodles Hahn," in *The Baseball Biography Project*.
26. Ibid.
27. Faber, *Baseball Ratings*, p. 215.
28. *Racine Daily Journal*, July 21, 1906.
29. *Washington Post*, January 5, 1906.
30. *Cedar Rapids Evening Gazette*, May 5, 1913.
31. *Logansport* (Ind.) *Pharos-Tribune*, February 22, 1995.
32. Ibid.
33. *Charleston Daily Mail*, March 29, 1961.
34. Rory Costello, "Ted Lewis," in *The Baseball Biography Project*.
35. Ibid.
36. *http://www.bigbenmcdonald.com*.
37. Faber, *Baseball Ratings*, p. 220.
38. *Syracuse Post-Standard*, May 9, 1978.
39. Jim Bouton, *Ball Four* (New York: Dell, 1970), p. 369.
40. *Portsmouth Times*, February 22, 1952.
41. Ibid.
42. Jim Sumner and Robert L. Tiemann, "Thomas A. Ramsey (Toad)" in *Nineteenth Century Stars*, p. 105.
43. Harry Metcalf, cited by the *Hamilton Sun*, March 30, 1906.
44. Palmer and Gillette, *The Baseball Encyclopedia*, p. 1668.
45. Cited in *http://www.astrodaily.com/files/team/richard/richard.html*.
46. *Oakland Tribune*, November 9, 1936.
47. Ring Lardner, *You Know Me Al* (Cleveland: World Publishing, 1945).
48. *Reno Evening Gazette*, October 23, 1920.
49. Ibid.
50. R. J. Lesch, "Jeff Tesreau" in *The Baseball Biography Project*.
51. Ibid.

Bibliography

Angell, Roger. *Five Seasons: A Baseball Companion*. New York: Simon and Schuster, 1988.
Asinof, Eliot. *Bleeding Between the Lines*. New York: Holt, Rinehart and Winston, 1979.
_____. *Eight Men Out*. New York: Henry Holt, 1963.
The Baseball Encyclopedia, 9th ed. New York: Macmillan, 1993.
Bevis, Charlie. *The New England League: A Baseball History 1885–1949*. Jefferson, NC: McFarland, 2008.
Bowman, John S., and Joel Zoss. *The Pictorial History of Baseball*. New York: W. H. Smith, 1986.
Boxerman, Burton A., and Benita W. Boxerman. *Jews and Baseball*, 2 vols. Jefferson, NC: McFarland, 2006, 2009.
Broeg, Bob. *Super Stars of Baseball: Their Lives, Their Loves, Their Laughs, Their Laments*. St. Louis: Sporting News, 1971.
College World Series Record Book. Fishers, IN: Madden, 2002.
Davids, L. Robert. *Great Hitting Pitchers*. Cleveland: Society for American Baseball Research, 1979.
Deveaux, Tom. *The Washington Senators, 1901–1971*. Jefferson, NC: McFarland, 2001.
Faber, Charles F. *Baseball Ratings: The All-Time Best Players at Each Position*. Jefferson, NC: McFarland, 2008.
_____, and Richard B. Faber. *Spitballers: The Last Legal Hurlers of the Wet One*. Jefferson, NC: McFarland, 2006.
Filichia, Peter. *Professional Baseball Franchises: From the Abbeville Athletics to the Zanesville Indians*. New York: Facts on File, 1993.
Fleitz, David L. *The Irish in Baseball*. Jefferson, NC: McFarland, 2009.
Frommer, Harvey. *Shoeless Joe and Ragtime Baseball*. Dallas: Taylor, 1992.
Gregory, Robert. *Diz: The Story of Dizzy Dean and Baseball During the Great Depression*. New York: Penguin, 1992.
Ivor-Campbell, Frederick, ed. *Baseball's First Stars*. Cleveland: Society for American Baseball Research, 1996.
James, Bill. *The Bill James Historical Baseball Abstract*. New York: Villard Books, 1988.
_____. *The New Bill James Historical Baseball Abstract*. New York: Simon and Schuster, 2003.
_____, and Rob Neyer. *The Neyer/James Guide to Pitching*. New York: Simon and Shuster, 2004.
Johnson, Lloyd, and Miles Wolff. *Encyclopedia of Minor League Baseball*, 3rd ed. Durham, NC: Baseball America, 2007.
Jones, David. *Deadball Stars of the American League*. Dulles, VA: Potomac Books, 2006.
Kahn, Roger. *The Era: 1947–1957 When the Yankees, the Giants, and the Dodgers Ruled the World*. New York: Ticknor & Fields, 1993.

Bibliography

Kavanagh, Jack, and Norman Macht. *Uncle Robbie.* Cleveland: Society for American Baseball Research, 1999.
Kelley, Brent. *The Early All-Stars: Conversations with Standout Baseball Players of the 1930s and 1940s.* Jefferson, NC: McFarland, 1997.
Koufax, Sandy, and Ed Linn. *Koufax.* New York: Viking Press, 1966.
Leavy, Jane. *Sandy Koufax: A Lefty's Legacy.* New York: HarperCollins, 2007.
Lieb, Frederick J. *The Baltimore Orioles.* New York: G. P. Putnam's Sons, 1955.
_____. *The Detroit Tigers.* New York: G. P. Putnam's Sons, 1946.
Light, Jonathan Fraser. *The Cultural Encyclopedia of Baseball.* Jefferson, NC: McFarland, 1997.
Lindberg, Richard. *The White Sox Encyclopedia.* Philadelphia: Temple University Press, 1997.
Longert, Scott. *Addie Joss: King of the Pitchers.* Cleveland: Society for American Baseball Research, 1998.
Lowry, Philip J. *Green Cathedrals.* New York: Walker and Company, 2006.
Maraniss, David. *Clemente: The Passion and Grace of Baseball's Last Hero.* New York: Simon and Schuster, 2006.
McKenna, Brian. *Early Exits: The Premature Endings of Baseball Careers.* Lanham, MD: Scarecrow Press, 2007.
Meany, Tom. *Baseball's Greatest Hitters.* New York: A. S. Barnes, 1950.
_____. *Baseball's Greatest Teams.* New York: A. S. Barnes, 1949.
Megdal, Howard. *The Baseball Talmud.* New York: HarperCollins, 2009.
Nash, Bruce, and Allan Zullo. *The Baseball Hall of Shame.* New York: Pocket Books, 1985.
Nemec, David. *The Baseball Challenge Quiz Book.* New York: Penguin Books, 1991.
_____. *The Beer and Whiskey League: The Illustrated History of the American Association — Baseball's Renegade Major League.* New York: Lyons and Burford, 1994.
_____. *The Official Rules of Baseball Illustrated:* Guilford, CT: Globe Pequot, 2006.
_____, et. al. *The Baseball Chronicle.* Lincolnwood, IL: Publications International, 2005.
Oliver, Ted C. *Kings of the Mound,* 2nd ed. Los Angeles: The Author, 1947.
O'Neal, Bill. *International League: A Baseball History, 1884–1981.* Austin, TX: Eakin Press, 1992.
Palmer, Pete, and Gary Gillette, eds. *The Baseball Encyclopedia.* New York: Barnes and Noble, 2004.
Petrocelli, Rico, and Chaz Scoggins. *Petrocelli's Tales from the Impossible Dream Red Sox.* Champaign, IL: Sports Publishing, 2007.
Ritter, Lawrence S. *The Glory of Their Times: The Story of the Early Days of Baseball Told by the Men Who Played It.* New York: HarperCollins, 1992.
_____, and Donald Honig. *The 100 Greatest Baseball Players of All Time.* New York: Crown Publishers, 1981.
Shatzkin, Mike, ed. *The Ballplayers: Baseball's Ultimate Biographical Reference:* New York: Arbor House and William Morrow, 1990.
Simon, Tom, ed. *Deadball Stars of the National League.* Washington, D.C.: Brassey's, 2004.
Snyder, John S. *Play Ball: Great Moments and Dubious Achievements in Baseball History.* San Francisco: Chronicle Books, 1991.
Solomon, Burt. *Where They Ain't.* New York: Free Press, 2000.
Sowell, Mike. *The Pitch That Killed.* New York: Macmillan, 1989.
Spatz, Lyle, ed. *The SABR Baseball List & Record Book: Baseball's Most Fascinating Records and Unusual Statistics.* New York: Scribner, 2007.
Stein, Irving. *The Ginger Kid: The Buck Weaver Story.* Dubuque, IA: Brown and Benchmark, 1992.
Stout, Glenn, and Richard A. Johnson. *Red Sox Century: One Hundred Years of Red Sox Baseball.* Boston: Houghton Mifflin, 2000.
Thorn, John, et al. *Total Baseball: The Ultimate Baseball Encyclopedia.* Wilmington, DE: Sports Media, 2004.

Bibliography

Wallace, Joseph. *World Series: An Opinionated Chronicle: 100 Years*. New York: Harry N. Abrams, 2003.
Will, George F. *Men at Work: The Craft of Baseball*. New York: Macmillan, 1990.
Williams, Ted, with John Underwood. *My Turn at Bat: The Story of My Life*. New York: Simon and Schuster, 1969.
Wright, Marshall D. *The American Association*. Jefferson, NC: McFarland, 1997.
_____. *The International League: Year by Year Statistics, 1884–1953*. Jefferson, NC: McFarland, 1998.
_____. *The Southern Association in Baseball, 1885–1961*. Jefferson, NC: McFarland, 2002.
Zoss, Joel, and John S. Bowman. *The History of Major League Baseball*. Greenwich, CT: Brompton, 1993.

Index

Aaron, Hank 32, 40, 201
Aaron, Tommie 40
Abreu, Bobby 120
Agee, Tommie 231
Aikens, Willie 82–83
Akin, William 11, 79
Alexander, Grover 58, 194, 239
Alger, Horatio 234
Allen, Lee 192
Anderson, John 68
Anderson, Sparky 242
Andrews, Mike 94–96
Ankiel, Rick 91
Anson, Cap 220
Armour, Bill 156
Asinof, Eliot 48, 123
Asnen, Bill 156
Ayers, Doc 260

Baird, Doug 123–124
Baker, Frank 167
Baker, Newton 45, 129, 201
Baldwin, Mark 183–184
Bancroft, Dave 17
Bang, Ed 37
Barber, Steve 205
Barry, Jack 172
Barry, Shad 172
Bartell, Dick 136
Bassett, Charley 94, 96
Becker, Beals 172, 173–174
Becker, Rich 158, 159
Bedient, Hugh 111
Bell, Les 123, 124–125
Bench, Johnny 137, 141, 242
Berra, Yogi 140
Birmingham, Joe 68, 158, 159–160
Blankenship, Ted 184
Blefary, Curt 172, 174, 273
Blyleven, Bert 31, 194

Bond, Tommy 49–50, 185–186, 273
Boros, Steve 235
Bottomley, Jim 28
Bouton, Jim 250
Boyer, Ken 30
Boyle, Henry 186
Bradley, Bill 68
Brain, Dave 123, 125–126
Branca, Ralph 186–187, 188
Braun, Evelyn 55
Braun, Jack 55
Braun, Sanford see Koufax, Sandy
Bresnahan, Roger 167
Brett, Ken 40
Brewer, Tom 187–188
Brock, Lou 188
Broglio, Ernie 188–189
Brouthers, Dan 147
Brown, Mace 113
Brown, Sam 148
Browne, Jerry 94, 97
Browning, Pete 4, 6–8, 215
Brush, John T. 50, 53
Buckley, Dick 51
Buddin, Don 112–113
Burke, Eddie 52
Burke, Jimmy 203
Burkett, Jesse 65
Burns, Britt 189
Burns, George 64
Burns, Jack 82, 83
Burns, Oyster 98
Bushong, Doc 71
Byrne, C.H. 72

Camilli, Dolph 89
Campanis, Al 57
Cantillon, Joe 208
Carey, Andy 123, 126–127
Carlton, Steve 217

Carpenter, Bill 77
Carpenter, Hick 114
Carroll, Fred 136–138, 273
Carsey, Kid 189–191
Caruthers, Bob 49, 70–75, 76–77, 191, 273
Caruthers, Flora 72
Caruthers, Mary Danks "Mamie" 73, 75
Casey, Dan 191–192
Cash, Dave 106
Cassidy, John 142, 143
Castino, John 123, 127–128
Chamberlain, Icebox 192–193
Chambliss, Chris 40
Chance, Dean 193–194
Chance, Frank 109, 219
Chaney, Darrell 242
Chapman, Barbara 34
Chapman, Everette 34
Chapman, Kathleen Daly 35
Chapman, Rae-Marie 38
Chapman, Ray 34–38, 112, 113, 273
Charboneau, Joe 274
Chase, Dick 195
Chase, Hal 24, 176
Chase, Ken 194–195
Chesbro, Jack 79, 209
Cicotte, Eddie 46, 48
Clarke, Nig 270
Clarkson, Arthu 190
Clemens, Doug 188
Cobb, Ty 11, 19, 20, 22, 23, 24, 48, 121
Coggins, Rich 40
Colbert, Nate 82, 84
Collins, Eddie 45, 46
Collins, Hub 94, 97–98, 273
Collins, Jimmy 270
Collins, Ray 195–196

285

Index

Comiskey, Charles 42, 45, 46, 183
Conigliaro, Billy 145
Conigliaro, Tony 142, 143–145, 150
Connelly, John 102
Connolly, Tommy 35, 37
Corbett, James 12
Corcoran, Larry 196–198
Corridon, Frank 198–199
Costello, Rory 233–234
Coughlin, Bill 123, 128
Cramer, Doc 134
Crandall, Doc 199–200
Crandall, Karl 200
Crane, Sam 51
Cronin, Jack 265
Crotty, Joe 4, 6
Cullen, Tim 94, 98–99
Cummings, Candy 185
Cusack, John 123

Danforth, Dave 24
Davenport, Dave 200–201
Davidson, Mordecai 8
Davis, Mike 142, 145
Deal, Charlie 123, 129, 133
Dean, Dizzy 217
Death Valley Scotty 260
Delahanty, Ed 15
De Mont, Gene 94, 99
Demontreville, Eugene see De Mont, Gene
Deveaux, Tom 79
Devore, Josh 111
Dexter, Charlie 158, 160–161
Dobbs, John 158, 161
Doheny, Ed 201–202
Dolan, Cozy 14
Dombrowski, Dave 151
Dooin, Charley 121
Doolan, Mickey 16, 17
Doubleday, Abner 182
Drysdale, Don 59
Du Pont, Alfred 65
Du Pont, Bessie 65
Durocher, Leo 118

Easterbrook, Dode 7, 8
Eckersley, Dennis 145
Edward VIII 9
Ehret, Red 202–203, 220
Elliott, Bob 233
Engle, Clyde 111
Esasky, Nick 82, 84–85
Esbacher, Charles see Esper, Duke
Esper, Duke 63, 203–204
Estrada, Chuck 205
Evans, Jake 142, 146

Evans, Steve 142, 146–148
Evers, Johnny 109

Faber, Red 23, 43, 45, 122, 184
Falcone, Pete 204–205
Feller, Bob 135
Felsch, Charles 42
Felsch, Happy 42–48, 158, 161–162
Felsch, Maria 42
Felsch, Marie Wagner 47, 48
Felsch, Oscar 48
Fennelly, Frank 112, 114
Ferguson, Bob 185
Fidrych, Mark 274
Finley, Charlie 95, 150
Fisher, Jack 205–206
Fitzsimmons, Bob 12
Ford, Whitey 75
Foreman, George 226
Foster, George 242
Foutz, Dave 71
Freeman, Andrew 53
Fricano, Mariano 105
Frick, Ford 19
Frisch, Frankie 30
Frommer, Harvey 46
Fuller, Shorty 112, 114–115
Fullmer, Brad 82, 85–86

Gaetti, Gary 127
Gandil, Chick 45, 46, 48, 260
Ganzel, Charlie 212
Gardner, Larry 111, 218
Garrelts, Scott 206–207
Garvin, Virgil 207–210
Geggus, Charlie 248
Gehrig, Lou 93
German, Les 210–211
Geronimo, Cesar 242
Gessler, Doc 142, 148–149
Getzien, Charlie 211–212
Gibson, Kirk 145
Giles, Brian 100
Giles, Marcus 84, 100
Gillette, Gary 6
Giselman, Anna 13
Giselman, William 13
Gleason, Bill 112, 115–116
Gleason, Jack 115
Goetzien, Charles see Getzein, Charlie
Golenbock, Peter 134
Gomez, Preston 231, 268
Goode, Wilbur 68
Gooden, Dwight 246
Graham, Charles 14
Graney, Jack 37
Gray, Ted 212–213

Green, Danny 142, 148–149
Griffin, Alfredo 127
Griffith, Clark 11, 27–28, 209
Grimes, Burleigh 29
Groh, Heinie 27, 28, 132
Grote, Jerry 95
Grove, Lefty 212, 238
Guerrero, Vladimir 101
Guerrero, Wilton 94, 101
Gullett, Don 213–214
Gumbert, Ad 214–215
Gustine, Frankie 94, 101–102

Haak, Howie 106
Hack, Stan 30
Haddock, George 215–216
Hahn, Noodles 49, 216–217
Halligan, Jocko 193
Hamilton, Jack 144
Hanlon, Ned 62–63
Hansen, Ron 98
Harper, Bessie Brewster 218
Harper, Harry 217–218
Harper, Jack 219–220
Harrelson, Ken 142, 150–151
Harris, Bucky 27
Hawley, Blue 220
Hawley, Camille 220
Hawley, Franc 220
Hawley, Pink 219–221
Healy, Frank 221
Healy, John 221–222
Hemming, George 222
Henderson, Rickey 188
Hendley, Bob 58
Hermann, Garry 88
Hernandez, Enzo 111, 116–117
Heydler, John 62
Higham, Dick 46
Hinchman, Bill 270
Hobbie, Glenn 222–223
Hobbs, Ken 274
Hoblitzell, Dick 82, 86–88, 273
Hodges, Russ 187
Hoernschemeyer, Leopold see Magee, Lee
Hogan, Shanty 169
Honig, Donald 20
Hooper, Harry 111
Horner, Bob 31–33, 123, 129–130
Horner, Chris 32
Horner, Trent 32
Horner, Tyler 32
Hornsby, Rogers 169, 192
Houtteman, Art 223–224
Houtteman, Sheryl 224
Howell, Roy 123, 130
Hubbell, Carl 212

Index

Hudson, Charles 224–226
Huff, Frank 240
Huggins, Miller 37
Hunter, Catfish 130
Hurst, Don 82, 88–89
Huskey, Butch 142, 151–152

Ivie, Mike 82, 90–91, 96, 165

Jackson, Joe 27, 45, 46, 160
Jackson, Sonny 112, 117
James, Bill 3, 12, 28, 30, 38, 40, 49, 58, 68, 75, 114, 116, 137, 152, 159–160, 163, 14–65, 169, 182, 185, 208, 273
Jamieson, Charlie 218
Jeffries, Jim 266
Jennings, Hughie 64
Jensen, Don 34
Johnson, Ban 13, 69, 170
Johnson, Lou 58
Johnson, Randy 183
Johnson, Walter 18, 27, 194
Johnston, Dick 158, 162
Jones, Andruw 100
Jones, Dalton 82, 90–91
Jones, Fielder 68, 201
Jones, Percy 226
Joss, Addie 14, 49, 65–70, 77, 79–80, 226–227, 273
Joss, Jacob 66
Joss, Lillian Shinavar 70
Joss, Theresa Staudenmeyer 66
Jurges, Billy 117, 124

Kauff, Benny 20–25, 158, 162–163, 273
Kauff, Hannah 20
Kauff, Hazel Cassley 25
Kauff, Robert 25
Kauff, William 20
Kawano, Nobe 55
Keefe, Tim 192
Keister, Bill 274
Kelley, Joe 63
Kelly, George 14, 17
Kelly, King 72
Kelly, Mary Lange 14
Kennedy, Joe 227
Kerlan, Robert 59
Kerr, Buddy 112, 118
Kerr, Dickie 45
Killen, Frank 227–228
Kilroy, Matt 196
King, Eric 228–229
King, Silver 49, 229–231, 273
Kinsella, Dick 16
Kirby, Clay 231–232
Knell, Phil 232

Knetzer, Elmer 147
Knoblauch, Chuck 96
Koenig, Charles *see* King, Silver
Koufax, Irving 55
Koufax, Sandy 49, 55–61, 196, 197, 232, 269, 273
Kruk, John 171
Kubek, Tony 112, 118–119
Kucks, Johnny 233
Kuenn, Harvey 56
Kuhn, Bowie 82, 91–92, 95
Kwietniewski, Casimir *see* Michaels, Cass

La Cock, Pete 82
Lajoie, Nap 17, 68, 160
Landis, Kenesaw M. 14, 18, 21, 24, 42, 44, 46, 93, 122
Lane, F.C. 184
Lange, Bill 9–15, 53, 158, 163, 273
Lange, Charles 9
Lange, Grace Giselman 13
Lange, Mary 9
Larkin, Barry 85
La Russa, Tony 151
Law, Rudy 158, 163–164
Leavy, Jane 232
Lee, Manny 112, 119–120
Lefebvre, Benny 102
Lefebvre, Gil 102
Lefebvre, Jim 84, 102–103, 273
Lefebvre, Tip 102
Lewis, Duffy 111
Lewis, Floyd 255
Lewis, Jack 147
Lewis, Ted 233–234
Lieb, Fred 79
Lindstrom, Andy 30
Lindstrom, Chuck 30
Lindstrom, Frances Udaloff 30
Lindstrom, Fred 25–30, 123, 131 272
Lindstrom, Fred C. 25
Lindstrom, Mary Sweeney 25
Linn, Ed 232
Listach, Pat 274
Longerts, Scott 79, 227
Lowe, Bobby 193
Lumley, Harry 142, 152–153
Lynn, Byrd 45
Lyons, Edward 262
Lyons, Ted 184

Mack, Connie 48, 65, 156, 204, 244, 251, 270
Mack, Earl 244

Madoff, Bernie 60
Magee, Lee 172, 175–176
Mancuso, Peter 265
Mantle, Mickey 12
Maris, Roger 266
Marlow, Lucy 127
Marshall, Peter 92
Mathewson, Christy 19, 53, 111, 194
May, Carlos 38–42, 172, 176–177, 273
May, Lee 39, 40
Mayer, Erskine 239–240
Mays, Al 240
Mays, Carl 34, 35, 37
Mays, Willie 40
Mazeroski, Bill 119, 242
McCormick, Barry 94, 103–104
McCovey, Willie 39
McDonald, Ben 234–235
McDowell, Sam 175
McElroy, Jim 248
McGann, Dan 219
McGeachy, Jack 142–143
McGill, Willie 50, 235–236
McGinnity, Joe 220
McGlothlin, Jim 236–237
McGraw, John 13, 14, 15, 19, 20, 23, 24, 28, 43, 51, 53, 62, 64, 122, 167, 250, 266, 267
McLain, Denny 183, 237–238
McLemore, Henry 29–30
McMahon, Nora 65
McMahon, Sadie 49, 61–65, 238–239, 273
McMullin, Fred 23
McNeeley, Earl 27
McPhee, Bid 114
McQuillan, Hugh 274
McRae, Hal 242
McTamany, Jim 158, 164–165
Meany, Tom 170
Meekin, Jouett 52
Mench, Kevin 172, 177–178
Menke, Denis 242
Menosky, Mike 172, 178
Mercer, Maggie 78–79
Mercer, Win 49, 76–80, 240–241
Merkle, Fred 111, 248
Metzger, Butch 274
Meyers, Chief 111, 167
Michaels, Cass 94, 104–105
Miley, Dave 214
Milner, John 95
Mitchell, Willie 241
Monday, Rick 91

Montefusco, John 204
Moose, Bob 241–243
More, Sir Thomas 233
Morgan, Joe 40, 255
Morris, Ed 137, 243–244, 248
Murdoch, Rupert 60
Murnane, Tim 11, 35, 234
Murphy, Dale 32, 91
Murray, Eddie 110
Murray, George 78
Musial, Stan 84
Myers, Al 94, 105–106
Myers, Elmer 244–245

Nagy, Mike 39
Nash, Billy 215
Nash, Bruce 77
Nash, Jim 245–246
Nehf, Art 239
Nemec, David 4, 186
Newhouser, Hal 212
Neyer, Rob 208
Niekro, Phil 39
Nilsson, Dave 136, 138–139
Nolan, Gary 246–247
Norman, Walter 253
Nuxhall, Joe 236

Oakley, Annie 210
O'Brien, Darby 172, 178–179
Ochoa, Alex 142, 153–154, 159
O'Connell, Jim 13–14, 16, 18
O'Connor, Jack 65
O'Day, Hank 247–248
Office, Rowland 158, 165
Oliva, Tony 144
Olson, Ivy 34
O'Neil, Mickey 136, 139–140
O'Neill, Paul 207
O'Neill, Steve 218
O'Neill, Tip 78, 190, 211
Orr, Dave 274
Ortega, Phil 248–249
Ortiz, Russ 85
O'Toole, Jim 249–250
Ott, Mel 118

Palmer, Pete 6
Pappas, Milt 205
Peckinpaugh, Roger 17, 34
Perez, Tony 242
Perritt, Pol 250–251
Petrocelli, Rico 144, 145
Piatt, Wiley 251–252
Piniella, Lou 39
Pipp, Wally 35
Plank, Eddie 270
Powell, Ab 7
Powell, Hosken 142, 154–155

Presley, Jim 123, 131
Prior, Mark 100
Pritchard, Joe 72

Ramsey, Toad 252–253
Reccius, Billy 4
Reccius, John 4, 6, 8
Reccius, Phil 4, 6
Reilly, Long John 114
Reitz, Ken 123, 132
Rhines, Billy 253–254
Richard, J.R. 254–255
Richards, Paul 141
Richie, Lew 255–256
Risberg, Swede 47, 48
Ritter, Lawrence 20
Robinson, Brooks 157
Robinson, Jackie 135
Robinson, Wilbert 61, 64
Rodriguez, Ellie 136, 140–141
Roseboro, Johnny 39
Roth, Bobby 143, 155–157
Ruel, Muddy 27, 35
Runyon, Damon 199, 256
Rusie, Amos 49, 50–55, 61, 78, 183, 251, 253, 256, 273
Rusie, Mary Donovan 50
Rusie, Susan Sloan 54
Rusie, William Asbury 50
Russell, Lillian 50
Ruth, Babe 19, 48, 93, 170, 206
Ryan, Jimmy 51
Ryan, Nolan 60, 141, 183

Saier, Vic 82, 92–93, 273
Sand, Heinie 14, 18
Sanders, Ben 182, 256–257
Sanguillen, Manny 242
Santo, Ron 30
Sax, Steve 96
Scanlan, Doc 257–258
Schalk, Ray 45
Schnabel, Gustav 259
Schneider, Pete 258–259
Schneider, Russell 37
Schoendienst, Red 212
Schumacher, Hal 215
Scoggins, Chaz 145
Score, Herb 274
Scott, Jim 258–261
Seaver, Tom 206, 246
Shamsky, Art 231
Shanks, Howard 260
Shannon, Dan 7
Shannon, Spike 172, 179–180
Shantz, Bobby 188
Sharrott, George 265
Sharrott, Jack 265
Shavers, Ernie 194

Shaw, Dupee 261–262
Sheckard, Jimmy 124
Sheen, Charlie 48
Sheridan, Jack 149
Sherry, Norm 57
Shotton, Burt 89
Sinclair, Harry 250
Sisler, George 93
Slagle, Jimmy 128
Smith, Ozzie 32
Smith, Red 123, 129, 132–133, 273
Smoot, Homer 158, 165–166
Snodgrass, Fred 111, 158, 166–168
Solomon, Burt 62
Somers, Charlie 160
Spalding, Albert 11, 221
Spaulding, Clarence 54
Spaulding, Jeannette Rusie 54
Speaker, Tris 11, 19, 23, 35, 37, 48, 93, 111
Spink, Al 11
Spring, Jack 188
Staley, Harry 262–263
Stargell, Willie 206
Start, Joe 185
Stein, Ed 263
Stein, Irving 123
Stein, Margaret 263
Steinfeldt, Harry 109
Stengel, Casey 29, 206
Stennett, Rennie 94, 106–107, 273
Stewart, Art 171
Stocker, Kevin 112, 120–121
Stovall, George 68, 69
Stratton, Scott 264
Strobel, Allie 148
Strobel, Charles 66
Sullivan, Haywood 151
Sweeney, Bill 88, 107–109
Swoboda, Ron 143, 159

Tabor, Jim 123, 134
Tannehill, Jesse 74
Taylor, Jack 264–265
Taylor, John W. 265
Tebeau, Patsy 62, 63, 228
Temple, William 52
Tenace, Gene 95
Tener, John 23
Terry, Bill 19, 28
Tesreau, Jeff 266–267
Thayer, Ernest 192
Thiemann, Robert L. 62
Thomas, Darrell 116
Thomasson, Gary 172, 180–181

Index

Thompson, Hank 123, 134–135
Thomson, Bobby 186–187, 188
Tinker, Joe 108–109
Todt, Phil 82, 93–94
Toth, Paul 188
Traynor, Pie 102
Trillo, Manny 95
Turner, Tuck 265

Veiock, Jack 23
Vergez, Johnny 123, 135–136
Viau, Lee 267–268
Virdon, Bill 119
von der Ahe, Chris 72, 183–184, 190, 204

Wagner, Honus 198, 268
Walsh, Ed 67–68, 79
Wambsganss, Bill 248
Ward, Monte 53
Weaver, Buck 112, 121–123, 147, 158
Weaver, Farmer 158, 168–169

Welch, Curt 61
Welsh, Jimmy 158, 169
Whitaker, E.G. 29
Widmark, Anne 60
Widmark, Richard 60
Williams, Dick 95
Williams, Earl 136, 141–142
Williams, Jimmy 74
Williams, Lefty 45, 46
Williams, Ted 195, 206
Wills, Bump 94, 109–110
Wills, Maury 110
Wilson, Alexander 269
Wilson, Bernice 269
Wilson, Don 268–269
Wilson, Jack 269–270
Wilson, Woodrow 239
Wingo, Ivy 147
Winter, George 270–271
Witt, Whitey 158, 169–170
Wittkowski, Waldemar *see* Witt, Whitey
Wolf, Andrew 4, 8
Wolf, Barbara 4
Wolf, Carrie 8

Wolf, Chicken 4–9, 143, 158, 273
Wolf, Milton 8
Wolf, William 8
Wood, Joe 111
Wright, Harry 257
Wynne, Marvel 158, 171
Wynne, Marvel, II 171

Yerkes, Steve 94, 111–112
Yost, Ed 30
Young, Pep *see* Youngs, Ross
Youngs, Caroline 18
Youngs, Dorothy Pienecke 18
Youngs, Henrietta Middlebrook 15
Youngs, Ross 15–20, 143, 158, 273
Youngs, Stonewall Jackson 15

Zimmerman, Heinie 24, 176
Zullo, Allan 77

www.ingramcontent.com/pod-product-compliance
Ingram Content Group UK Ltd.
Pitfield, Milton Keynes, MK11 3LW, UK
UKHW041927140426
5217IPUK00014B/353